# THE ULTIMATE DIABETIC COOKBOOK FOR BEGINNERS

602 EASY AND TASTY RECIPES FOR THE NEWLY DIAGNOSED. MANAGING PREDIABETES AND TYPE 2 DIABETES AND STAY HEALTHY WITH 31-DAY MEAL PLAN. INCLUDING FOOD DISHES WITH AIR FRYER

## JESSICA MEAL

# TABLE OF CONTENTS

# Introduction

## Basics of diabetes

Diabetes is a chronic disease that causes too much sugar in the blood. It can lead to nerve and kidney damage, blindness, heart disease, and poor circulation in your fingers and toes. You can keep your diabetes under control with proper diet and exercise. If you're a diabetic, then it's important that you remember to take care of yourself and your condition. That being said, there are a lot of pitfalls that can derail your self-care regimen.

For example, your blood sugar levels fluctuate, so it's not always easy to figure out if you're within the normal range. This is why it's important to keep track of your sugar levels.

You can use a variety of methods to monitor your blood glucose:

You can also try using new devices that monitor both glucose and ketone levels in order to help you make more informed decisions about your health and wellness.

It's also important to remember that depression is common among diabetics.

The good news is that there are lots of steps you can take to combat this. Traditional counseling techniques are also helpful.

Treatment for diabetes includes taking one or more pills or shots of insulin each day to control blood sugar levels. Most people with type 2 diabetes can control the disease by following a healthy lifestyle that includes exercise and weight loss. For some people, only a few lifestyle changes are needed to control their blood sugar levels well enough so they don't need insulin therapy. These people often continue to take oral medication even though they may be able to stop it in time. Several studies show that people with type 2 diabetes who are able to stop taking insulin have better blood sugar control and fewer complications than those who continue to use the drug.

## Differences between type 1 and type 2 diabetes

-Type 1 diabetes is called insulin dependent diabetes mellitus. In this type of diabetes, the body does not produce insulin, a hormone necessary for the breakdown of glucose. The reason that some people develop this disease is not known.

-Type 2 diabetes is called non-insulin dependent or adult onset diabetes mellitus. In this type of diabetes, the body produces enough insulin but it does not work properly due to problems with cells in the pancreas or other organs involved in the production or use of insulin.

## Prevention and control of diabetes

Diabetes is often controlled by diet, exercise and weight management. While type 1 diabetes cannot be prevented, type 2 can be controlled in many cases. For those of us who are diabetic, the new year often brings resolutions to make life-long changes. For some, that means going vegan. Or quitting smoking. Or losing weight. But for those of us with diabetes, making a resolution to lose weight may seem impossible. Let's break it down:

1) Life expectancy for those who have been diagnosed with diabetes is 10 years shorter than it is for people who do not have diabetes. If you have been diagnosed with diabetes, you are likely much more concerned about managing your disease than looking good.

2) Every 10 pounds of weight lost reduces the chances of a heart attack by 25%. By keeping

your current weight, you will save yourself from a potentially deadly heart attack.

3) Having a normal risk for diabetes impairs your ability to sleep more, which is associated with fewer calories burned during sleep. This means that losing weight could help reduce your risk for developing new, or worsening existing diabetes symptoms.

4) For people with diabetes (type 1/type 2), shedding just a few pounds can reduce blood-sugar levels and decrease the risk for complications such as kidney disease.

5) For those living with diabetes, weight loss is linked to better quality of life.

6) 75% of people who lose weight can lower their blood sugar levels without drugs.

7) In a study, healthy but obese individuals saw an increase in their insulin sensitivity over a 6-month period.

8 ) For people with diabetes, there is no benefit to taking blood-sugar medications for weight loss. A study found that there was no difference in weight loss between people who took insulin (briefly) and those who did not.

9) Having diabetes is associated with a higher risk for cancer. Obesity is a well-known risk factor for developing cancer. Being overweight or obese significantly increases the risk of developing several types of cancer including: diabetes, breast, endometrial, colon and rectal, gallbladder and liver.

10) Having diabetes increases your risk for heart disease as much as smoking.

11) For people with diabetes, losing even slightly more weight could lower their blood sugar levels by 10% .

12) Research shows that when diabetic patients lose weight, they can reduce their amount of diabetes medication and/or change their medications.

13) Another study found that when diabetic patients lost weight, they were able to reduce their risk for complications from diabetes.

14) Having diabetes increases your risk for developing other conditions such as gallbladder disorder, angina pectoris (non-smokers), erectile dysfunction, and osteoporosis. These conditions can be improved by losing weight.

## Symptoms of Type 2 Diabetes, that are Rarely Present in Type 1 Diabetes

Due to the delayed onset of type 2 diabetes, symptoms may be present that are rarely seen in type 1 diabetes.

### *Acanthosis Nigricans (dark patches)*

Dark patches can be present around the neck, the underarms, and other parts of the body. This is due to insulin resistance and the skin's inability to control the production of melanin.

However, many experts suggest acanthosis nigricans may be a coincidental symptom, as many type 2 diabetics are obese. Obesity often causes the folds in the skin to become darker.

### Hair Loss or Thinning

New studies show that hair loss, or thinning, may be an indication of type 2 diabetes. The hair follicles weaken, and new ones develop slower, due to a lack of fuel in the cells. This symptom is more visible in females than males.

Symptoms of Type 2 Diabetes

The symptoms of type 2 diabetes are almost the same as Type 1 diabetes. However, how the symptoms develop, and progress differ:

In type 2 diabetes, the symptoms usually start to manifest upwards of the age of thirty. Whereas, in type 1 diabetes, the symptoms start as early as at 7 years old.

The symptoms of type 2 diabetes occur gradually. While on the other hand, the symptoms of type 1 diabetes, as mentioned before, are sudden and are easier to identify. This is the reason a type 2 diabetic discovers the disease later in life. Statistics show that type 2 diabetics are routinely diagnosed five to ten years after the initial symptoms have occurred.

# Breakfast Recipes

### 1. Hash Browns

**Preparation Time:** 15 minutes
**Cooking Time:** 15 minutes
**Servings:** 4
**Ingredients:**
- 1 pound Russet potatoes, peeled, processed using a grater
- Pinch of sea salt
- Pinch of black pepper, to taste
- 3 Tbsp. olive oil

**Directions:**
1. Line a microwave safe-dish with paper towels. Spread shredded potatoes on top. Microwave veggies on the highest heat setting for 2 minutes. Remove from heat.
2. Pour 1 tablespoon of oil into a non-stick skillet set over medium heat.
3. Cooking in batches, place a generous pinch of potatoes into the hot oil. Press down using the back of a spatula.
4. Cook for 3 minutes every side, or until brown and crispy. Drain on paper towels. Repeat step for remaining potatoes. Add more oil as needed.
5. Season with salt and pepper. Serve.

**Nutrition:**
Calories: 200 kcal
Protein: 4.03 g
Fat: 11.73 g
Carbohydrates: 20.49 g

### 2. Sun-Dried Tomato Garlic Bruschetta

**Preparation Time:** 10 minutes
**Cooking Time:** 5 minutes
**Servings:** 6
**Ingredients:**
- 2 slices sourdough bread, toasted
- 1 tsp. chives, minced
- 1 garlic clove, peeled
- 2 tsp. sun-dried tomatoes in olive oil, minced
- 1 tsp. olive oil

**Directions:**
1. Vigorously rub garlic clove on 1 side of each of the toasted bread slices
2. Spread equal portions of sun-dried tomatoes on the garlic side of bread. Sprinkle chives and drizzle olive oil on top.
3. Pop both slices into oven toaster, and cook until well heated through.
4. Place bruschetta on a plate. Serve warm.

**Nutrition:**
Calories: 149 kcal
Protein: 6.12 g
Fat: 2.99 g
Carbohydrates: 24.39 g

### 3. Mushroom Crêpes

**Preparation Time:** 1 hour 30 minutes
**Cooking Time:** 30 minutes
**Servings:** 6
**Ingredients:**
- 2 eggs
- 3/4 cup milk
- 1/2 cup all-purpose flour
- 1/4 teaspoon salt
- For the filling
- 3 tablespoons all-purpose flour
- 2 cups of cremini mushrooms, sliced
- 3/4 cup chicken broth
- 1/2 cup Parmesan cheese, grated
- 1/8 teaspoon cayenne
- 1/8 teaspoon nutmeg
- ¾ cup milk
- 3 garlic cloves, minced
- 2 tablespoons of parsley (chopped)
- 6 slices of deli-sliced cooked lean ham

•1/4 teaspoon of salt
•Freshly ground pepper

**Directions:**
1.Put and combine the salt and flour in a bowl. In another bowl, whisk the eggs and milk. Gradually combine the two mixtures until smooth. Leave for 15 minutes.
2.Spray a skillet using non-stick cooking spray and put over medium heat. Stir the batter a little. Add 1/4 of the batter into the skillet. Tilt the skillet to form a thin and even crêpe. Cook for 1-2 minutes or until the bottom is golden and the top is set. Flip and cook for 20 seconds. Transfer to a plate.
3.Repeat the steps with the remaining batter. Loosely cover the cooked crêpes with plastic wrap.
4.For the filling. Put all together the ingredients for filling in a saucepan on medium heat – flour, milk, cayenne, nutmeg, and pepper. Constantly whisk until thick or around 7 minutes. Remove from the stove. Stir in a tablespoon of parsley and cheese. Loosely cover to keep warm.
5.Spray a skillet using non-stick cooking spray and put over medium heat. Cook the garlic and mushrooms. Season with salt. Cook for 6 minutes or until the mushrooms are soft. Add 2 tablespoons of sherry. Cook for a couple of minutes. Remove from the stove. Add the remaining parsley and stir.
6.Put the crêpes side by side on a flat surface. Spread a tablespoon of the sauce and 2 tablespoons of the cooked mushrooms. Roll up the crêpes and transfer them to a greased baking dish. Put all the sauce on top. Bake in the oven at 450°F for 15 minutes.
**Nutrition:**
Calories: 232 kcal

Protein: 16.51 g
Fat: 10.8 g
Carbohydrates: 16.25 g

### 4.Oat Porridge with Cherry & Coconut
**Preparation Time:** 10 minutes
**Cooking Time:** 0 minutes
**Servings:** 3
**Ingredients:**
•1 ½ cups regular oats
•3 cups coconut milk
•4 tbsp. chia seed
•3 tbsp. raw cacao
•Coconut shavings
•Dark chocolate shavings
•Fresh or frozen tart cherries
•A pinch of stevia, optional
•Maple syrup, to taste (optional)

**Directions:**
1.Combine the oats, milk, stevia, and cacao in a medium saucepan over medium heat and bring to a boil. Lower the heat, then simmer until the oats are cooked to desired doneness.
2.Divide the porridge among 3 serving bowls and top with dark chocolate and coconut shavings, cherries, and a little drizzle of maple syrup.
**Nutrition:**
Calories: 343 kcal
Protein: 15.64 g
Fat: 12.78 g
Carbohydrates: 41.63 g

### 5.Gingerbread Oatmeal Breakfast
**Preparation Time:** 10 minutes
**Cooking Time:** 0 minutes
**Servings:** 4

**Ingredients:**

- 1 cup steel-cut oats
- 4 cups drinking water
- Organic Maple syrup, to taste
- 1 tsp ground cloves
- 1 ½ tbsp. ground cinnamon
- 1/8 tsp nutmeg
- ¼ tsp ground ginger
- ¼ tsp ground coriander
- ¼ tsp ground allspice
- ¼ tsp ground cardamom
- Fresh mixed berries

**Directions:**

1. Cook the oats based on the package instructions. When it comes to a boil, reduce heat and simmer.
2. Stir in all the spices and continue cooking until cooked to desired doneness.
3. Serve in four serving bowls and drizzle with maple syrup and top with fresh berries.
4. Enjoy!

**Nutrition:**

Calories: 87 kcal

Protein: 5.82 g

Fat: 3.26 g

Carbohydrates: 18.22 g

## 6. Apple, Ginger, and Rhubarb Muffins

**Preparation Time**: 15 minutes

**Cooking Time:** 25 minutes

**Servings:** 4

**Ingredients:**

- ½ cup finely ground almonds
- ¼ cup brown rice flour
- ½ cup buckwheat flour
- 1/8 cup unrefined raw sugar
- 2 tbsp. arrowroot flour
- 1 tbsp. linseed meal
- 2 tbsp. crystallized ginger, finely chopped
- ½ tsp. ground ginger
- ½ tsp. ground cinnamon
- 2 tsp. gluten-free baking powder
- A pinch of fine sea salt
- 1 small apple, peeled and finely diced
- 1 cup finely chopped rhubarb
- 1/3 cup almond/ rice milk
- 1 large egg
- ¼ cup extra virgin olive oil
- 1 tsp. pure vanilla extract

**Directions:**

1. Set your oven to 350Fgrease an eight-cup muffin tin and line with paper cases.
2. Combine the almond four, linseed meal, ginger and sugar in a mixing bowl. Sieve this mixture over the other flours, spices and baking powder and use a whisk to combine well.
3. Stir in the apple and rhubarb in the flour mixture until evenly coated.
4. In a separate bowl, whisk the milk, vanilla, and egg then pour it into the dry mixture. Stir until just combined – don't overwork the batter as this can yield very tough muffins.
5. Scoop the mixture into the arrange muffin tin and top with a few slices of rhubarb. Bake for at least 25 minutes, till they start turning golden or when an inserted toothpick emerges clean.
6. Take off from the oven and let sit for at least 5 minutes before transferring the muffins to a wire rack for further cooling.
7. Serve warm with a glass of squeezed juice.
8. Enjoy!

**Nutrition:**

Calories: 325 kcal

Protein: 6.32 g

Fat: 9.82 g

Carbohydrates: 55.71 g

# 7. Anti-Inflammatory Breakfast Frittata

**Preparation Time:** 10 minutes
**Cooking Time:** 40 minutes
**Servings:** 4
**Ingredients:**

- 4 large eggs
- 6 egg whites
- 450g button mushrooms
- 450g baby spinach
- 125g firm tofu
- 1 onion, chopped
- 1 tbsp. minced garlic
- ½ tsp. ground turmeric
- ½ tsp. cracked black pepper
- ¼ cup water
- Kosher salt to taste

**Directions:**

1. Set your oven to 350F.
2. Sauté the mushrooms in a little bit of extra virgin olive oil in a large non-stick ovenproof pan over medium heat. Add the onions once the mushrooms start turning golden and cook for 3 minutes until the onions become soft.
3. Stir in the garlic then cook for at least 30 seconds until fragrant before adding the spinach. Pour in water, cover, and cook until the spinach becomes wilted for about 2 minutes.
4. Take off the lid and continue cooking up to the water evaporates. Now, combine the eggs, egg whites, tofu, pepper, turmeric, and salt in a bowl. When all the liquid has evaporated, pour in the egg mixture, let cook for about 2 minutes until the edges start setting, then transfer to the oven and bake for about 25 minutes or until cooked.
5. Take off from the oven then let sit for at least 5 minutes before cutting it into quarters and serving.
6. Enjoy!
7. Baby spinach and mushrooms boost the nutrient profile of the eggs to provide you with amazing anti-inflammatory benefits.

**Nutrition:**
Calories: 521 kcal
Protein: 29.13 g
Fat: 10.45 g
Carbohydrates: 94.94 g

# 8. Breakfast Sausage and Mushroom Casserole

**Preparation Time:** 20 minutes
**Cooking Time:** 45 minutes
**Servings:** 4
**Ingredients:**

- 450g of Italian sausage, cooked and crumbled
- Three-fourth cup of coconut milk
- 8 ounces of white mushrooms, sliced
- 1 medium onion, finely diced
- 2 Tablespoons of organic ghee
- 6 free-range eggs
- 600g of sweet potatoes
- 1 red bell pepper, roasted
- 3/4 tsp. of ground black pepper, divided
- 1 ½ tsp. of sea salt, divided

**Directions:**

1. Peel and shred the sweet potatoes.
2. Take a bowl, fill it with ice-cold water, and soak the sweet potatoes in it. Set aside.
3. Peel the roasted bell pepper, remove its seeds and finely dice it.
4. Set the oven 375°F.
5. Get a casserole baking dish and grease it with the organic ghee.

6.Put a skillet over medium flame and cook the mushrooms in it. Cook until the mushrooms are crispy and brown.

7.Take the mushrooms out and mix them with the crumbled sausage.

8.Now sauté the onions in the same skillet. Cook up to the onions are soft and golden. This should take about 4 – 5 minutes.

9.Take the onions out and mix them in the sausage-mushroom mixture.

10.Add the diced bell pepper to the same mixture.

11.Mix well and set aside for a while.

12.Now drain the soaked shredded potatoes, put them on a paper towel, and pat dry.

13.Bring the sweet potatoes in a bowl and add about a teaspoon of salt and half a teaspoon of ground black pepper to it. Mix well and set aside.

14.Now take a large bowl and crack the eggs in it.

15.Break the eggs and then blend in the coconut milk.

16.Stir in the remaining black pepper and salt.

17.Take the greased casserole dish and spread the seasoned sweet potatoes evenly in the base of the dish.

18.Next, spread the sausage mixture evenly in the dish.

19.Finally, spread the egg mixture.

20.Now cover the casserole dish using a piece of aluminum foil.

21.Bake for 20 - 30 minutes. To check if the casserole is baked properly, insert a tester in the middle of the casserole, and it should come out clean.

22.Uncover the casserole dish and bake it again, uncovered for 5 - 10 minutes, until the casserole is a little golden on the top.

23.Allow it to cool for 10 minutes.

24.Enjoy!

26

**Nutrition:**
Calories: 598 kcal
Protein: 28.65 g
Fat: 36.75 g
Carbohydrates: 48.01 g

## 9. Steak Muffins

**Preparation Time:** 10 minutes
**Cooking Time:** 20 minutes
**Servings:** 4
**Ingredients:**
- 1 cup red bell pepper, diced
- 2 Tablespoons of water
- 8 ounce thin steak, cooked and finely chopped
- ¼ teaspoon of sea salt
- Dash of freshly ground black pepper
- 8 free-range eggs
- 1 cup of finely diced onion

**Directions:**
1.Set the oven to 350°F
2.Take 8 muffin tins and line then with parchment paper liners.
3.Get a large bowl and crack all the eggs in it.
4.Beat well the eggs.
5.Blend in all the remaining ingredients.
6.Spoon the batter into the arrange muffin tins. Fill three-fourth of each tin.
7.Put the muffin tins in the preheated oven for about 20 minutes, until the muffins are baked and set in the middle.
8.Enjoy!

**Nutrition:**
Calories: 151 kcal
Protein: 17.92 g
Fat: 7.32 g
Carbohydrates: 3.75 g

## 10.White and Green Quiche

**Preparation Time:** 10 minutes
**Cooking Time:** 40 minutes

**Servings:** 3
**Ingredients:**
- 3 cups of fresh spinach, chopped
- 15 large free-range eggs
- 3 cloves of garlic, minced
- 5 white mushrooms, sliced
- 1 small sized onion, finely chopped
- 1 ½ teaspoon of baking powder
- Ground black pepper to taste
- 1 ½ cups of coconut milk
- Ghee, as required to grease the dish
- Sea salt to taste

**Directions:**
1. Set the oven to 350°F.
2. Get a baking dish then grease it with the organic ghee.
3. Break all the eggs in a huge bowl then whisk well.
4. Stir in coconut milk. Beat well
5. While you are whisking the eggs, start adding the remaining ingredients in it.
6. When all the ingredients are thoroughly blended, pour all of it into the prepared baking dish.
7. Bake for at least 40 minutes, up to the quiche is set in the middle.
8. Enjoy!

**Nutrition:**
Calories: 608 kcal
Protein: 20.28 g
Fat: 53.42 g
Carbohydrates: 16.88 g

## 11. Cheddar and Chive Souffles

**Preparation Time:** 10 minutes
**Cooking Time:** 25 minutes
**Servings:** 8
**Ingredients:**
- ½ cup almond flour
- ¼ cup chopped chives

- 1 tsp salt
- ½ tsp xanthan gum
- 1 tsp ground mustard
- ¼ tsp cayenne pepper
- ½ tsp cracked black pepper
- ¾ cup heavy cream
- 2 cups shredded cheddar cheese
- ½ cup baking powder
- 6 organic eggs, separated

**Directions:**
1. Switch on the oven, then set its temperature to 350°F and let it preheat.
2. Take a medium bowl, add flour in it, add remaining ingredients, except for baking powder and eggs, and whisk until combined.
3. Separate egg yolks and egg whites between two bowls, add egg yolks in the flour mixture and whisk until incorporated.
4. Add baking powder into the egg whites and beat with an electric mixer until stiff peaks form and then stir egg whites into the flour mixture until well mixed.
5. Divide the batter evenly between eight ramekins and then bake for 25 minutes until done.
6. Serve straight away or store in the refrigerator until ready to eat.

**Nutrition:**
Calories 288
Total Fat 21g
Total Carbs 3g
Protein 14g

## 12. Beef Breakfast Casserole

**Preparation Time:** 10 minutes
**Cooking Time:** 30 minutes
**Servings:** 5
**Ingredients:**
- 1 pound of ground beef, cooked
- 10 eggs

•½ cup Pico de Gallo

•1 cup baby spinach

•¼ cup sliced black olives

•Freshly ground black pepper

**Directions:**

1.Preheat oven to 350 degrees Fahrenheit. Prepare a 9" glass pie plate with non-stick spray.

2.Whisk the eggs until frothy. Season with salt and pepper.

3.Layer the cooked ground beef, Pico de Gallo, and spinach in the pie plate.

4.Slowly pour the eggs over the top.

5.Top with black olives.

6.Bake for at least 30 minutes, until firm in the middle.

7.Slice into 5 pieces and serve.

**Nutrition:**

Calories: 479 kcal

Protein: 43.54 g

Fat: 30.59 g

Carbohydrates: 4.65 g

## 13.Blueberry & Cashew Waffles

**Preparation Time:** 15 minutes

**Cooking Time:** 4-5 minutes

**Servings:** 5

**Ingredients:**

•1 cup raw cashews

•3 tablespoons coconut flour

•1 tsp baking soda

•Salt, to taste

•½ cup unsweetened almond milk

•3 organic eggs

•¼ cup coconut oil, melted

•3 tablespoons organic honey

•½ teaspoon organic vanilla flavor

•1 cup fresh blueberries

**Directions:**

1.Preheat the waffle iron after which grease it.

2.In a mixer, add cashews and pulse till flour-like consistency forms.

3.Transfer the cashew flour in a big bowl.

4.Add almond flour, baking soda and salt and mix well.

5.In another bowl, put the remaining ingredients and beat till well combined.

6.Put the egg mixture into the flour mixture then mix till well combined.

7.Fold in blueberries.

8.In preheated waffle iron, add the required amount of mixture.

9.Cook for around 4-5 minutes.

10.Repeat with the remaining mixture.

**Nutrition:**

Calories: 432

 Fat: 32

 Carbohydrates: 32g

Protein: 13g

## 14.Cheesy Flax and Hemp Seeds Muffins

**Preparation Time:** 5 minutes

 **Cooking Time:** 30 minutes

 **Servings:** 2

**Ingredients:**

•1/8 cup flax seeds meal

•¼ cup raw hemp seeds

•¼ cup almond meal

•Salt, to taste

•¼ tsp baking powder

•3 organic eggs, beaten

•1/8 cup nutritional yeast flakes

•¼ cup cottage cheese, low-fat

•¼ cup grated parmesan cheese

•¼ cup scallion, sliced thinly

•1 tbsp. olive oil

**Directions:**

1.Switch on the oven, then set it 360°F and let it preheat.

2.Meanwhile, take two ramekins, grease them with oil, and set aside until required.

3.Take a medium bowl, add flax seeds, hemp seeds, and almond meal, and then stir in salt and baking powder until mixed.

4.Crack eggs in another bowl, add yeast, cottage cheese, and parmesan, stir well until combined, and then stir this mixture into the almond meal mixture until incorporated.

5.Fold in scallions, then distribute the mixture between prepared ramekins and bake for 30 minutes until muffins are firm and the top is nicely golden brown.

6.When done, take out the muffins from the ramekins and let them cool completely on a wire rack.

7.For meal prepping, wrap each muffin with a paper towel and refrigerate for up to thirty-four days.

8.When ready to eat, reheat muffins in the microwave until hot and then serve.

**Nutrition:**
Calories 179
 Total Fat 10.9g
Total Carbs 6.9g
Protein 15.4g
Sugar 2.3g
Sodium 311mg

## 15.Ham and Veggie Frittata Muffins

**Preparation Time:** 10 minutes
**Cooking Time:** 25 minutes
**Servings:** 12
**Ingredients:**
- 5 ounces thinly sliced ham
- 8 large eggs
- 4 tablespoons coconut oil
- ½ yellow onion, finely diced
- 8 oz. frozen spinach, thawed and drained
- 8 oz. mushrooms, thinly sliced
- 1 cup cherry tomatoes, halved
- ¼ cup coconut milk (canned)
- 2 tablespoons coconut flour
- Sea salt and pepper to taste

**Directions:**
1.Preheat oven to 375 degrees Fahrenheit.

2.In a medium skillet, warm the coconut oil on medium heat. Add the onion and cook until softened.

3.Add the mushrooms, spinach, and cherry tomatoes. Season with salt and pepper. Cook until the mushrooms have softened. About 5 minutes. Remove from heat and set aside.

4.In a huge bowl, beat the eggs together with the coconut milk and coconut flour. Stir in the cooled the veggie mixture.

5.Line each cavity of a 12 cavity muffin tin with the thinly sliced ham. Pour the egg mixture into each one and bake for 20 minutes.

6.Remove from oven and allow to cool for about 5 minutes before transferring to a wire rack.

7.To maximize the benefit of a vegetable-rich diet, it's important to eat a variety of colors, and these veggie-packed frittata muffins do just that. The onion, spinach, mushrooms, and cherry tomatoes provide a wide range of vitamins and nutrients and a healthy dose of fiber.

**Nutrition:**
Calories: 125 kcal
Protein: 5.96 g
Fat: 9.84 g
Carbohydrates: 4.48 g

## 16.Shirataki Pasta with Avocado and Cream

**Preparation Time:** 10 minutes
 **Cooking Time:** 6 minutes

Servings: 2

**Ingredients:**

- ½ packet of shirataki noodles, cooked
- ½ of an avocado
- ½ tsp cracked black pepper
- ½ tsp salt
- ½ tsp dried basil
- 1/8 cup heavy cream

**Directions:**

1.Place a medium pot half full with water over medium heat, bring it to boil, then add noodles and cook for 2 minutes.

2.Then drain the noodles and set aside until required.

3.Place avocado in a bowl, mash it with a fork,

4.Mash avocado in a bowl, transfer it in a blender, add remaining ingredients, and pulse until smooth.

5.Take a frying pan, place it over medium heat and when hot, add noodles in it, pour in the avocado mixture, stir well and cook for 2 minutes until hot.

6.Serve straight away.

**Nutrition:**

Calories 131

Total Fat 12.6g

Total Carbs 4.9g

Protein 1.2g

Sugar 0.3g

Sodium 588mg

## 17.Spaghetti Squash with Cheese and Basil Pesto

**Preparation Time:** 10 minutes

**Cooking Time:** 35 minutes

**Servings:** 2

**Ingredients:**

- 1 cup cooked spaghetti squash, drained
- Salt, to taste
- Freshly cracked black pepper, to taste
- ½ tbsp. olive oil
- ¼ cup ricotta cheese, unsweetened
- 2oz fresh mozzarella cheese, cubed
- 1/8 cup basil pesto

**Directions:**

1.Switch on the oven, then set its temperature to 375 °F and let it preheat.

2.Meanwhile, take a medium bowl, add spaghetti squash in it and then season with salt and black pepper.

3.Take a casserole dish, grease it with oil, add squash mixture in it, top it with ricotta cheese and mozzarella cheese and bake for 10 minutes until cooked.

4.When done, remove the casserole dish from the oven, drizzle pesto on top and serve immediately.

**Nutrition:**

Calories 169

Total Fat 11.3g

Total Carbs 6.2g

Protein 11.9g

Sugar 0.1g

Sodium 217mg

## 18.Tomato and Avocado Omelet

**Preparation Time:** 5 minutes

**Cooking Time:** 5 minutes

**Servings:** 1

**Ingredients:**

- 2 eggs
- ¼ avocado, diced
- 4 cherry tomatoes, halved
- 1 tablespoon cilantro, chopped
- Squeeze of lime juice
- Pinch of salt

**Directions:**

1.Put together the avocado, tomatoes, cilantro, lime juice, and salt in a small bowl, then mix well and set aside.

2.Warm a medium nonstick skillet on medium heat. Whisk the eggs until frothy and add to the pan. Move the eggs around gently with a rubber spatula until they begin to set.

3.Scatter the avocado mixture over half of the omelet. Remove from heat, and slide the omelet onto a plate as you fold it in half.

4.Serve immediately.

**Nutrition:**

Calories: 433 kcal

Protein: 25.55 g

Fat: 32.75 g

Carbohydrates: 10.06 g

## 19.Vegan-Friendly Banana Bread

**Preparation Time:** 15 minutes

**Cooking Time:** 40 minutes

**Servings:** 4-6

**Ingredients:**

- 2 ripe bananas, mashed
- 1/3 cup brewed coffee
- 3 tbsp. chia seeds
- 6 tbsp. water
- ½ cup soft vegan butter
- ½ cup maple syrup
- 2 cups flour
- 2 tsp. baking powder
- 1 tsp. cinnamon powder
- 1 tsp. allspice
- ½ tsp. salt

**Directions:**

1.Set oven at 350F.

2.Bring the chia seeds in a small bowl then soak it with 6 tbsp. of water. Stir well and set aside.

3.In a mixing bowl, mix using a hand mixer the vegan butter and maple syrup until it turns fluffy. Add the chia seeds along with the mashed bananas.

4.Mix well and then add the coffee.

5.Meanwhile, sift all the dry ingredients (flour, baking powder, cinnamon powder, all spice, and salt) and then gradually add into the bowl with the wet ingredients.

6.Combine the ingredients well and then pour over a baking pan lined with parchment paper.

7.Place in the oven to bake for at least 30-40 minutes, or until the toothpick comes out clean after inserting in the bread.

8.Allow the bread to cool before serving.

**Nutrition:**

Calories: 371 kcal

Protein: 5.59 g

Fat: 16.81 g

Carbohydrates: 49.98 g

## 20.Mango Granola

**Preparation Time:** 10 minutes

**Cooking Time:** 30 minutes

**Servings:** 4

**Ingredients:**

- 2 cups rolled oats
- 1 cup dried mango, chopped
- ½ cup almonds, roughly chopped
- ½ cup nuts
- ½ cup dates, roughly chopped
- 3 tbsp. sesame seeds
- 2 tsp. cinnamon
- 2/3 cup agave nectar
- 2 tbsp. coconut oil
- 2 tbsp. water

**Directions:**

1.Set oven at 320F

2.In a large bowl, put the oats, almonds, nuts, sesame seeds, dates, and cinnamon then mix well.

3.Meanwhile, heat a saucepan over medium heat, pour in the agave syrup, coconut oil, and water.

4.Stir and let it cook for at least 3 minutes or until the coconut oil has melted.

5.Gradually pour the syrup mixture into the bowl with the oats and nuts and stir well, ensure that all the ingredients are coated with the syrup.

6.Transfer the granola on a baking sheet lined with parchment paper and place in the oven to bake for 20 minutes.

7.After 20 minutes, take off the tray from the oven and lay the chopped dried mango on top. Put back in the oven then bake again for another 5 minutes.

8.Let the granola cool to room temperature before serving or placing it in an airtight container for storage. The shelf life of the granola will last up to 2-3 weeks.

**Nutrition:**

Calories: 434 kcal

Protein: 13.16 g

Fat: 28.3 g

Carbohydrates: 55.19 g

## 21.Pumpkin & Banana Waffles

**Preparation Time:** 15 minutes

**Cooking Time:** 5 minutes

**Servings:** 4

**Ingredients:**

- ½ cup almond flour
- ½ cup coconut flour
- 1 tsp baking soda
- 1½ teaspoons ground cinnamon
- ¾ teaspoon ground ginger
- ½ teaspoon ground cloves
- ½ teaspoon ground nutmeg
- Salt, to taste
- 2 tablespoons olive oil
- 5 large organic eggs
- ¾ cup almond milk
- ½ cup pumpkin puree
- 2 medium bananas, peeled and sliced

**Directions:**

1.Preheat the waffle iron, and after that, grease it.

2.In a sizable bowl, mix together flours, baking soda, and spices.

3.In a blender, put the remaining ingredients and pulse till smooth.

4.Add flour mixture and pulse till

5.In preheated waffle iron, add the required quantity of mixture.

6.Cook approximately 4-5 minutes.

7.Repeat using the remaining mixture.

**Nutrition:**

Calories: 357.2

Fat: 28.5g

Carbohydrates: 19.7g

Fiber: 4g

Protein: 14g

## 22.Flaxseed Porridge with Cinnamon

**Preparation Time:** 10 minutes

**Cooking Time:** 5 minutes

**Servings:** 4

**Ingredients:**

- 1 tsp cinnamon
- 1½ tsp stevia
- 1 tbsp. unsalted butter
- 2 tbsp. flaxseed meal
- 2 tbsp. flaxseed oatmeal
- ½ cup shredded coconut
- 1 cup heavy cream
- 2 cups of water

**Directions:**

1.Take a medium pot, place it over low heat, add all the ingredients in it, stir until mixed and bring the mixture to boil.

2.When the mixture has boiled, remove the pot from heat, stir it well and divide it evenly between four bowls.

3.Let porridge rest for 10 minutes until slightly thicken and then serve.

**Nutrition:**

Calories 171

Total Fat 16g

 Total Carbs 6g

Protein 2g

## 23.Cinnamon Pancakes with Coconut

**Preparation Time:** 5 minutes

 **Cooking Time:** 18 minutes

 **Servings:** 2

**Ingredients:**

- 2 organic eggs
- 1 tbsp. almond flour
- 2oz cream cheese
- ¼ cup shredded coconut and more for garnishing
- ½ tbsp. erythritol
- 1/8 tsp salt
- 1 tsp cinnamon
- 4 tbsp. stevia
- ½ tbsp. olive oil

**Directions:**

1.Crack eggs in a bowl, beat until fluffy and then beat in flour and cream cheese until smooth.

2.Add remaining ingredients and then stir until well combined.

3.Take a frying pan, place it over medium heat, grease it with oil, then pour in half of the batter and cook for 3 to 4 minutes per side until the pancake has cooked and nicely golden brown.

4.Transfer pancake to a plate and cook another pancake in the same manner by using the remaining batter.

5.Sprinkle coconut on top of cooked pancakes and serve.

**Nutrition:**

Calories 575

 Total Fat 51g

 Total Carbs 3.5g

Protein 19g

## 24.Banana Cashew Toast

**Preparation Time:** 10 minutes

 **Cooking Time:** 0 minutes

 **Servings:** 3

**Ingredients:**

- 1 cup roasted cashews (unsalted)
- 4 pieces oat bread
- 2 ripe medium-sized bananas
- Dash of salt
- Pinch of cinnamon
- 2 tsp. flax meals
- 2 tsp. honey

**Directions:**

1.Peel and slice the bananas into ½-inch pieces. Toast the bread. In a food processor, puree the salt and cashews until they are smooth. Use the puree as a spread on the toasts. On top of the spread, arrange a layer of bananas. Add flax meals and a dash of cinnamon on top of the bananas. Top the toast with honey.

**Nutrition:**

Calories: 634 kcal

Protein: 13.42 g

Fat: 47.6 g

Carbohydrates: 48.02 g

## 25. Strawberry-Oat-Chocolate Chip Muffins

**Preparation Time:** 10 minutes
**Cooking Time:** 23 minutes
**Servings:** 12
**Ingredients:**
- 1¼ c. whole wheat pastry flour
- 1 c. rolled oats
- ¾ tsp. Baking soda
- ½ tsp. Baking powder
- ¼ tsp. salt
- 1 heaping cup bananas (about 2 to 3 large very ripe bananas)
- 1 tbsp. extra virgin olive oil
- 1 tbsp. honey or agave nectar
- 1 tsp. vanilla
- 1 egg
- 1 egg white
- 1/3 c. nonfat plain Greek yogurt
- ½ c. unsweetened vanilla almond milk
- 1/3 c. mini chocolate chips
- 2/3 c. diced strawberries
- 12 thin slices of strawberries (about 3-4 strawberries) for garnish, if desired

**Directions:**
1. Set the oven to 350°F and lightly grease a standard 12-cup muffin pan or grease with paper liners. In a large-sized mixing bowl, combine flour, oats, baking powder, baking soda, and salt. Stir to blend. Set aside the 2 tbsp. of the mixture.
2. In a separate huge mixing bowl, combine together the mashed banana, olive oil, honey, and vanilla. Next, beat in the egg and egg white and beat until combined. Now add in Greek yogurt and almond milk and beat with an electric mixer on low until smooth.
3. Gradually put wet ingredients to dry ingredients and blend until just combined, but don't over mix the batter as it will make the muffins firm.
4. Fill each muffin cup 2/3 full of batter. Gently tap the pan on the counter to even out the batter. Place a thin slice of strawberry onto each muffin, if desired. Put the pan in the oven, then cook for 18 to 23 minutes, up to a toothpick place in the middle of the muffins, and comes out clean. Take off from the oven and let sit for 5 to 10 minutes in the pan before placing on a cooling rack.

**Nutrition:**
Calories: 91 kcal
Protein: 4.02 g
Fat: 2.63 g
Carbohydrates: 16.31 g

## 26. Huevos Rancheros

**Preparation Time:** 5 minutes
**Cooking Time:** 5 minutes
**Servings:** 2
**Ingredients:**
- (2) 8-inch whole wheat tortillas
- 2 hard-boiled eggs, sliced
- 2 slices of Canadian bacon or ham
- 1-ounce slice of cheddar cheese
- 2 tbsp. salsa

**Directions:**
1. Prepare the hardboiled eggs.
2. Put 1 tortilla on a plate, top with a slice of Canadian bacon or ham, the sliced egg, and a slice of cheddar cheese. Roll the tortilla up. Repeat with the remaining ingredients to prepare the second burrito.
3. Serve immediately with 1 tbsp. Salsa.

**Nutrition:**
Calories: 741 kcal
Protein: 36.12 g
Fat: 30.75 g
Carbohydrates: 79.37 g

# 27.Oatmeal-Applesauce Muffins

**Preparation Time:** 15 minutes
**Cooking Time:** 25 minutes
**Servings:** 12
**Ingredients:**
- Topping
- 1/4 cup rolled oats
- 1 tbsp. brown sugar
- 1/8 tsp. cinnamon
- 1 tbsp. unsalted butter, melted
- Muffins
- 1 c. old fashioned rolled oats (not instant)
- 1 c. nonfat milk
- 1 c. whole wheat flour
- ½ c. unsweetened applesauce
- 2 egg whites
- 1 tsp. Baking powder
- ½ tsp. Baking soda
- ½ tsp. Salt
- ½ tsp. Cinnamon
- raisins or nuts (opt.)

**Directions:**

1. To begin, first, presoak the oats in milk for 1 hour,
2. Set the oven to 400°F then grease a standard 12-cup muffin pan with cooking spray or use paper liners.
3. In a mixing bowl, combine oat-milk mixture, applesauce, and egg whites. Blend well and set aside.
4. In a separate bowl, put together the whole wheat flour, brown sugar, baking powder, baking soda, salt, and cinnamon then mix.
5. Gradually put wet ingredients to dry ingredients and blend until just combined, but don't over mix the batter as it will make the muffins firm. Add raisins or nuts (opt.).
6. Prepare topping: In a small bowl, whisk together the oats, and cinnamon. Add in melted butter and toss gently with a fork to coat ingredients.
7. Fill each muffin cup 2/3 full of batter. Sprinkle topping on the top of each batter-filled muffin cup. Tap the pan gently on the counter to even out the batter. Place muffin pan in preheated oven and cook for 20 to 25 minutes or until a toothpick put in the middle of one of the muffins comes out clean. Take off from the oven and let sit for 5 minutes before serving.

**Nutrition:**
Calories: 115 kcal
Protein: 5.06 g
Fat: 2.57 g
Carbohydrates: 22.33 g

# 28.Barley Breakfast Bowl with Lemon Yogurt Sauce

**Preparation Time:** 10 minutes
**Cooking Time:** 0 minutes
**Servings:** 2
**Ingredients:**
- 1½ c. cooked barley, keep warm
- 1 c. mung bean sprouts (or preferred variety)
- 1/3 c. Cotija cheese or queso fresco - crumbled
- ¼ c. sliced almonds, toasted
- ¼ tsp. kosher salt
- 1 small avocado – peeled/pitted, and flesh diced or sliced
- ½ tsp. Sea salt
- ¼ tsp. fresh ground black pepper
- Lemon Yogurt Sauce
- 1 c. Greek plain yogurt
- 1 tsp. lemon zest, finely grated
- 1 tsp. Fresh lemon juice
- ¼ c. fresh mint or parsley, chopped
- Sea salt, to taste

•Fresh ground black pepper, to taste

**Directions:**

1.First, prepare the Lemon Yogurt Sauce: Combine the plain yogurt, lemon zest and juice, fresh mint or parsley, and salt & pepper in a bowl and stir to blend well. Cover and refrigerate until ready to serve.

2.Next, prepare the barley bowl: In a small mixing bowl, combine the barley, bean sprouts, cheese, almonds, and salt. Stir to mix well.

3.Divide barley mixture into 2 serving bowls. Top each barley bowl with 2 tbsp. lemon yogurt sauce and avocado. Put a pinch of salt and pepper to taste, serve, and enjoy!

**Nutrition:**

Calories: 432 kcal

Protein: 13.6 g

Fat: 23.37 g

Carbohydrates: 47.62 g

## 29.Apple Oatmeal

**Preparation Time:** 10 minutes

**Cooking Time:** 5 minutes

**Servings:** 2

**Ingredients:**

•2/3 cups rolled oats

•1 cup water

•1 teaspoon ground cinnamon

•1 cup of any non-fat milk, coconut milk or almond milk (optional)

•¼ cup fresh apple juice

•1 chopped apple, (unpeeled or peeled)

**Directions:**

1.Place the water, juice, and the apple in a deep pot. Bring to boil over medium heat.

2.Add the oats and cinnamon. Bring to another boil. Lower the heat temperature and let it simmer for 3 minutes or until it is thick.

3.Divide the serving into two and serve with milk.



**Nutrition:**

Calories: 277 kcal

Protein: 12.69 g

Fat: 7.69 g

Carbohydrates: 52.71 g

## 30.Blueberry-Bran Breakfast Sundae

**Preparation Time:** 10 minutes

**Cooking Time:** 0 minutes

**Servings:** 2

**Ingredients:**

•2 c. vanilla or lemon-flavored low-fat yogurt (preferably Greek yogurt) or flavor of choice.

•2 c. bran flakes

•1/4 c. fresh blueberries

•2 tbsp. sliced almonds (or nuts of choice)

•2 tbsp. chopped pecans (or nuts of choice)

•2 tbsp. dried cranberries (or dried or fresh fruit of choice)

**Directions:**

1.In a bowl, place 1 c. yogurt, and one c. bran flakes.

2.Top with 1/8 c. fresh blueberries, followed by 1 tbsp. Each of sliced almonds, chopped pecans, and dried cranberries.

3.Repeat using the remaining ingredients to make a second serving. Serve immediately.

**Nutrition:**

Calories: 420 kcal

Protein: 21.12 g

Fat: 13.58 g

Carbohydrates: 59.8 g

## 31.Greek Yogurt with Cherry-Almond Syrup Parfait

**Preparation Time:** 25 minutes

**Cooking Time:** 5 minutes

**Servings:** 2

**Ingredients:**

•1 c. fresh black or red cherries, pitted

- 2 tbsp. almond syrup
- 2 tbsp. coconut palm sugar
- 1 tsp. fresh-squeezed lemon juice
- 2 c. Greek plain yogurt, stir to loosen
- 2 tbsp. sliced almonds, to garnish
- 4 tbsp. granola of choice, to garnish (opt.)

**Directions:**

1. Place a saucepan over medium-high heat and combine cherries, almond syrup, sugar, lemon juice, and 1 tbsp. of water. Stir to combine, then place it to simmer, constantly stirring until sugar is dissolved. Continue to simmer for further 5 minutes, until liquid starts to turn into a syrupy mixture, but the cherries are still holding firm. Place the mixture to a bowl and let cool for 5 minutes at room temperature, then bring it in the refrigerator to chill until it is completely cold.

2. Place 1 cup of Greek yogurt into 2 serving bowls and spoon ½ of the cherries and their syrupy juices over the yogurt. Garnish with sliced almonds or granola, if desired. Serve immediately.

**Nutrition:**

Calories: 185 kcal

Protein: 4.75 g

Fat: 4.88 g

Carbohydrates: 33.07 g

## 32. Cinnamon-Apple Granola with Greek Yogurt

**Preparation Time:** 5 minutes

**Cooking Time:** 10 minutes

**Servings:** 2

**Ingredients:**

- 1/2 c. raw almonds, chopped (or raw nuts of choice)
- 1/2 c. raw walnuts, chopped (or raw nuts of choice)
- 1/2 apple, peeled and diced
- 1 tbsp. almond flour
- 2 tbsp. vanilla protein powder
- 1 tsp. ground cinnamon
- 1/8 c. applesauce, unsweetened preferred
- 2 tsp. honey
- 2 tsp. almond butter
- 1/16 tsp. vanilla extract
- dash of sea salt
- 1 cup Greek plain or vanilla yogurt (or flavor of choice)

**Directions:**

1. In a mixing bowl, combine the chopped almonds, chopped walnuts (or preferred raw nuts), diced apple, vanilla protein powder, almond flour, lucuma (opt), and cinnamon and salt in a bowl. Mix well.

2. In a second bowl, combine the apple sauce, almond butter, honey, and vanilla extract. Mix well. Pour the bowl with the nuts into the bowl with the wet ingredients and blend together thoroughly. Make sure all dry ingredients get coated.

3. Place the granola mixture onto a parchment paperlined baking sheet and bake until the desired crunch is obtained approximately 8 to 10 minutes. Take off from oven and let cool or eat hot. Place 1/2 cup each Greek yogurt into two bowls. Divide the granola and sprinkle over the yogurt in each bowl. Serve immediately.

**Nutrition:**

Calories: 312 kcal

Protein: 11.72 g

Fat: 22.37 g

Carbohydrates: 19.92 g

## 33. Peanut Butter-Banana Muffins

**Preparation Time:** 15 minutes

**Cooking Time:** 25 minutes

**Servings:** 12

**Ingredients:**
- 1½ c. all-purpose flour
- 1 c. old-fashioned oats
- 1 tsp. Baking powder
- ½ tsp. Baking soda
- ½ tsp. salt
- 2 tbsp. Applesauce
- ¾ c. light brown sugar
- 2 large eggs
- 1 c. mashed banana (about 3 bananas)
- 6 tbsp. creamy peanut butter
- 1 c. low-fat buttermilk

**Directions:**

1. Bring a small nonstick skillet on medium heat and spray lightly with cooking spray. Add in the bell pepper and onion and sauté for 1 to 2 minutes, or until both are tender and the onion translucent.

2. In a small bowl, crack in eggs and whisk. Add in milk; whisk until well-blended. Pour eggs into the pan and cook, frequently stirring until eggs are scrambled to your liking.

3. To serve, spoon half the egg mixture into each tortilla, wrap, and serve. Try serving with a side of fresh fruit for a complete meal.

**Nutrition:**

Calories: 187 kcal

Protein: 8.12 g

Fat: 6.25 g

Carbohydrates: 27.82 g

## 34. Banana-Oatmeal Vegan Pancakes

**Preparation Time:** 5 minutes

**Cooking Time:** 5 minutes

**Servings:** 12

**Ingredients:**
- 1¼ c. old fashioned oats
- ½ c. organic whole wheat flour
- 2 tsp. Baking powder
- ½ tsp. sea salt
- 1½ c. soymilk
- 2 ripe bananas

**Directions:**

1. To begin, heat griddle or skillet over medium heat.

2. Next, place all ingredients, except for banana, into a blender and process until smooth. Add the bananas to blender and blend until smooth.

3. Lightly grease griddle with olive or coconut oil, then pour ¼ c. of batter onto griddle and cook for at least 2 to 3 minutes, then flip and cook for about 2 minutes or up to the pancake is golden brown and cooked through.

4. Repeat process with remaining batter.

**Nutrition:**

Calories: 59 kcal

Protein: 3.49 g

Fat: 1.48 g

Carbohydrates: 11.52 g

## 35. Strawberry Yogurt treat

**Preparation Time:** 10 minutes

**Cooking Time:** 0 minutes

**Servings:** 2

**Ingredients:**
- 4 cups 0% fat plain yogurt
- 1 cup sliced strawberries
- 8 tbsp. of flax meal
- 4 tbsp. honey
- 8 tbsp. walnuts (chopped)

**Directions:**

1. Distribute 2 cups of the yogurt into your serving bowls. Neatly layer the flax meal and the walnut in the middle. Add a drizzle of half of the honey before covering with the last layer of yogurt. Add the honey on top of the yogurt to add color when you serve.

**Nutrition:**

Calories: 733 kcal

Protein: 38.42 g
Fat: 30.57 g
Carbohydrates: 83.44 g

### 36.Omelette Margherita

**Preparation Time:** 10 minutes
**Cooking Time:** 20 minutes
**Servings:** 2
**Ingredients:**
- 3 eggs
- 50 g parmesan cheese
- 2 tbsp heavy cream
- 1 tbsp olive oil
- 1 teaspoon oregano
- nutmeg
- salt
- pepper
- For covering:
- 3 - 4 stalks of basil
- 1 tomato
- 100 g grated mozzarella

**Directions:**
1.Mix the cream and eggs in a medium bowl.
2.Add the grated parmesan, nutmeg, oregano, pepper and salt and stir everything.
3.Heat the oil in a pan.
4.Add 1/2 of the egg and cream to the pan.
5.Let the omelette set over medium heat, turn it, and then remove it.
6.Repeat with the second half of the egg mixture.
7.Cut the tomatoes into slices and place them on top of the omelets.
8.Scatter the mozzarella over the tomatoes.
9.Place the omelets on a baking sheet.
10.Cook at 180 degrees for 5 to 10 minutes.
11.Then take the omelets out and decorate them with the basil leaves.

**Nutrition:**
kcal: 402

Carbohydrates: 7 g
Protein: 21 g
Fat: 34 g

### 37.Omelette With Tomatoes And Spring Onions

**Preparation Time:** 5 minutes
**Cooking Time:** 20 minutes
**Servings:**
**Ingredients:**
- 6 eggs
- 2 tomatoes
- 2 spring onions
- 1 shallot
- 2 tbsp butter
- 1 tbsp olive oil
- 1 pinch of nutmeg
- salt
- pepper

**Directions:**
1.Whisk the eggs in a bowl.
2.Mix them together and season them with salt and pepper.
3.Peel the shallot and chop it up.
4.Clean the onions and cut them into rings.
5.Wash the tomatoes and cut them into pieces.
6.Heat butter and oil in a pan.
7.Braise half of the shallots in it.
8.Add half the egg mixture.
9.Let everything set over medium heat.
10.Scatter a few tomatoes and onion rings on top.
11.Repeat with the second half of the egg mixture.
12.At the end, spread the grated nutmeg over the whole thing.

**Nutrition:**
kcal: 263
Carbohydrates: 8 g

Protein: 20.3 g

Fat: 24 g

### 38.Breakfast Pitas

**Preparation Time:** 4 minutes

**Cooking Time:** 6 minutes

**Servings:** 4

**Ingredients:**

•8 egg whites

•2 c. bell peppers, chopped (any color)

•1 tsp. garlic powder

•1 tsp. onion powder

•1 c. raw spinach (cook if you prefer)

•2 tsp. extra virgin olive oil

•4 whole-wheat pita pockets

**Directions:**

1.Put the olive oil to a large sauté pan and place over medium heat. When the oil is hot in glistening, toss in the bell pepper and sauté for about 3 minutes or until tender. Add in the spinach now (if you want it cooked) and sauté for about 1 to 3 minutes or just up to the sides starts to wilt.

2.Place the egg whites into a small bowl, whisk well. Add in spices; whisk well. Pour the egg mixture into the sauté pan and scramble everything together.

3.Remove from heat and stuff ½ to 1 c. mixture into a pita pocket and serve.

**Nutrition:**

Calories: 153 kcal

Protein: 12.4 g

Fat: 3.41 g

Carbohydrates: 19.32 g

### 39.Omega-3-rich Cold Banana Breakfast

**Preparation Time:** 10 minutes

**Cooking Time:** 0 minutes

**Servings:** 2

**Ingredients:**

•½ cup cold milk

•4 tbsp. sesame seeds

•2 tbsp. flaxseeds

•4 tbsp. sunflower seeds

•2 tbsp. ground coconut

•1 large sliced Banana

**Directions:**

1.Mix the milk and honey on your breakfast bowl. Use your coffee grinder to grind all the seeds. Add the ground seeds to the honey and milk mixture. Place the sliced bananas neatly on top. Sprinkle the ground coconuts for added flavor.

**Nutrition:**

Calories: 393 kcal

Protein: 14.85 g

Fat: 27.63 g

Carbohydrates: 27.37 g

### 40.Swiss Chard and Spinach with Egg

**Preparation Time:** 5 minutes

**Cooking Time:** 10 minutes

**Servings:** 4

**Ingredients:**

•4 egg whites

•4 pieces of rice bread

•20 pieces spinach leaves

•20 pieces Swiss chard leaves

•4 tbsp. parsley (fresh)

•1 tsp. olive oil

•Sea salt, ground pepper, and dried mint

**Directions:**

1.Bring to a boil 2 cups of water in a pan just below the boiling point. Open an egg, separate the whites from the yolks. Put the whites in a small bowl. Lower the bowl towards the heated water, and gently pour the egg into the pan. Do the same with the other eggs. Poach the eggs for 4 minutes. After that, gently take the eggs, one at a time and transfer them into a plate. Do the same with the remaining 2 eggs.

2.Chop the parsley and sauté the leaves in a pan for 6 minutes. Toast the bread while doing this. When done, make a layer of the sautéed greens and the chopped parsley on top of the toasted rice bread. Put the poached eggs above the bed of greens. Sprinkle each serving with ground pepper, sea salt, and dried mint.

**Nutrition:**

Calories: 49 kcal

Protein: 5.31 g

Fat: 2.73 g

Carbohydrates: 0.48 g

## 41.Pancakes With Berries

**Preparation Time:** 5 minutes

**Cooking Time:** 20 minutes

**Servings:** 2

**Ingredients:**

•Pancake:

•1 egg

•50 g spelled flour

•50 g almond flour

•15 g coconut flour

•150 ml of water

•salt

Filling:

•40 g mixed berries

•10 g chocolate

•5 g powdered sugar

•4 tbsp yogurt

**Directions:**

1.Put the flour, egg, and some salt in a blender jar.

2.Add 150 ml of water.

3.Mix everything with a whisk.

4.Mix everything into a batter.

5.Heat a coated pan.

6.Put in half of the batter.

7.Once the pancake is firm, turn it over.

8.Take out the pancake, add the second half of the batter to the pan and repeat.

9.Melt chocolate over a water bath.

10.Let the pancakes cool.

11.Brush the pancakes with the yogurt.

12.Wash the berry and let it drain.

13.Put berries on the yogurt.

14.Roll up the pancakes.

15.Sprinkle them with the powdered sugar.

16.Decorate the whole thing with the melted chocolate.

**Nutrition:**

kcal: 298

Carbohydrates: 26 g

Protein: 21 g

Fat: 9 g

## 42.Coconut Chia Pudding With Berries

**Preparation Time:** 20 minutes

**Cooking Time:** 45 minutes

**Servings:** 2

**Ingredients:**

•150 g raspberries and blueberries

•60 g chia seeds

•500 ml coconut milk

•1 teaspoon agave syrup

•½ teaspoon ground bourbon vanilla

**Directions:**

1.Put the chia seeds, agave syrup, and vanilla in a bowl.

2.Pour in the coconut milk.

3.Mix thoroughly and let it soak for 30 minutes.

4.Meanwhile, wash the berries and let them drain well.

5.Divide the coconut chia pudding between two glasses.
6.Put the berries on top.
**Nutrition:**
kcal: 662
Carbohydrates: 18 g
Protein: 8 g
Fat: 55 g

### 43.Eel On Scrambled Eggs And Bread

**Preparation Time:** 5 minutes
**Cooking Time:** 10 minutes
**Servings:** 2
**Ingredients:**
●4 eggs
●1 shallot
●4 slices of low carb bread
●2 sticks of dill
●200 g smoked eel
●1 tbsp oil
●salt
●White pepper
**Directions:**
1.Mix the eggs in a bowl and season with salt and pepper.
2.Peel the shallot and cut it into fine cubes.
3.Chop the dill.
4.Remove the skin from the eel and cut it into pieces.
5.Heat the oil in a pan and steam the shallot in it.
6.Add in the eggs in and let them set.
7.Use the spatula to turn the eggs several times.
8.Reduce the heat and add the dill.
9.Stir everything.
10.Spread the scrambled eggs over four slices of bread.
11.Put the eel pieces on top.

12.Add some fresh dill and serve everything.
**Nutrition:**
kcal: 830
Carbohydrates: 8 g
Protein: 45 g
Fat: 64 g

### 44.Chia Seed Gel With Pomegranate And Nuts

**Preparation Time:** 5 minutes
**Cooking Time:** 10 minutes
**Servings:** 3
**Ingredients:**
●20 g hazelnuts
●20 g walnuts
●120 ml almond milk
●4 tbsp chia seeds
●4 tbsp pomegranate seeds
●1 teaspoon agave syrup
●Some lime juice
**Directions:**
1.Finely chop the nuts.
2.Mix the almond milk with the chia seeds.
3.Let everything soak for 10 to 20 minutes.
4.Occasionally stir the mixture with the chia seeds.
5.Stir in the agave syrup.
6.Pour 2 tablespoons of each mixture into a dessert glass.
7.Layer the chopped nuts on top.
8.Cover the nuts with 1 tablespoon each of the chia mass.
9.Sprinkle the pomegranate seeds on top and serve everything.
**Nutrition:**
kcal: 248
Carbohydrates: 7 g
Protein: 1 g
Fat: 19 g

### 45. Lavender Blueberry Chia Seed Pudding

**Preparation Time:** 1 hour 10 minutes
**Cooking Time:** 0 minutes
**Servings:** 4
**Ingredients:**
- 100 g blueberries
- 70 g organic quark
- 50 g soy yogurt
- 30 g hazelnuts
- 200 ml almond milk
- 2 tbsp chia seeds
- 2 teaspoons agave syrup
- 2 teaspoons of lavender

**Directions:**
1. Bring the almond milk to a boil along with the lavender.
2. Let the mixture simmer for 10 minutes at a reduced temperature.
3. Let them cool down afterwards.
4. If the milk is cold, add the blueberries and puree everything.
5. Mix the whole thing with the chia seeds and agave syrup.
6. Let everything soak in the refrigerator for an hour.
7. Mix the yogurt and curd cheese together.
8. Add both to the crowd.
9. Divide the pudding into glasses.
10. Finely chop the hazelnuts and sprinkle them on top.

**Nutrition:**
kcal: 252
Carbohydrates: 12 g
Protein: 1 g
Fat: 11 g

### 46. Yogurt With Granola And Persimmon

**Preparation Time:** 5 minutes
**Cooking Time:** 5 minutes
**Servings:** 1
**Ingredients:**
- 150g Greek style yogurt
- 20g oatmeal
- 60g fresh persimmons
- 30 ml of tap water

**Directions:**
1. Put the oatmeal in the pan without any fat.
2. Toast them, stirring constantly, until golden brown.
3. Then put them on a plate and let them cool down briefly.
4. Peel the persimmon and put it in a bowl with the water. Mix the whole thing into a fine puree.
5. Put the yogurt, the toasted oatmeal, and the puree in layers in a glass and serve.

**Nutrition:**
kcal: 286
Carbohydrates: 29 g
Protein: 1 g
Fat: 11 g

### 47. Smoothie Bowl With Spinach, Mango And Muesli

**Preparation Time:** 10 minutes
**Cooking Time:** 0 minutes
**Servings:** 1
**Ingredients:**
- 150g yogurt
- 30g apple
- 30g mango
- 30g low carb muesli
- 10g spinach
- 10g chia seeds

**Directions:**
1. Soak the spinach leaves and let them drain.
2. Peel the mango and cut it into strips.
3. Remove apple core and cut it into pieces.

4.Put everything except the mango together with the yogurt in a blender and make a fine puree out of it.
5.Put the spinach smoothie in a bowl.
6.Add the muesli, chia seeds, and mango.
7.Serve the whole thing
**Nutrition:**
kcal: 362
Carbohydrates: 21 g
Protein: 12 g
Fat: 21 g

## 48.Fried Egg With Bacon

**Preparation Time:** 5 minutes
**Cooking Time:** 10 minutes
**Servings:** 1
**Ingredients:**
- 2 eggs
- 30 grams of bacon
- 2 tbsp olive oil
- salt
- pepper

**Directions:**
1.Heat oil in the pan and fry the bacon.
2.Reduce the heat and beat the eggs in the pan.
3.Cook the eggs and season with salt and pepper.
4.Serve the fried eggs hot with the bacon.
**Nutrition:**
kcal: 405
Carbohydrates: 1 g
Protein: 19 g
Fat: 38 g

## 49. Blueberry Muffins

**Preparation Time:** 5 Minutes
**Cooking Time:** 20 minutes
**Servings:** 3
**Ingredients:**
- 1 cup Coconut Milk
- 3/4 cup Spelt Flour
- 3/4 Teff Flour
- 1/2 cup Blueberries
- 1/3 cup Agave
- 1/4 cup Sea Moss Gel
- 1/2 tsp. Sea Salt
- Grapeseed Oil

**Directions:**
1.Adjust the temperature of the oven to 365 degrees.
2.Grease 6 regular-size muffin cups with muffin liners.
3.In a bowl, mix together sea salt, sea moss, agave, coconut milk, and flour gel until they are properly blended.
4.You then crimp in blueberries.
5.Coat the muffin pan lightly with the grapeseed oil.
6.Pour in the muffin batter.
7.Bake for at least 30 minutes until it turns golden brown.
8.Serve.
**Nutrition:**
Calories: 160 kcal
Fat: 5g
Carbs: 25g
Proteins: 2g

## 50.Quinoa Porridge

**Preparation Time:** 5 minutes
**Cooking Time:** 25 minutes
**Servings:** 2
**Ingredients:**
- 2 cups coconut milk
- 1 cup rinsed quinoa
- 1/8 tsp. ground cinnamon
- 1 cup fresh blueberries

**Directions:**
1.In a saucepan, boil the coconut milk over high heat.

2.Add the quinoa to the milk then bring the mixture to a boil.

3.You then let it simmer for 15 minutes on medium heat until the milk is reduces.

4.Add the cinnamon then mix it properly in the saucepan.

5.Cover the saucepan and cook for at least 8 minutes until milk is completely absorbed.

6.Add in the blueberries then cook for 30 more seconds.

7.Serve.

**Nutrition:**

Calories: 271 kcal

Fat: 3.7g

Carbs: 54g

Protein:6.5g

### 51.Coconut Pancakes

**Preparation Time:** 5 minutes

**Cooking Time:** 15 minutes

**Servings:** 4

**Ingredients:**

- 1 cup coconut flour
- 2 tbsps. arrowroot powder
- 1 tsp. baking powder
- 1 cup coconut milk
- 3 tbsps. coconut oil

**Directions:**

1.In a medium container, mix in all the dry ingredients.

2.Add the coconut milk and 2 tbsps. of the coconut oil then mix properly.

3.In a skillet, melt 1 tsp. of coconut oil.

4.Pour a ladle of the batter into the skillet then swirl the pan to spread the batter evenly into a smooth pancake.

5.Cook it for like 3 minutes on medium heat until it becomes firm.

6.Turn the pancake to the other side then cook it for another 2 minutes until it turns golden brown.

7.Cook the remaining pancakes in the same process.

8.Serve.

**Nutrition:**

Calories: 377 kcal

Fat: 14.9g

Carbs: 60.7g

Protein: 6.4g

### 52.Banana Barley Porridge

**Preparation Time:** 15 minutes

**Cooking Time:** 5 minutes

**Servings:** 2

**Ingredients:**

- 1 cup divided unsweetened coconut milk
- 1 small peeled and sliced banana
- 1/2 cup barley
- 3 drops liquid stevia
- 1/4 cup chopped coconuts

**Directions:**

1.In a bowl, properly mix barley with half of the coconut milk and stevia.

2.Cover the mixing bowl then refrigerate for about 6 hours.

3.In a saucepan, mix the barley mixture with coconut milk.

4.Cook for about 5 minutes on moderate heat.

5.Then top it with the chopped coconuts and the banana slices.

6.Serve.

**Nutrition:**

Calories: 159kcal

Fat: 8.4g

Carbs: 19.8g

Proteins: 4.6g

### 53.Millet Porridge

**Preparation Time:** 10 minutes
**Cooking Time:** 20 minutes
**Servings:** 2
**Ingredients:**
•Sea salt
•1 tbsp. finely chopped coconuts
•1/2 cup unsweetened coconut milk
•1/2 cup rinsed and drained millet
•1-1/2 cups alkaline water
•3 drops liquid stevia
**Directions:**
1.Sauté the millet in a non-stick skillet for about 3 minutes.
2.Add salt and water then stir.
3.Let the meal boil then reduce the amount of heat.
4.Cook for 15 minutes then add the remaining ingredients. Stir.
5.Cook the meal for 4 extra minutes.
6.Serve the meal with toping of the chopped nuts.
**Nutrition:**
Calories: 219 kcal
Fat: 4.5g
Carbs: 38.2g
Protein: 6.4g

### 54.Zucchini Muffins

**Preparation Time:** 10 minutes
**Cooking Time:** 25 minutes
**Servings:** 16
**Ingredients:**
•1 tbsp. ground flaxseed
•3 tbsps. alkaline water
•1/4 cup walnut butter
•3 medium over-ripe bananas
•2 small grated   zucchinis
•1/2 cup coconut milk
•1 tsp. vanilla extract
•2 cups coconut flour
•1 tbsp. baking powder
•1 tsp. cinnamon
•1/4 tsp. sea salt
**Directions:**
1.Tune the temperature of your oven to 375ºF.
2.Grease the muffin tray with the cooking spray.
3.In a bowl, mix the flaxseed with water.
4.In a glass bowl, mash the bananas then stir in the remaining ingredients.
5.Properly mix and then divide the mixture into the muffin tray.
6.Bake it for 25 minutes.
7.Serve.
**Nutrition:**
Calories: 127 kcal
Fat: 6.6g
Carbs: 13g
Protein: 0.7g

### 55. Vegetable Fry

**Preparation Time:** 5 minutes
**Cooking Time:** 5 minutes
**Servings:** 6
**Ingredients:**
•2 finely chopped small onions
•2 cups finely chopped cherry tomatoes
•1/8 tsp. ground turmeric
•1 tbsp. olive oil
•2 seeded and chopped red bell peppers
•3 cups seeded and chopped firm jackfruit
•1/8 tsp. cayenne pepper
•2 tbsps. chopped fresh basil leaves
•Salt
**Directions:**
1.In a greased skillet, sauté the onions and bell peppers for about 5 minutes.

2.Add the tomatoes then stir.

3.Cook for 2 minutes.

4.Then add the jackfruit, cayenne pepper, salt, and turmeric.

5.Cook for about 8 minutes.

6.Garnish the meal with basil leaves.

7.Serve warm.

**Nutrition:**

Calories: 236 kcal

Fat: 1.8g

Carbs: 48.3g

Protein: 7g

## 56.Zucchini Pancakes

**Preparation Time:** 15 minutes

**Cooking Time:** 8 minutes

**Servings:** 8

**Ingredients:**

•12 tbsps. alkaline water

•6 large grated zucchinis

•Sea salt

•4 tbsps. ground Flax Seeds

•2 tsps. olive oil

•2 finely chopped jalapeño peppers

•1/2 cup finely chopped scallions

**Directions:**

1.In a bowl, mix together water and the flax seeds then set it aside.

2.Pour oil in a large non-stick skillet then heat it on medium heat.

3.The add the black pepper, salt, and zucchini.

4.Cook for 3 minutes then transfer the zucchini into a large bowl.

5.Add the flax seed and the scallion's mixture then properly mix it.

6.Preheat a griddle then grease it lightly with the cooking spray.

7.Pour 1/4 of the zucchini mixture into griddle then cook for 3 minutes.

8.Flip the side carefully then cook for 2 more minutes.

9.Repeat the procedure with the remaining mixture in batches.

10.Serve.

**Nutrition:**

Calories: 71 kcal

Fat: 2.8g

Carbs: 9.8g

Protein: 3.7g

## 57.Crunchy Quinoa Meal

**Preparation Time:** 5 minutes

**Cooking Time:** 25 minutes

**Servings:** 2

**Ingredients:**

•3 cups coconut milk

•1 cup rinsed quinoa

•1/8 tsp. ground cinnamon

•1 cup raspberry

•1/2 cup chopped coconuts

**Directions:**

1.In a saucepan, pour milk and bring to a boil over moderate heat.

2.Add the quinoa to the milk and then bring it to a boil once more.

3.You then let it simmer for at least 15 minutes on medium heat until the milk is reduced.

4.Stir in the cinnamon then mix properly.

5.Cover it then cook for 8 minutes until the milk is completely absorbed.

6.Add the raspberry and cook the meal for 30 seconds.

7.Serve and enjoy.

**Nutrition:**

Calories: 271 kcal

Fat: 3.7g

Carbs: 54g

Proteins: 6.5g

## 58. Blueberry Spelt Pancakes

**Preparation Time:** 6 minutes
**Cooking Time:** 20 minutes
**Servings:** 3
**Ingredients:**

- 2 cups Spelt Flour
- 1 cup Coconut Milk
- 1/2 cup Alkaline Water
- 2 tbsps. Grapeseed Oil
- 1/2 cup Agave
- 1/2 cup Blueberries
- 1/4 tsp. Sea Moss

**Directions:**

1. Mix the spelt flour, agave, grapeseed oil, hemp seeds, and the sea moss together in a bowl.
2. Add in 1 cup of hemp milk and alkaline water to the mixture, until you get the consistency mixture you like.
3. Crimp the blueberries into the batter.
4. Heat the skillet to moderate heat then lightly coat it with the grapeseed oil.
5. Pour the batter into the skillet then let them cook for approximately 5 minutes on every side.
6. Serve and Enjoy.

**Nutrition:**

Calories: 203 kcal
Fat: 1.4g
Carbs: 41.6g
Proteins: 4.8g

## 59. Breakfast Donuts

**Preparation Time:** 5 minutes
**Cooking Time:** 5 minutes
**Servings:** 4
**Ingredients:**

- 43 grams cream cheese
- 2 eggs
- 2 tablespoons almond flour
- 2 tablespoons erythritol
- 1 ½ tablespoons coconut flour
- ½ teaspoon baking powder
- ½ teaspoon vanilla extract
- 5 drops Stevia (liquid form)
- 2 strips bacon, fried until crispy

**Directions:**

1. Rub coconut oil over donut maker and turn on.
2. Mix all ingredients except bacon in a blender or food processor until smooth (should take around 1 minute).
3. Pour batter into donut maker, leaving 1/10 in each round for rising.
4. Leave for 3 minutes before flipping each donut. Leave for another 2 minutes or until a fork comes out clean when piercing them.
5. Take donuts out and let cool.
6. Repeat steps 1-5 until all batter is used.
7. Crumble bacon into bits and use to top donuts.

**Nutrition:**

Calories: 60
Fat: 5 g
Carbs: 1 g
Fiber: 0 g
Protein: 3 g

## 60. Cheesy Spicy Bacon Bowls

**Preparation Time:** 10 minutes
**Cooking Time:** 22 minutes
**Servings:** 12
**Ingredients:**

- 6 strips Bacon, pan-fried until cooked but still malleable
- 4 eggs
- 60 grams' cheddar cheese
- 40 grams' cream cheese, grated
- 2 Jalapenos, sliced and seeds removed

•2 tablespoons coconut oil
•¼ teaspoon onion powder
•¼ teaspoon garlic powder
•Dash of salt and pepper
**Directions:**
1.Preheat oven to 375 degrees Fahrenheit
2.In a bowl, beat together eggs, cream cheese, jalapenos (minus 6 slices), coconut oil, onion powder, garlic powder, and salt and pepper.
3.Using leftover bacon grease on a muffin tray, rubbing it into each insert. Place bacon-wrapped inside the parameters of each insert.
4.Pour beaten mixture halfway up each bacon bowl.
5.Garnish each bacon bowl with cheese and leftover jalapeno slices (placing one on top of each).
6.Leave in the oven for about 22 minutes, or until the egg is thoroughly cooked and cheese is bubbly.
7.Remove from oven and let cool until edible.
8.Enjoy!
**Nutrition:**
Calories: 259
Fat: 24g
Carbs: 1g
Fiber: 0g
Protein: 10g

## 61.Porridge With Walnuts

**Preparation Time:** 5 minutes
**Cooking Time:** 10 minutes
**Servings:** 1
**Ingredients:**
•50 g raspberries
•50 g blueberries
•25 g of ground walnuts
•20 g of crushed flaxseed
•10 g of oatmeal
•200 ml nut drink
•Agave syrup
•½ teaspoon cinnamon
•salt
**Directions:**
1.Warm the nut drink in a small saucepan.
2.Add the walnuts, flaxseed, and oatmeal, stirring constantly.
3.Stir in the cinnamon and salt.
4.Simmer for 8 minutes.
5.Keep stirring everything.
6.Sweet the whole thing.
7.Put the porridge in a bowl.
8.Wash the berries and let them drain.
9.Add them to the porridge and serve everything.
**Nutrition:**
kcal: 378
Carbohydrates: 11 g
Protein: 18 g
Fat: 27 g

## 62.Squash Hash

**Preparation Time:** 2 minutes
**Cooking Time:** 10 minutes
**Servings:** 2
**Ingredients:**
•1 tsp. onion powder
•1/2 cup finely chopped onion
•2 cups spaghetti squash
•1/2 tsp. sea salt
**Directions:**
1.Using paper towels, squeeze extra moisture from spaghetti squash.
2.Place the squash into a bowl then add the salt, onion, and the onion powder.
3.Stir properly to mix them.

4.Spray a non-stick cooking skillet with cooking spray then place it over moderate heat.

5.Add the spaghetti squash to pan.

6.Cook the squash for about 5 minutes.

7.Flip the hash browns using a spatula.

8.Cook for 5 minutes until the desired crispness is reached.

9.Serve.

**Nutrition:**

Calories: 44 kcal

Fat: 0.6g

Carbs: 9.7g

Protein: 0.9g

### 63.Goat, Cheese, Zucchini, and Kale Quiche

**Preparation Time**: 35 minutes

**Cooking Time:** 1 hour 10 minutes

**Servings:** 4

**Ingredients:**

- 4 large eggs
- 8 ounces fresh zucchini, sliced
- 10 ounces kale
- 3 garlic cloves (minced)
- 1 cup of soy milk
- 1-ounce goat cheese
- 1 cup grated parmesan
- 1 cup shredded cheddar cheese
- 2 teaspoons olive oil
- Salt and pepper, to taste

**Directions:**

1.Preheat oven to 350°F.

2.Heat 1 tsp of olive oil in a saucepan over medium-high heat. Sauté garlic for 1 minute until flavored.

3.Add the zucchini and cook for another 5-7 minutes until soft.

4.Beat the eggs and then add a little milk and Parmesan cheese.

5.Meanwhile, heat the remaining olive oil in another saucepan and add the kale. Cover and cook for 5 minutes until dry.

6.Slightly grease a baking dish with cooking spray and spread the kale leaves across the bottom. Add the zucchini and top with goat cheese.

7.Pour the egg, milk, and parmesan mixture evenly over the other ingredients. Top with cheddar cheese.

8.Bake for 50–60 minutes until golden brown. Check the center of the quiche, it should have a solid consistency.

9.Let chill for a few minutes before serving.

**Nutrition:**

Total Carbohydrates: 15g

Dietary Fiber: 2 g

Net Carbs: 13 g

Protein: 19 g

Total Fat: 18 g

Calories: 290

### 64.Cream Cheese Egg Breakfast

**Preparation Time**: 5 minutes

**Cooking Time:** 5 minutes

**Servings:** 4

**Ingredients:**

- 2 eggs, beaten
- 1 tablespoon butter
- 2 tablespoons soft cream cheese with chives

**Directions:**

1.Melt the butter in a small skillet.

2.Add the eggs and cream cheese.

3.Stir and cook to desired doneness.

**Nutrition:**

Calories: 341

Fat: 31 g

Protein: 15 g

Carbohydrate: 0 g

Dietary Fiber: 3 g

## 65.Avocado Red Peppers Roasted Scrambled Eggs

**Preparation Time**: 10 minutes
**Cooking Time:** 12 minutes
**Servings:** 3
**Ingredients:**
- 1/2 tablespoon butter
- Eggs, 2
- 1/2 roasted red pepper, about 1 1/2 ounces
- 1/2 small avocado, coarsely chopped, about 2 1/4 ounces
- Salt, to taste

**Directions:**
1.In a nonstick skillet, heat the butter over medium heat. Break the eggs into the pan and break the yolks with a spoon. Sprinkle with a little salt.
2.Stir to stir and continue stirring until the eggs start to come out. Quickly add the bell peppers and avocado.
3.Cook and stir until the eggs suit your taste. Adjust the seasoning, if necessary.

**Nutrition:**
Calories: 317
Fat: 26g
Protein: 14g
Dietary Fiber: 5g
Net Carbs: 4g

## 66.Pumpkin Spice Quinoa

**Preparation Time:** 10 minutes
**Cooking Time:** 0 minutes
**Servings:** 2
**Ingredients:**
- 1 cup cooked quinoa
- 1 cup unsweetened coconut milk
- 1 large mashed banana
- 1/4 cup pumpkin puree
- 1 tsp. pumpkin spice
- 2 tsps. chia seeds

**Directions:**
1.In a container, mix all the ingredients.
2.Seal the lid then shake the container properly to mix.
3.Refrigerate overnight.
4.Serve.

**Nutrition:**
Calories: 212 kcal
Fat: 11.9g
Carbs: 31.7g
Protein: 7.3g

## 67.Mushroom Quickie Scramble

**Preparation Time**: 10 minutes
**Cooking Time:** 10 minutes
**Servings:** 4
**Ingredients:**
- 3 small-sized eggs, whisked
- 4 pcs. Bella mushrooms
- ½ cup of spinach
- ¼ cup of red bell peppers
- 2 deli ham slices
- 1 tablespoon of ghee or coconut oil
- Salt and pepper to taste

**Directions:**
1.Chop the ham and veggies.
2.Put half a tbsp. of butter in a frying pan and heat until melted.
3.Sauté the ham and vegetables in a frying pan then set aside.
4.Get a new frying pan and heat the remaining butter.
5.Add the whisked eggs into the second pan while stirring continuously to avoid overcooking.
6.When the eggs are done, sprinkle with salt and pepper to taste.

7.Add the ham and veggies to the pan with the eggs.

8.Mix well.

9.Remove from burner and transfer to a plate.

**Nutrition:**

Calories: 350

Total Fat: 29 g

Protein: 21 g

Total Carbs: 5 g

## 68.Coconut Coffee and Ghee

**Preparation Time**: 10 minutes

**Cooking Time:** 10 minutes

**Servings:** 5

**Ingredients:**

•½ Tbsp. of coconut oil

•½ Tbsp. of ghee

•1 to 2 cups of preferred coffee (or rooibos or black tea, if preferred)

•1 Tbsp. of coconut or almond milk

**Directions:**

1.Place the almond (or coconut) milk, coconut oil, ghee, and coffee in a blender (or milk frother).

2.Mix for around 10 seconds or until the coffee turns creamy and foamy.

3.Pour contents into a coffee cup.

4.Serve immediately and enjoy.

**Nutrition:**

Calories: 150

Total Fat: 15 g

Protein: 0 g

Total Carbs: 0 g

Net Carbs: 0 g

## 69.Yummy Veggie Waffles

**Preparation Time**: 10 minutes

**Cooking Time:** 9 minutes

**Servings:** 3

**Ingredients:**

•3 cups raw cauliflower, grated

•1 cup cheddar cheese

•1 cup mozzarella cheese

•½ cup parmesan

•1/3 cup chives, finely sliced

•6 eggs

•1 teaspoon garlic powder

•1 teaspoon onion powder

•½ teaspoon chili flakes

•Dash of salt and pepper

**Directions:**

1.Turn waffle maker on.

2.In a bowl, mix all the listed ingredients very well until incorporated.

3.Once the waffle maker is hot, distribute the waffle mixture into the insert.

4.Let cook for about 9 minutes, flipping at 6 minutes.

5.Remove from waffle maker and set aside.

6.Serve and enjoy!

**Nutrition:**

Calories: 390

Fat: 28 g

Carbs: 6 g

Fiber: 2 g

Protein: 30 g

## 70.Amaranth Porridge

**Preparation Time**: 5 minutes

**Cooking Time:** 30 minutes

**Servings:** 2.

**Ingredients:**

•2 cups coconut milk

•2 cups alkaline water

•1 cup amaranth

•2 tbsps. coconut oil

•1 tbsp. ground cinnamon

**Directions:**
1.In a saucepan, mix in the milk with water, then boil the mixture.
2.You stir in the amaranth, then reduce the heat to medium.
3.Cook on the medium heat, then simmer for at least 30 minutes as you stir it occasionally.
4.Turn off the heat.
5.Add in cinnamon and coconut oil then stir.
6.Serve.
**Nutrition:**
Calories: 434 kcal
Fat: 35g
Carbs: 27g
Protein: 6.7g

### 71.Fried Zucchini
**Preparation Time**: 10 minutes
**Cooking Time:** 8 minutes
**Servings:** 4
**Ingredients:**
•2 medium zucchinis, cut into strips 19 mm. thick
•60 g all-purpose flour
•12 g of salt
•2 g black pepper
•2 beaten eggs
•15 ml. of milk
•84 g Italian seasoned breadcrumbs
•25 g grated Parmesan cheese
•Nonstick spray oil
•Ranch sauce, to serve
**Directions:**
1.Cut the zucchini into strips 19 mm thick.
2.Mix the flour, salt, and pepper on a plate.
3.Mix the eggs and milk in a separate dish.
4.Put breadcrumbs and Parmesan cheese in another dish.

5.Cover each piece of zucchini with flour, then dip them in egg and milk mixture, and pass them through the crumbs. Leave aside.
6.Preheat the air fryer, set it to 175°C.
7.Place the covered zucchini in the preheated air fryer and spray with oil spray. Set the timer to 8 minutes and press Start / Pause.
8.Be sure to shake the baskets in the middle of cooking.
9.Serve with tomato sauce or ranch sauce.
**Nutrition:**
Calories: 68
Carbs: 2 g
Fat: 11 g
Protein: 4 g
Fiber: 143 g

### 72.Blueberry Cantaloupe Avocado
**Preparation Time:** 5 minutes
**Cooking Time:** 0 minutes
**Servings:** 2
**Ingredients:**
•1 diced cantaloupe
•2–3 chopped avocados
•1 package of blueberries
•¼ cup olive oil
•1/8 cup balsamic vinegar
**Directions:**
1.Mix all ingredients.
**Nutrition:**
Calories: 406
Protein: 9g
Carbohydrate: 32g
Fat: 5 g

### 73.Omega 3 Breakfast Shake
**Preparation Time**: 5 minutes
**Cooking Time:** 5 minutes
**Servings:** 2

**Ingredients:**
- 1 cup vanilla almond milk (unsweetened)
- 2 tablespoons blueberries
- 1 ½ tablespoons flaxseed meal
- 1 tablespoon MCT Oil
- ¾ tablespoon banana extract
- ½ tablespoon chia seeds
- 5 drops Stevia (liquid form)
- 1/8 tablespoon Xanthan gum

**Directions:**
1. In a blender, mix vanilla almond milk, banana extract, Stevia, and three ice cubes.
2. When smooth, add blueberries and pulse.
3. Once blueberries are thoroughly incorporated, add flaxseed meal and chia seeds.
4. Let sit for 5 minutes.
5. After 5 minutes, pulse again until all ingredients are nicely distributed. Serve and enjoy

**Nutrition:**
Calories: 264
Fats: 25 g
Carbs: 7 g
Protein: 4 g

## 74. Lime Bacon Thyme Muffins

**Preparation Time**: 10 minutes
**Cooking Time:** 20 minutes
**Servings:** 3
**Ingredients:**
- 3 cups of almond flour
- 4 medium-sized eggs
- 1 cup of bacon bits
- 2 tsp. of lemon thyme
- ½ cup of melted ghee
- 1 tsp. of baking soda
- ½ tsp. of salt, to taste

**Directions:**

1. Pre-heat oven to 3500 F.
2. Put ghee in mixing bowl and melt.
3. Add baking soda and almond flour.
4. Put the eggs in.
5. Add the lemon thyme (if preferred, other herbs or spices may be used).
6. Drizzle with salt.
7. Mix all ingredients well.
8. Sprinkle with bacon bits
9. Line the muffin pan with liners.
10. Spoon mixture into the pan, filling the pan to about ¾ full.
11. Bake for about 20 minutes. Test by inserting a toothpick into a muffin. If it comes out clean, then the muffins are done.

**Nutrition:**
Calories: 300
Total Fat: 28 g
Protein: 11 g
Total Carbs: 6 g
Fiber: 3 g

## 75. Fried Avocado

**Preparation Time**: 15 minutes
**Cooking Time:** 10 minutes
**Servings:** 2
**Ingredients:**
- 2 avocados cut into wedges 25 mm. thick
- 50 g breadcrumbs
- 2 g garlic powder
- 2 g onion powder
- 1 g smoked paprika
- 1 g cayenne pepper
- Salt and pepper to taste
- 60 g all-purpose flour
- 2 eggs, beaten
- Nonstick spray oil
- Tomato sauce or ranch sauce, to serve

**Directions:**

1.Cut the avocados into 25 mm. thick pieces.
2.Combine the crumbs, garlic powder, onion powder, smoked paprika, cayenne pepper, and salt in a bowl.
3.Separate each wedge of avocado in the flour, then dip the beaten eggs and stir in the breadcrumb mixture.
4.Preheat the air fryer.
5.Place the avocados in the preheated air fryer baskets, spray with oil spray, and cook at 205°C for 10 minutes. Turn the fried avocado halfway through cooking and sprinkle with cooking oil.
6.Serve with tomato sauce or ranch sauce.

**Nutrition:**
Calories: 123
Carbs: 2 g
Fat: 11 g
Protein: 4 g
Fiber: 0 g

## 76.Gluten-Free Pancakes

**Preparation Time**: 5 minutes
**Cooking Time:** 2 minutes
**Servings:** 2
**Ingredients:**
•6 eggs
•1 cup low-fat cream cheese
•1 1/12; teaspoons baking powder
•1 scoop protein powder
•1/4 cup almond meal
•¼ teaspoon salt
**Directions:**
1.Combine dry ingredients in a food processor. Add the eggs one after another and then the cream cheese. Mix it well.
2.Lightly grease a skillet with cooking spray and place over medium-high heat.
3.Pour the batter into the pan. Turn the pan gently to create round pancakes.

4.Cook for about 2 minutes on each side.
5.Serve pancakes with your favorite topping.
**Nutrition:**
Dietary Fiber: 1 g
Net Carbs: 5 g
Protein: 25 g
Total Fat: 14 g
Calories: 288

# Lunch Recipes

### 77. Pizza Hack

**Preparation Time**: 5-10 minutes
**Cooking Time:** 15-20 minutes
**Servings:** 1
**Ingredients:**

- 1/4 fueling of garlic mashed potato
- 1/2 egg whites
- 1/4 tablespoon of baking powder
- 3/4 oz. of reduced-fat shredded mozzarella
- 1/8 cup of sliced white mushrooms
- 1/16 cup of pizza sauce
- 3/4 oz. of ground beef
- 1/4 sliced black olives
- You also need a sauté pan, baking sheets, and parchment paper

**Directions:**

1. Start by preheating the oven to 400°.
2. Mix your baking powder and garlic potato packet.
3. Add egg whites to your mixture and stir well until it blends.
4. Line the baking sheet with parchment paper and pour the mixed batter onto it.
5. Put another parchment paper on top of the batter and spread out the batter to a 1/8-inch circle.
6. Then place another baking sheet on top; this way, the batter is between two baking sheets.
7. Place into an oven and bake for about 8 minutes until the pizza crust is golden brown.
8. For the toppings, place your ground beef in a sauté pan and fry till it's brown and wash your mushrooms very well.
9. After the crust is baked, remove the top layer of parchment paper carefully to prevent the foam from sticking to the pizza crust.
10. Put your toppings on top of the crust and bake for an extra 8 minutes.
11. Once ready, slide the pizza off the parchment paper and onto a plate.

**Nutrition:**

Calories: 478
Protein: 30 g
Carbohydrates: 22 g
Fats: 29 g

### 78. Meat in Lettuce

**Preparation Time**: 5 minutes
**Cooking Time:** 15 minutes
**Servings:** 1
**Ingredients:**

- 5 ounces of lean ground beef
- Two tablespoons of diced white or yellow onion.
- 1/8 teaspoon of onion powder
- 1/8 teaspoon of white vinegar
- 1 ounce of dill pickle slices
- One teaspoon sesame seed
- 3 cups of shredded Romaine lettuce
- Cooking spray
- Two tablespoons reduced-fat shredded cheddar cheese
- Two tablespoons of Wish-Bone light thousand island as dressing

**Directions:**

1. Place a lightly greased small skillet on fire to heat.
2. Add your onion to cook for about 2-3 minutes.
3. Next, add the beef and allow cooking until it's brown.
4. Next, mix your vinegar and onion powder with the dressing.

5.Finally, top the lettuce with the cooked meat and sprinkle cheese on it, add your pickle slices.

6.Drizzle the mixture with the sauce and sprinkle the sesame seeds.

7.Your dish is ready for consumption.

**Nutrition:**

Calories: 150

Protein: 21 g

Carbohydrates: 32 g

Fats: 19 g

## 79.Plant-Powered Pancakes

**Preparation Time**: 5 minutes

**Cooking Time:** 15 minutes

**Servings:** 8

**Ingredients:**

- 1 cup whole-wheat flour
- 1 teaspoon baking powder
- 1/2 teaspoon ground cinnamon
- 1 cup plant-based milk
- 1/2 cup unsweetened applesauce
- 1/4 cup maple syrup
- 1 teaspoon vanilla extract

**Directions:**

1.In a large bowl, combine the flour, baking powder, and cinnamon.

2.Stir in the milk, applesauce, maple syrup, and vanilla until no dry flour is left, and the batter is smooth.

3.Heat a large, nonstick skillet or griddle over medium heat. For each pancake, pour 1/4 cup of batter onto the hot skillet. Once bubbles form over the top of the pancake and the sides begin to brown, flip and cook for 1 or 2 minutes more.

4.Repeat until all of the batter is used, and serve.

**Nutrition:**

Fat: 2 g

Carbohydrates: 44 g

Fiber: 5 g

Protein: 5 g

## 80.Hemp Seed Porridge

**Preparation Time**: 5 minutes

**Cooking Time:** 5 minutes

**Servings:** 6

**Ingredients:**

- 3 cups cooked hemp seed
- 1 packet Stevia
- 1 cup coconut milk

**Directions:**

1.In a saucepan, mix the rice and the coconut milk over moderate heat for about 5 minutes as you stir it constantly.

2.Remove the pan from the burner then add the Stevia. Stir.

3.Serve in 6 bowls.

4.Enjoy.

**Nutrition:**

Calories: 236 kcal

Fat: 1.8 g

Carbs: 48.3 g

Protein: 7 g

## 81.Mushroom & Spinach Omelet

**Preparation Time**: 20 minutes

**Cooking Time:** 20 minutes

**Servings:** 3

**Ingredients:**

- 2 tablespoons butter, divided
- 6-8 fresh mushrooms, sliced, 5 ounces
- Chives, chopped, optional
- Salt and pepper, to taste
- 1 handful baby spinach, about 1/2 ounce
- Pinch garlic powder

•4 eggs, beaten
•1-ounce shredded Swiss cheese
**Directions:**
1.In a very large saucepan, sauté the mushrooms in one tablespoon of butter until soft. Season with salt, pepper, and garlic.
2.Remove the mushrooms from the pan and keep warm. Heat the remaining tablespoon of butter in the same skillet over medium heat.
3.Beat the eggs with a little salt and pepper and add to the hot butter. Turn the pan over to coat the entire bottom of the pan with egg. Once the egg is almost out, place the cheese over the middle of the tortilla.
4.Fill the cheese with spinach leaves and hot mushrooms. Let cook for about a minute for the spinach to start to wilt. Fold the empty side of the tortilla carefully over the filling and slide it onto a plate and sprinkle with chives, if desired.
5.Alternatively, you can make two tortillas using half the mushroom, spinach, and cheese filling in each.
**Nutrition:**
Calories: 321
Fat: 26 g
Protein: 19 g
Carbohydrate: 4 g
Dietary Fiber: 1 g

## 82.Walnut Crunch Banana Bread

**Preparation Time**: 5 minutes
**Cooking Time:** 1 hour and 30 minutes
**Servings:** 1
**Ingredients:**
•4 ripe bananas
•1/4 cup maple syrup
•1 tablespoon apple cider vinegar
•1 teaspoon vanilla extract
•11/2 cups whole-wheat flour
•1/2 teaspoon ground cinnamon



•1/2 teaspoon baking soda
•1/4 cup walnut pieces (optional)
**Directions:**
1.Preheat the oven to 350°F.
2.In a large bowl, use a fork or mixing spoon to mash the bananas until they reach a puréed consistency (small bits of banana are acceptable). Stir in the maple syrup, apple cider vinegar, and vanilla.
3.Stir in the flour, cinnamon, and baking soda. Fold in the walnut pieces (if using).
4.Gently pour the batter into a loaf pan, filling it no more than three-quarters of the way full. Bake for 1 hour, or until you can stick a knife into the middle and it comes out clean.
5.Remove from the oven and allow cooling on the countertop for a minimum of 30 minutes before serving.
**Nutrition:**
Fat: 1g
Carbohydrates: 40 g
Fiber: 5 g
Protein: 4 g

## 83.Sweet Cashew Cheese Spread

**Preparation Time**: 5 minutes
**Cooking Time:** 5 minutes
**Servings:** 10 servings
**Ingredients:**
•Stevia (5 drops)
•Cashews (2 cups, raw)
•Water (1/2 cup)
**Directions:**
1.Soak the cashews overnight in water.
2.Next, drain the excess water then transfer cashews to a food processor.
3.Add in the stevia and the water.
4.Process until smooth.
5.Serve chilled. Enjoy.
**Nutrition:**
Fat: 5 g

Cholesterol: 0 mg
Sodium: 12.6 mg
Carbohydrates: 5.7 g

## 84.Mini Zucchini Bites

**Preparation Time**: 10 minutes
**Cooking Time:** 10 minutes
**Servings:** 6
**Ingredients:**
•1 zucchini, cut into thick circles
•3 cherry tomatoes, halved
•1/2 cup parmesan cheese, grated
•Salt and pepper to taste
•1 tsp. chives, chopped
**Directions:**
1.Preheat the oven to 390 degrees F.
2.Add wax paper on a baking sheet.
3.Arrange the zucchini pieces.
4.Add the cherry halves on each zucchini slice.
5.Add parmesan cheese, chives, and sprinkle with salt and pepper.
6.Bake for 10 minutes. Serve.
**Nutrition:**
Fat: 1.0 g
Cholesterol: 5.0 mg
Sodium: 400.3 mg
Potassium: 50.5 mg
Carbohydrates: 7.3 g

## 85.Shake Cake

**Preparation Time**: 5 minutes
**Cooking Time:** 0 minutes
**Servings:** 1
**Ingredients:**
•One packet of Shakes
•1/4 teaspoon of baking powder

•Two tablespoons of eggbeaters or egg whites
•Two tablespoons of water
•Other options that are not compulsory include sweetener, reduced-fat cream cheese, etc.
**Directions:**
1.Begin by preheating the oven.
2.Mix all the ingredients. Begin with the dry ingredients, and then add the wet ingredients.
3.After the mixture/batter is ready, pour gently into muffin cups.
4.Inside the oven, place, and bake for about 16-18 minutes or until it is baked and ready. Allow it to cool completely.
5.Add additional toppings of your choice and ensure your delicious shake cake is refreshing.
**Nutrition:**
Calories: 203
Fat: 22 g
Carbohydrate: 12.5 g
Protein: 34 g

## 86.Whole-Wheat Blueberry Muffins

**Preparation Time**: 5 minutes
**Cooking Time:** 25 minutes
**Servings:** 8
**Ingredients:**
•1/2 cup plant-based milk
•1/2 cup unsweetened applesauce
•1/2 cup maple syrup
•1 teaspoon vanilla extract
•2 cups whole-wheat flour
•1/2 teaspoon baking soda
•1 cup blueberries
**Directions:**
1.Preheat the oven to 375°F.

2.In a large bowl, mix the milk, applesauce, maple syrup, and vanilla.

3.Stir in the flour and baking soda until no dry flour is left, and the batter is smooth.

4.Gently fold in the blueberries until they are evenly distributed throughout the batter.

5.In a muffin tin, fill eight muffin cups with three-quarters full of batter.

6.Bake for 25 minutes, or until you can stick a knife into the center of a muffin and it comes out clean. Allow cooling before serving.

Tip: both frozen and fresh blueberries will work great in this recipe. The only difference will be that muffins using fresh blueberries will cook slightly quicker than those using frozen.

**Nutrition:**

Fat: 1 g

Carbohydrates: 45 g

Fiber: 2 g

Protein: 4 g

## 87. Biscuit Pizza

**Preparation Time**: 5 minutes

**Cooking Time:** 15-20 minutes

**Servings:** 1

**Ingredients:**

•1/4 sachet of  buttermilk cheddar and herb biscuit

•1/4 tablespoon of tomato sauce

•1/4 tablespoon of low-fat shredded cheese

•¼ bottle of water

•Parchment paper

**Directions:**

1.Begin by preheating the oven to about 350°F

2.Mix the biscuit and water and stir properly.

3.In the parchment paper, pour the mixture and spread it into a thin circle. Allow cooking for 10 minutes.

4.Take it out and add the tomato sauce and shredded cheese.

5.Bake it for a few more minutes.

**Nutrition:**

Calories: 478

Protein: 30 g

Carbohydrates: 22 g

Fats: 29 g

## 88.Green Smoothie 1

**Preparation Time**: 5 minutes

**Cooking Time:** 0 minutes

**Servings:** 1

**Ingredients:**

•2 1/2 cups of kale leaves

•3/4 cup of chilled apple juice

•1 cup of cubed pineapple

•1/2 cup of frozen green grapes

•1/2 cup of chopped apple

**Directions:**

1.Place the pineapple, apple juice, apple, frozen seedless grapes, and kale leaves in a blender.

2.Cover and blend until it's smooth.

3.Smoothie is ready and can be garnished with halved grapes if you wish.

**Nutrition:**

Calories: 81

Protein: 2 g

Carbohydrates: 19 g

Fats: 1 g

## 89.Green Smoothie 2

**Preparation Time**: 5 minutes

**Cooking Time:** 0 minutes

**Servings:** 1

**Ingredients:**

•Six kale leaves

•Two peeled oranges

•2 cups of mango kombucha

•2 cups of chopped pineapple
•2 cups of water
**Directions:**
1.Break up the oranges, place in the blender.
2.Add the mango kombucha, chopped pineapple, and kale leaves into the blender.
3.Blend everything until it is smooth.
4.Smoothie is ready to be taken.
**Nutrition:**
Calories: 81
Protein: 2 g
Carbohydrates: 19 g
Fats: 1 g

## 90.Easiest Tuna Cobbler Ever

**Preparation Time:** 15 minutes
**Cooking Time:** 25 minutes
**Servings:** 4
**Ingredients:**
•Water, cold (1/3 cup)
•Tuna, canned, drained (10 ounces)
•Sweet pickle relish (2 tablespoons)
•Mixed vegetables, frozen (1 ½ cups)
•Soup, cream of chicken, condensed (10 ¾ ounces)
•Pimientos, sliced, drained (2 ounces)
•Lemon juice (1 teaspoon)
•Paprika
**Directions:**
1.Preheat the air fryer at 375 degrees Fahrenheit.
2.Mist cooking spray into a round casserole (1 ½ quarts).
3.Mix the frozen vegetables with milk, soup, lemon juice, relish, pimientos, and tuna in a saucepan. Cook for 8 minutes over medium heat.
4.Fill the casserole with the tuna mixture.

5.Mix the biscuit mix with cold water to form a soft dough. Beat for half a minute before dropping by four spoonfuls into the casserole.
6.Dust the dish with paprika before air-frying for twenty to twenty-five minutes.
**Nutrition:**
Calories 320
Fat 10 g
Protein 20 g
Carbohydrates 30 g

## 91.Yogurt Garlic Chicken

**Preparation Time:** 30 minutes
**Cooking Time:** 60 min
**Servings:** 6
**Ingredients:**
•Pita bread rounds, halved (6 pieces)
•English cucumber, sliced thinly, w/ each slice halved (1 cup)
Chicken & vegetables:
•Olive oil (3 tablespoons)
•Black pepper, freshly ground (1/2 teaspoon)
•Chicken thighs, skinless, boneless (20 ounces)
•Bell pepper, red, sliced into half-inch portions (1 piece)
•Garlic cloves, chopped finely (4 pieces)
•Cumin, ground (1/2 teaspoon)
•Red onion, medium, sliced into half-inch wedges (1 piece)
•Yogurt, plain, fat free (1/2 cup)
•Lemon juice (2 tablespoons)
•Salt (1 ½ teaspoons)
•Red pepper flakes, crushed (1/2 teaspoon)
•Allspice, ground (1/2 teaspoon)
•Bell pepper, yellow, sliced into half-inch portions (1 piece)
Yogurt sauce:
•Olive oil (2 tablespoons)

•Salt (1/4 teaspoon)
•Parsley, flat leaf, chopped finely (1 tablespoon)
•Yogurt, plain, fat free (1 cup)
•Lemon juice, fresh (1 tablespoon)
•Garlic clove, chopped finely (1 piece)
**Directions:**
1.Mix the yogurt (1/2 cup), garlic cloves (4 pieces), olive oil (1 tablespoon), salt (1 teaspoon), lemon juice (2 tablespoons), pepper (1/4 teaspoon), allspice, cumin, and pepper flakes. Stir in the chicken and coat well. Cover and marinate in the fridge for two hours.
2.Preheat the air fryer at 400 degrees Fahrenheit.
3.Grease a rimmed baking sheet (18x13-inch) with cooking spray.
4.Toss the bell peppers and onion with remaining olive oil (2 tablespoons), pepper (1/4 teaspoon), and salt (1/2 teaspoon).
5.Arrange veggies on the baking sheet's left side and the marinated chicken thighs (drain first) on the right side. Cook in the air fryer for twenty-five to thirty minutes.
6.Mix the yogurt sauce ingredients.
7.Slice air-fried chicken into half-inch strips.
8.Top each pita round with chicken strips, roasted veggies, cucumbers, and yogurt sauce.
**Nutrition:**
Calories 380
Fat 10 g
Protein 20 g
Carbohydrates 30 g

### 92. Tuna Spinach Casserole
**Preparation Time:** 30 minutes
**Cooking Time:** 25 minutes
**Servings:** 8
**Ingredients:**

•Mushroom soup, creamy (18 ounces)
•Milk (1/2 cup)
•White tuna, solid, in-water, drained (12 ounces)
•Crescent dinner rolls, refrigerated (8 ounces)
•Egg noodles, wide, uncooked (8 ounces)
•Cheddar cheese, shredded (8 ounces)
•Spinach, chopped, frozen, thawed, drained (9 ounces)
•Lemon peel grated (2 teaspoons)
**Directions:**
1.Preheat the oven at 350 degrees Fahrenheit.
2.Mist cooking spray onto a glass baking dish (11x7-inch).
3.Follow package directions in cooking and draining the noodles.
4.Stir the cheese (1 ½ cups) and soup together in a skillet heated on medium. Once cheese melts, stir in your noodles, milk, spinach, tuna, and lemon peel. Once bubbling, pour into the prepped dish.
5.Unroll the dough and sprinkle with remaining cheese (1/2 cup). Roll up dough and pinch at the seams to seal. Slice into 8 portions and place over the tuna mixture.
6.Air-fry for twenty to twenty-five minutes.
**Nutrition:**
Calories 400
Fat 10 g
Protein 20 g
Carbohydrates 30 g

### 93. Lean Chicken Pesto Pasta
**Preparation Time:** 5 minutes
**Cooking Time:** 15 minutes
**Servings:** 1
**Ingredients:**
•3 cups of raw kale leaves
•2 tbsp. of olive oil

•2 cups of fresh basil
•1/4 teaspoon salt
•3 tbsp. lemon juice
•Three garlic cloves
•2 cups of cooked chicken breast
•1 cup of baby spinach
•6 ounces of uncooked chicken pasta
•3 ounces of diced fresh mozzarella
•Basil leaves or red pepper flakes to garnish
**Directions:**
1.Start by making the pesto; add the kale, lemon juice, basil, garlic cloves, olive oil, and salt to a blender and blend until it's smooth.
2.Add salt and pepper to taste.
3.Cook the pasta and strain off the water. Reserve 1/4 cup of the liquid.
4.Get a bowl and mix everything, the cooked pasta, pesto, diced chicken, spinach, mozzarella, and the reserved pasta liquid.
5.Sprinkle the mixture with additional chopped basil or red paper flakes (optional).
6.Now your salad is ready. You may serve it warm or chilled. Also, it can be taken as a salad mix-ins or as a side dish. Leftovers should be stored in the refrigerator inside an air-tight container for 3-5 days.
**Nutrition:**
Calories: 244
Protein: 20.5 g
Carbohydrates: 22.5 g
Fats: 10 g

## 94.Open-Face Egg Sandwiches with Cilantro-Jalapeño Spread
**Preparation Time**: 20 minutes
**Cooking Time:** 10 minutes
**Servings:** 2
**Ingredients:**
For the cilantro and jalapeño spread

•1 cup filled up fresh cilantro leaves and stems (about a bunch)
•1 jalapeño pepper, seeded and roughly chopped
•½ cup extra-virgin olive oil
•¼ cup pepitas (hulled pumpkin seeds), raw or roasted
•2 garlic cloves, thinly sliced
•1 tablespoon freshly squeezed lime juice
•1 teaspoon kosher salt
For the eggs
•4 large eggs
•¼ cup milk
•¼ to ½ teaspoon kosher salt
•2 tablespoons butter
For the sandwich
•2 slices bread
•1 tablespoon butter
•1 avocado, halved, pitted, and divided into slices
•Microgreens or sprouts, for garnish
**Directions:**
To make the cilantro and jalapeño spread
1.In a food processor, combine the cilantro, jalapeño, oil, pepitas, garlic, lime juice, and salt. Whirl until smooth. Refrigerate if making in advance; otherwise set aside.
To make the eggs
2.In a medium bowl, whisk the eggs, milk, and salt.
3.Dissolve the butter in a skillet over low heat, swirling to coat the bottom of the pan. Pour in the whisked eggs.
4.Cook until they begin to set then, using a heatproof spatula, push them to the sides, allowing the uncooked portions to run into the bottom of the skillet.
5.Continue until the eggs are set.
To assemble the sandwiches

1.Toast the bed and spread with butter.
2.Spread a spoonful of the cilantro-jalapeño spread on each piece of toast. Top each with scrambled eggs.
3.Arrange avocado over each sandwich and garnish with microgreens.
**Nutrition:**
Calories: 311
Total fat: 4 g
Cholesterol: 54 mg
Fiber: 12 g
Protein: 12 g
Sodium: 327 mg

## 95.Homemade Pork Buns

**Preparation Time:** 20 minutes
**Cooking Time:** 25 minutes
**Servings:** 8
**Ingredients:**
•Green onions, sliced thinly (3 pieces)
•Egg, beaten (1 piece)
•Pulled pork, diced, w/ barbecue sauce (1 cup)
•Buttermilk biscuits, refrigerated (16 1/3 ounces)
•Soy sauce (1 teaspoon)
**Directions:**
1.Preheat the air fryer at 325 degrees Fahrenheit.
2.Use parchment paper to line your baking sheet.
3.Combine pork with green onions.
4.Separate and press the dough to form 8 four-inch rounds.
5.Fill each biscuit round's center with two tablespoons of pork mixture. Cover with the dough edges and seal by pinching. Arrange the buns on the sheet and brush with a mixture of soy sauce and egg.

6.Cook in the air fryer for twenty to twenty-five minutes.
**Nutrition:**
Calories 240
Fat 0 g
Protein 0 g
Carbohydrates 20 g

## 96.Lemony Parmesan Salmon

**Preparation Time:** 10 minutes
**Cooking Time:** 25 minutes
**Servings:** 4
**Ingredients:**
•Butter, melted (2 tablespoons)
•Green onions, sliced thinly (2 tablespoons)
•Breadcrumbs, white, fresh (3/4 cup)
•Thyme leaves, dried (1/4 teaspoon)
•Salmon fillet, 1 ¼-pound (1 piece)
•Salt (1/4 teaspoon)
•Parmesan cheese, grated (1/4 cup)
•Lemon peel, grated (2 teaspoons)
**Directions:**
1.Preheat the oven at 350 degrees Fahrenheit.
2.Mist cooking spray onto a baking pan (shallow). Fill with pat-dried salmon. Brush salmon with butter (1 tablespoon) before sprinkling with salt.
3.Combine the breadcrumbs with onions, thyme, lemon peel, cheese, and remaining butter (1 tablespoon).
4.Cover salmon with the breadcrumb mixture. Air-fry for fifteen to twenty-five minutes.
**Nutrition:**
Calories 290
Fat 10 g
Protein 30 g
Carbohydrates 0 g

## 97.Tuna Melts

**Preparation Time:** 15 minutes
**Cooking Time:** 20 minutes
**Servings:** 8
**Ingredients:**
•Salt (1/8 teaspoon)
•Onion, chopped (1/3 cup)
•Biscuits, refrigerated, flaky layers (16 1/3 ounces)
•Tuna, water packed, drained (10 ounces)
•Mayonnaise (1/3 cup)
•Pepper (1/8 teaspoon)
•Cheddar cheese, shredded (4 ounces)
•Tomato, chopped
•Sour cream
•Lettuce, shredded
**Directions:**
1.Preheat the air fryer at 325 degrees Fahrenheit.
2.Mist cooking spray onto a cookie sheet.
3.Mix tuna with mayonnaise, pepper, salt, and onion.
4.Separate dough so you have 8 biscuits; press each into 5-inch rounds.
5.Arrange 4 biscuit rounds on the sheet. Fill at the center with tuna mixture before topping with cheese. Cover with the remaining biscuit rounds and press to seal.
6.Air-fry for fifteen to twenty minutes. Slice each sandwich into halves. Serve each piece topped with lettuce, tomato, and sour cream.
**Nutrition:**
Calories 320
Fat 10 g
Protein 10 g
Carbohydrates 20 g

## 98.Almond Pancakes

**Preparation Time:** 10 minutes
**Cooking Time:** 13 minutes
**Servings:** 12
**Ingredients:**
•6 eggs
•1/4 cup almonds; toasted
•2 ounces' cocoa chocolate
•1 teaspoon almond extract
•1/3 cup coconut; shredded
•1/2 teaspoon baking powder
•1/4 cup coconut oil
•1/2 cup coconut flour
•1/4 cup stevia
•1 cup almond milk
•Cooking spray
•A pinch of salt
**Directions:**
1.Mix coconut flour with stevia, baking powder, salt and coconut and stir.
2.Add coconut oil, eggs, almond milk and the almond extract and stir well again.
3.Add chocolate and almonds and whisk well again.
4.Heat up a pan and add cooking spray; add 2 tablespoons batter, spread into a circle, cook until it's golden, flip, cook again until it's done and transfer to a pan.
5.Do the same for rest of the batter and serve your pancakes right away.
**Nutrition:**
Calories: 266
Fat: 13
Fiber: 8
Carbs: 10
Protein: 11

## 99.Mouth-watering Pie

**Preparation Time:** 15 minutes
**Cooking Time:** 45 minutes
**Servings:** 8
**Ingredients:**
•3/4-pound beef; ground

- 1/2 onion; chopped.
- 1 pie crust
- 3 tablespoons taco seasoning
- 1 teaspoon baking soda
- Mango salsa for serving
- 1/2 red bell pepper; chopped.
- A handful cilantro; chopped.
- 8 eggs
- 1 teaspoon coconut oil
- Salt and black pepper to the taste.

**Directions:**

1. Heat up a pan, add oil, beef, cook until it browns and mixes with salt, pepper and taco seasoning.
2. Stir again, transfer to a bowl and leave aside for now.
3. Heat up the pan again over medium heat with cooking juices from the meat, add onion and pepper; stir and cook for 4 minutes
4. Add eggs, baking soda and some salt and stir well.
5. Add cilantro; stir again and take off heat.
6. Spread beef mix in pie crust, add veggies mix and spread over meat, heat oven oven at 350 degrees F and bake for 45 minutes
7. Leave the pie to cool down a bit, slice, divide between plates and serve with mango salsa on top.

**Nutrition:**

Calories: 198
Fat: 11
Fiber: 1
Carbs: 12
Protein: 12

## 100. Chicken Omelet

**Preparation Time:** 5 minutes
**Cooking Time:** 15 minutes
**Servings:** 1
**Ingredients:**

- 2 bacon slices; cooked and crumbled
- 2 eggs
- 1 tablespoon homemade mayonnaise
- 1 tomato; chopped.
- 1-ounce rotisserie chicken; shredded
- 1 teaspoon mustard
- 1 small avocado; pitted, peeled and chopped.
- Salt and black pepper to the taste.

**Directions:**

1. In a bowl, mix eggs with some salt and pepper and whisk gently.
2. Heat up a pan over medium heat; spray with some cooking oil, add eggs and cook your omelet for 5 minutes
3. Add chicken, avocado, tomato, bacon, mayo and mustard on one half of the omelet.
4. Fold omelet, cover pan and cook for 5 minutes more
5. Transfer to a plate and serve

**Nutrition:**

Calories: 300
Fat: 32
Fiber: 6
Carbs: 4
Protein: 25

## 101. Family Fun Pizza

**Preparation Time:** 30 minutes
**Cooking Time:** 25 minutes
**Servings:** 16
**Ingredients:**

Pizza crust:

- Water, warm (1 cup)
- Salt (1/2 teaspoon)
- Flour, whole wheat (1 cup)
- Olive oil (2 tablespoons)
- Dry yeast, quick active (1 package)
- Flour, all purpose (1 ½ cups)
- Cornmeal

•Olive oil
Filling:
•Onion, chopped (1 cup)
•Mushrooms, sliced, drained (4 ounces)
•Garlic cloves, chopped finely (2 pieces)
•Parmesan cheese, grated (1/4 cup)
•Ground lamb, 80% lean (1 pound)
•Italian seasoning (1 teaspoon)
•Pizza sauce (8 ounces)
•Mozzarella cheese, shredded (2 cups)
**Directions:**
1.Mix yeast with warm water. Combine with flours, oil (2 tablespoons), and salt by stirring and then beating vigorously for half a minute. Let the dough sit for twenty minutes.
2.Preheat oven at 350 degrees Fahrenheit.
3.Prep 2 square pans (8-inch) by greasing with oil before sprinkling with cornmeal.
4.Cut the rested dough in half; place each half inside each pan. Set aside, covered, for thirty to forty-five minutes. Cook in the air fryer for twenty to twenty-two minutes.
5.Sauté the onion, beef, garlic, and Italian seasoning until beef is completely cooked. Drain and set aside.
6.Cover the air-fried crusts with pizza sauce before topping with beef mixture, cheeses, and mushrooms.
7.Return to oven and cook for twenty minutes.
**Nutrition:**
Calories 215
Fat 0 g
Protein 10 g
Carbohydrates 20.0 g

## 102.Bacon Wings
**Preparation Time:** 15 minutes
**Cooking Time:** 1 hour 15 minutes
**Servings:** 12

**Ingredients:**
•Bacon strips (12 pieces)
•Paprika (1 teaspoon)
•Black pepper (1 tablespoon)
•Oregano (1 teaspoon)
•Chicken wings (12 pieces)
•Kosher salt (1 tablespoon)
•Brown sugar (1 tablespoon)
•Chili powder (1 teaspoon)
•Celery sticks
•Blue cheese dressing
**Directions:**
1.Preheat the air fryer at 325 degrees Fahrenheit.
2.Mix sugar, salt, chili powder, oregano, pepper, and paprika. Coat chicken wings with this dry rub.
3.Wrap a bacon strip around each wing. Arrange wrapped wings in the air fryer basket.
4.Cook for thirty minutes on each side in the air fryer. Let cool for five minutes.
5.Serve and enjoy with celery and blue cheese.
**Nutrition:**
Calories 100
Fat 0 g
Protein 0 g
Carbohydrates 0 g

## 103.Pepper Pesto Lamb
**Preparation Time:** 15 minutes
**Cooking Time:** 1 hour 15 minutes
**Servings:** 12
**Ingredients:**
Pesto:
•Rosemary leaves, fresh (1/4 cup)
•Garlic cloves (3 pieces)
•Parsley, fresh, packed firmly (3/4 cup)
•Mint leaves, fresh (1/4 cup)

•Olive oil (2 tablespoons)

Lamb:

•Red bell peppers, roasted, drained (7 ½ ounces)

•Leg of lamb, boneless, rolled (5 pounds)

•Seasoning, lemon pepper (2 teaspoons)

**Directions:**

1.Preheat the oven at 325 degrees Fahrenheit.

2.Mix the pesto ingredients in the food processor.

3.Unroll the lamb and cover the cut side with pesto. Top with roasted peppers before rolling up the lamb and tying with kitchen twine.

4.Coat lamb with seasoning (lemon pepper) and air-fry for one hour.

**Nutrition:**

Calories 310

Fat 10 g

Protein 40.0 g

Carbohydrates 0 g

## 104.Greek Style Mini Burger Pies

**Preparation Time:** 15 minutes

**Cooking Time:** 40 minutes

**Servings:** 6

**Ingredients:**

Burger mixture:

•Onion, large, chopped (1 piece)

•Red bell peppers, roasted, diced (1/2 cup)

•Ground lamb, 80% lean (1 pound)

•Red pepper flakes (1/4 teaspoon)

•Feta cheese, crumbled (2 ounces)

Baking mixture:

•Milk (1/2 cup)

•Biscuit mix, classic (1/2 cup)

•Eggs (2 pieces)

**Directions:**

1.Preheat oven at 350 degrees Fahrenheit.

2.Grease 12 muffin cups using cooking spray.

3.Cook the onion and beef in a skillet heated on medium-high. Once beef is browned and cooked through, drain and let cool for five minutes. Stir together with feta cheese, roasted red peppers, and red pepper flakes.

4.Whisk the baking mixture ingredients together. Fill each muffin cup with baking mixture (1 tablespoon).

5.Air-fry for twenty-five to thirty minutes. Let cool before serving.

**Nutrition:**

Calories 270

Fat 10 g

Protein 10 g

Carbohydrates 10 g

## 105.Almond Cereal

**Preparation Time:** 5 minutes

**Cooking Time:** 5 minutes

**Servings:** 1

**Ingredients:**

•2 tablespoons almonds; chopped.

•1/3 cup coconut milk

•1 tablespoon chia seeds

•2 tablespoon pepitas; roasted

•A handful blueberries

•1 small banana; chopped.

•1/3 cup water

**Directions:**

1.In a bowl, mix chia seeds with coconut milk and leave aside for 5 minutes

2.In your food processor, mix half of the pepitas with almonds and pulse them well.

3.Add this to chia seeds mix.

4.Also add the water and stir.

5.Top with the rest of the pepitas, banana pieces and blueberries and serve

**Nutrition:**

Calories: 200

Fat: 3

Fiber: 2

Carbs: 5

Protein: 4

## 106. Avocado Muffins

**Preparation Time:** 10 minutes

**Cooking Time:** 20 minutes

**Servings:** 12

**Ingredients:**

- 6 bacon slices; chopped.
- 1 yellow onion; chopped.
- 1/2 teaspoon baking soda
- 1/2 cup coconut flour
- 1 cup coconut milk
- 2 cups avocado; pitted, peeled and chopped.
- 4 eggs
- Salt and black pepper to the taste.

**Directions:**

1. Heat up a pan, add onion and bacon; stir and brown for a few minutes
2. In a bowl, mash avocado pieces with a fork and whisk well with the eggs
3. Add milk, salt, pepper, baking soda and coconut flour and stir everything.
4. Add bacon mix and stir again.
5. Add coconut oil to muffin tray, divide eggs and avocado mix into the tray, heat oven at 350 degrees F and bake for 20 minutes
6. Divide muffins between plates and serve them for breakfast.

**Nutrition:**

Calories: 200

Fat: 7

Fiber: 4

Carbs: 7

Protein: 5

## 107. Pancakes

**Preparation Time:** 12 minutes

**Cooking Time:** 3 minutes

**Servings:** 4

**Ingredients:**

- 2 ounces' cream cheese
- 1 teaspoon stevia
- 1/2 teaspoon cinnamon; ground
- 2 eggs
- Cooking spray

**Directions:**

1. Mix the eggs with the cream cheese, stevia, and cinnamon In a blender, and mix well.
2. Heat pan with cooking spray over medium high heat. add 1/4 of the batter, spread well, cook 2 minutes, invert and cook 1 minute more
3. Move to a plate and repeat with the rest of the dough.
4. Serve them right away.

**Nutrition:**

Calories: 344

Fat: 23

Fiber: 12

Carbs: 3

Protein: 16

## 108. Salad in A Jar

**Preparation Time:** 10 minutes

**Cooking Time:** 5 minutes

**Servings:** 1

**Ingredients:**

- 1 ounce favorite greens
- 1-ounce red bell pepper; chopped.
- 4 ounces' rotisserie chicken; roughly chopped.
- 4 tablespoons extra virgin olive oil
- 1/2 scallion; chopped.
- 1-ounce cucumber; chopped.
- 1-ounce cherry tomatoes; halved
- Salt and black pepper to the taste.

**Directions:**

1.In a bowl, mix greens with bell pepper, tomatoes, scallion, cucumber, salt, pepper and olive oil and toss to coat well.

2.Transfer this to a jar, top with chicken pieces and serve for breakfast.

**Nutrition:**

Calories: 180

Fat: 12

Fiber: 4

Carbs: 5

Protein: 17

### 109. Breakfast Cereal

**Preparation Time:** 10 minutes

**Cooking Time:** 3 minutes

**Servings:** 2

**Ingredients:**

•1/2 cup coconut; shredded

•1/3 cup macadamia nuts; chopped.

•4 teaspoons ghee

•2 cups almond milk

•1 tablespoon stevia

•1/3 cup walnuts; chopped.

•1/3 cup flax seed

•A pinch of salt

**Directions:**

1.Heat a pot of mistletoe over medium heat. Add the milk, coconut, salt, macadamia nuts, walnuts, flax seeds, and stevia and mix well.

2.Cook for 3 minutes. Stir again, remove from heat for 10 minutes.

3.Divide into 2 bowls and serve

**Nutrition:**

Calories: 140

Fat: 3

Fiber: 2

Carbs: 1. 5

Protein: 7

### 110. Smoked Salmon

**Preparation Time:** 10 minutes

**Cooking Time:** 10 minutes

**Servings:** 3

**Ingredients:**

•4 eggs; whisked

•1/2 teaspoon avocado oil

•4 ounces smoked salmon; chopped.

For the sauce:

•1/2 cup cashews; soaked; drained

•1/4 cup green onions; chopped.

•1 teaspoon garlic powder

•1 cup coconut milk

•1 tablespoon lemon juice

•Salt and black pepper to the taste.

**Directions:**

1.In your blender, mix cashews with coconut milk, garlic powder and lemon juice and blend well.

2.Add salt, pepper and green onions, blend again well, transfer to a bowl and keep in the fridge for now.

3.Heat up a pan with the oil over medium-low heat; add eggs, whisk a bit and cook until they are almost done

4.Introduce in your preheated broiler and cook until eggs set.

5.Divide eggs on plates, top with smoked salmon and serve with the green onion sauce on top.

**Nutrition:**

Calories: 200

Fat: 10

Fiber: 2

Carbs: 11

Protein: 15

### 111.Almond Coconut Cereal

**Preparation Time:** 5 minutes

**Cooking Time:** 5 minutes

**Servings:** 2

**Ingredients:**

•Water, 1/3 cup.

•Coconut milk, 1/3 cup.

•Roasted sunflower seeds, 2 tbsps.

•Chia seeds, 1 tbsp.

•Blueberries, ½ cup.

•Chopped almonds, 2 tbsps.

**Directions:**

1.Set a medium bowl in position to add coconut milk and chia seeds then reserve for five minutes

2.Plug in and set the blender in position to blend almond with sunflower seeds

3.Stir the combination to chia seeds mixture then add water to mix evenly.

4.Serve topped with the remaining sunflower seeds and blueberries

**Nutrition:**

Calories: 181

Fat: 15.2

Fiber: 4

Carbs: 10.8

Protein: 3.7

## 112.Almond Porridge

**Preparation Time:** 10 minutes

**Cooking Time:** 5 minutes

**Servings:** 1

**Ingredients:**

•Ground cloves, ¼ tsp.

•Nutmeg, ¼ tsp.

•Stevia, 1 tsp.

•Coconut cream, ¾ cup.

•Ground almonds, ½ cup.

•Ground cardamom, ¼ tsp.

•Ground cinnamon, 1 tsp.

**Directions:**

1.Set your pan over medium heat to cook the coconut cream for a few minutes

2.Stir in almonds and stevia to cook for 5 minutes

3.Mix in nutmeg, cardamom, and cinnamon

4.Enjoy while still hot

**Nutrition:**

Calories: 695

Fat: 66.7

Fiber: 11.1

Carbs: 22

Protein: 14.3

## 113.Asparagus Frittata

**Preparation Time:** 20 minutes

**Cooking Time:** 20 minutes

**Servings:** 4

**Ingredients:**

•Bacon slices, chopped: 4

•Salt and black pepper

•Eggs (whisked): 8

•Asparagus (trimmed and chopped): 1 bunch

**Directions:**

1.Heat a pan, add bacon, stir and cook for 5 minutes.

2.Add asparagus, salt, and pepper, stir and cook for another 5 minutes.

3.Add the chilled eggs, spread them in the pan, let them stand in the oven and bake for 20 minutes at 350° F.

4.Share and divide between plates and serve for breakfast.

**Nutrition:**

Calories 251

carbs 16

fat 6

fiber 8

protein 7

## 114.Avocados Stuffed with Salmon

**Preparation Time:** 5 minutes

**Cooking Time:** 5 minutes

**Servings:** 2

**Ingredients:**

•Avocado (pitted and halved): 1
•Olive oil: 2 tablespoons
•Lemon juice: 1
•Smoked salmon (flaked): 2 ounces
•Goat cheese (crumbled): 1 ounce
•Salt and black pepper
**Directions:**
1.Combine the salmon with lemon juice, oil, cheese, salt, and pepper in your food processor and pulsate well.
2.Divide this mixture into avocado halves and serve.
3.Dish and Enjoy!
**Nutrition:**
Calories: 300
Fat: 15
Fiber: 5
Carbs: 8
Protein: 16

## 115.Buffalo Chicken Sliders

**Preparation Time**: 10 minutes
**Cooking Time:** 15 minutes
**Servings:** 12
**Ingredients:**
•Chicken breasts (2 lb., cooked, shredded)
•Wing sauce (1 cup)
•Ranch dressing mix (1 pack)
•Blue cheese dressing (1/4 cup, low fat)
•Lettuce (for topping)
•Buns (12, slider)
**Directions:**
1.Add the chicken breasts (shredded, cooked) in a large bowl along with the ranch dressing and wing sauce.
2.Stir well to incorporate, then place a piece of lettuce onto each slider roll.
3.Top off using the chicken mixture.
4.Drizzle blue cheese dressing over chicken then top off using top buns of slider rolls

5.                    Serve.
**Nutrition:**
Calories: 300 Cal
Fat: 14 g
Cholesterol: 25 mg

## 116.Bacon and Brussels Sprout Breakfast

**Preparation Time:** 10 minutes
**Cooking Time:** 15 minutes
**Servings:** 3
**Ingredients:**
•Apple cider vinegar, 1½ tbsps.
•Salt
•Minced shallots, 2
•Minced garlic cloves, 2
•Medium eggs, 3
•Sliced Brussels sprouts, 12 oz.
•Black pepper
•Chopped bacon, 2 oz.
•Melted butter, 1 tbsp.
**Directions:**
1.Over medium heat, quick fry the bacon until crispy then reserve on a plate
2.Set the pan on fire again to fry garlic and shallots for 30 seconds
3.Stir in apple cider vinegar, Brussels sprouts, and seasoning to cook for five minutes
4.Add the bacon to cook for five minutes then stir in the butter and set a hole at the center
5.Crash the eggs to the pan and let cook fully
6.Enjoy
**Nutrition:**
Calories: 275
Fat: 16.5
Fiber: 4.3
Carbs: 17.2
Protein: 17.4

### 117. Bacon and Lemon spiced Muffins

**Preparation Time:** 10 minutes
**Cooking Time:** 20 minutes
**Servings:** 12
**Ingredients:**
•Lemon thyme, 2 tsps.
•Salt
•Almond flour, 3 cup.
•Melted butter, ½ cup.
•Baking soda, 1 tsp.
•Black pepper
•Medium eggs, 4
•Diced bacon, 1 cup.
**Directions:**
1.Set a mixing bowl in place and stir in the eggs and baking soda to incorporate well.
2.Whisk in the seasonings, butter, bacon, and lemon thyme
3.Set the mixture in a well-lined muffin pan.
4.Set the oven for 20 minutes at 3500F, allow to bake
5.Allow the muffins to cool before serving
**Nutrition:**
Calories: 186
Fat: 17.1
Fiber: 0.8
Carbs: 1.8
Protein: 7.4

### 118. Tropical Greens Smoothie

**Preparation Time:** 5 Minutes
**Cooking Time:** 0 Minutes
**Servings:** 1
**Ingredients:**
•One banana
•1/2 large navel orange, peeled and segmented
•1/2 cup frozen mango chunks
•1 cup frozen spinach
•One celery stalk, broken into pieces
•One tablespoon cashew butter or almond butter
•1/2 tablespoon spiraling
•1/2 tablespoon ground flaxseed
•1/2 cup unsweetened nondairy milk
•Water, for thinning (optional)
**Directions:**
1.In a high-speed blender or food processor, combine the bananas, orange, mango, spinach, celery, cashew butter, spiraling (if using), flaxseed, and milk.
2.Blend until creamy, adding more milk or water to thin the smoothie if too thick. Serve immediately—it is best served fresh.
**Nutrition:**
Calories: 391
Fat: 12g
Protein: 13g
Carbohydrates: 68g
Fiber: 13g

### 119. Vitamin C Smoothie Cubes

**Preparation Time:** 5 minutes
**Cooking Time:** 8 hours to chill
**Servings:** 1
**Ingredients:**
•1/8 large papaya
•1/8 mango
•1/4 cups chopped pineapple, fresh or frozen
•1/8 cup raw cauliflower florets, fresh or frozen
•1/4 large navel oranges, peeled and halved
•1/4 large orange bell pepper stemmed, seeded, and coarsely chopped
**Directions:**

1.Halve the papaya and mango, remove the pits, and scoop their soft flesh into a high-speed blender.

2.Add the pineapple, cauliflower, oranges, and bell pepper. Blend until smooth.

3.Evenly divide the puree between 2 (16-compartment) ice cube trays and place them on a level surface in your freezer. Freeze for at least 8 hours.

4.The cubes can be left in the ice cube trays until use or transferred to a freezer bag. The frozen cubes are good for about three weeks in a standard freezer, or up to 6 months in a chest freezer.

**Nutrition:**

Calories: 96

Fat: 1 g

Protein: 2 g

Carbohydrates: 24 g

Fiber: 4 g

## 120.Bok Choy with Tofu Stir Fry

**Preparation Time**: 15 minutes

**Cooking Time:** 15 minutes

**Servings:** 4

**Ingredients:**

•Super-firm tofu: 1 lb. (drained and pressed)

•Coconut oil: one tablespoon

•Clove of garlic: 1 (minced)

•Baby bok choy: 3 heads (chopped)

•Low-sodium vegetable broth;

•Maple syrup: 2 teaspoons

•Braggs liquid aminos

•Sambal oelek: 1 to 2 teaspoons (similar chili sauce)

•Scallion or green onion: 1 (chopped)

•Freshly grated ginger: 1 teaspoon

•Quinoa/rice, for serving

**Directions:**

1.With paper towels, pat the tofu dry and cut into tiny pieces of bite-size around 1/2 inch wide.

2.Heat coconut oil in a wide skillet over medium heat.

3.Remove tofu and stir-fry until painted softly.

4.Stir-fry for 1-2 minutes, before the choy of the Bok starts to wilt.

5.When this occurs, you'll want to apply the vegetable broth and all the remaining ingredients to the skillet.

6.Hold the mixture stir-frying until all components are well coated, and the bulk of the liquid evaporates, around 5-6 min.

7.Serve over brown rice or quinoa.

**Nutrition:**

Calories: 263.7 Cal

Fat 4.2 g

Cholesterol: 0.3 mg

Sodium: 683.6 mg

Potassium: 313.7 mg

Carbohydrate: 35.7 g

## 121.High Protein Chicken Meatballs

**Preparation Time**: 5 minutes

**Cooking Time:** 25 minutes

**Servings:** 2

**Ingredients:**

•Chicken (1 lbs., lean, ground)

•Oats (3/4 cup, rolled)

•Onions (2, grated)

•Allspice (2 tsp. ground)

•Salt and black pepper (dash)

**Directions:**

1.Heat a skillet (large) over medium heat then grease using cooking spray.

2.Add in the onions (grated), chicken (lean, ground), oats (rolled), allspice (earth), and a dash of salt and black pepper in a large-sized bowl, stir well to incorporate.

3.Shape mixture into meatballs (small).

4.Place into the skillet (greased). Cook for roughly 5 minutes until golden brown on all sides.

5.Remove meatballs from heat then serve immediately.

**Nutrition:**

Calories: 519 Cal

Protein: 57g

Carbohydrates: 32 g

Fat: 15 g

## 122.Three-Bean Medley

**Preparation Time**: 15 minutes

**Cooking Time:** 6 to 8 hours

**Servings:** 8

**Ingredients:**

•11/4 cups dried kidney beans, rinsed and drained

•11/4 cups dried black beans, rinsed and drained

•11/4 cups dried black-eyed peas, rinsed and drained

•1 onion, chopped

•1 leek, chopped

•2 garlic cloves, minced

•2 carrots, peeled and chopped

•6 cups low-sodium vegetable broth

•11/2 cups water

•1/2 teaspoon dried thyme leaves

**Directions:**

1.In a 6-quart slow cooker, mix all of the ingredients.

2.Cover and cook on low for 6 to 8 hours, or until the beans are tender and the liquid is absorbed.

**Nutrition:**

Calories: 284 Cal

Carbohydrates: 56 g

Sugar: 6 g

Fiber: 19 g

Fat: 0 g

Saturated Fat: 0 g

Protein: 19 g

Sodium: 131 mg

## 123.Zucchini Fritters

**Preparation Time**: 15 minutes

**Cooking Time:** 10 minutes

**Servings:** 4

**Ingredients:**

•1 1/2 pound of grated zucchini

•1 tsp. of salt

•1/4 cup of grated Parmesan

•1/4 cup of flour

•2 cloves of minced garlic

•2 tbsp. of olive oil

•1 large egg

•Freshly ground black pepper and kosher salt to taste

**Directions:**

1.Put the grated zucchini into a colander over the sink

2.Add your salt and toss it to mix properly, then leave it to settle for about 10 minutes.

3.Next, use a clean cheesecloth to drain the zucchini completely.

4.Combine drained zucchini, Parmesan, garlic, flour, and the beaten egg in a large bowl, mix, and season with pepper and salt.

5.Next, heat the olive oil in a skillet applying medium-high heat.

6.Use a tablespoon to scoop batter for each cake, put in the oil, and flatten using a spatula.

7.Allow to cook until the underside is richly golden brown, then flip over to the other side and cook.

8.Your delicious zucchini fritters are ready to be served.

**Nutrition:**

Total Fat: 12.0 g

Cholesterol: 101.9 mg

Sodium: 728.9 mg

Total Carbohydrate: 11.9 g

Dietary Fiber: 1.9 g

Sugars: 4.6 g

Protein: 8.6 g

## 124. Chocolate Chia Pudding

**Preparation Time**: 2 minutes

**Cooking Time:** overnight to chill

**Servings:** 1

**Ingredients:**

•1/8 cup chia seeds

•1/2 cup unsweetened nondairy milk

•One tablespoon raw cocoa powder

•1/2 teaspoon vanilla extract

•1/2 teaspoon pure maple syrup

**Directions:**

1.Stir together the chia seeds, milk, cacao powder, vanilla, and maple syrup in a large bowl.

2.Divide between two (1/2-pint) covered glass jars or containers.

3.Refrigerate overnight.

4.Stir before serving.

**Nutrition:**

Calories: 213

Fat: 10 g

Protein: 9 g

Carbohydrates: 20 g

Fiber: 15 g

## 125.Slow Cooker Savory Butternut Squash Oatmeal

**Preparation Time**: 15 minutes

**Cooking Time:** 6 to 8 hours

**Servings:** 1

**Ingredients:**

•1/4 cup steel-cut oats

•1/2 cups cubed (1/2-inch pieces), peeled butternut squash (freeze any leftovers after preparing a whole squash for future meals)

•3/4 cups of water

•1/16 cup unsweetened nondairy milk

•1/4 tablespoon chia seeds

•1/2 teaspoons yellow miso paste

•3/4 teaspoons ground ginger

•1/4 tablespoon sesame seeds, toasted

•1/4 tablespoon chopped scallion, green parts only

•Shredded carrot, for serving (optional)

**Directions:**

1.In a slow cooker, combine the oats, butternut squash, and water.

2.Cover the slow cooker and cook on low for 6 to 8 hours, or until the squash is fork-tender.

3.Using a potato masher or heavy spoon, roughly mash the cooked butternut squash.

4.Stir to combine with the oats.

5.Whisk together the milk, chia seeds, miso paste, and ginger in a large bowl. Stir the mixture into the oats.

6.Top your oatmeal bowl with sesame seeds and scallion for more plant-based fiber, top with shredded carrot (if using).

**Nutrition:**

Calories: 230

Fat: 5 g

Protein: 7 g

Carbohydrates: 40 g

Fiber: 9 g

## 126.Maple Lemon Tempeh Cubes

**Preparation Time**: 10 minutes
**Cooking Time**: 30 to 40 minutes
**Servings**: 4
**Ingredients:**
•Tempeh: 1 packet
•Coconut oil: 2 to 3 teaspoons
•Lemon juice: 3 tablespoons
•Maple syrup; 2 teaspoons
•Bragg's Liquid Aminos or low-sodium tamari or (optional): 1 to 2 teaspoons
•Water: 2 teaspoons
•Dried basil: 1/4 teaspoon
•Powdered garlic: 1/4 teaspoon
•Black pepper (freshly grounded): to taste
**Directions:**
1.Heat your oven to 400 ° C.
2.Cut your tempeh block into squares in bite form.
3.Heat coconut oil over medium to high heat in a non-stick skillet.
4.When melted and heated, add the tempeh and cook on one side for 2-4 minutes, or until the tempeh turns down into a golden-brown color.
5.Flip the tempeh bits, and cook for 2-4 minutes.
6.Mix the lemon juice, tamari, maple syrup, basil, water, garlic, and black pepper while the tempeh is browning.
7.Drop the mixture over tempeh, then swirl to cover the tempeh.
8.Sauté for 2-3 minutes, then turn the tempeh and sauté 1-2 minutes more.
9.The tempeh, on both sides, should be soft and orange.
**Nutrition:**
Carbohydrates: 22 Cal
Fats: 17 g
Sugar: 5 g
Protein: 21 g
Fiber: 9 g

## 127.Carrot Cake Oatmeal

**Preparation Time**: 10 minutes
**Cooking Time**: 15 minutes
**Servings**: 1
**Ingredients:**
•1/8 cup pecans
•1/2 cup finely shredded carrot
•1/4 cup old-fashioned oats
•5/8 cups unsweetened nondairy milk
•1/2 tablespoon pure maple syrup
•1/2 teaspoon ground cinnamon
•1/2 teaspoon ground ginger
•1/8 teaspoon ground nutmeg
•One tablespoon chia seed
**Directions:**
1.Over medium-high heat in a skillet, toast the pecans for 3 to 4 minutes, often stirring, until browned and fragrant (watch closely, as they can burn quickly).
2.Pour the pecans onto a cutting board and coarsely chop them. Set aside.
3.In an 8-quart pot over medium-high heat, combine the carrot, oats, milk, maple syrup, cinnamon, ginger, and nutmeg.
4.When it is already boiling, reduce the heat to medium-low.
5.Cook, uncovered, for 10 minutes, stirring occasionally.
6.Stir in the chopped pecans and chia seeds. Serve immediately.
**Nutrition:**
Calories: 307
Fat: 17 g
Protein: 7 g
Carbohydrates: 35 g

Fiber: 11 g

### 128.Bacon Spaghetti Squash Carbonara

**Preparation Time**: 20 minutes
**Cooking Time:** 40 minutes
**Servings:** 4
**Ingredients:**
•1 small spaghetti squash
•6 ounces' bacon (roughly chopped)
•1 large tomato (sliced)
•2 chives (chopped)
•1 garlic clove (minced)
•6 ounces low-fat cottage cheese
•1 cup Gouda cheese (grated)
•2 tablespoons olive oil
•Salt and pepper, to taste
**Directions:**
1.Preheat the oven to 350°F.
2.Cut the squash spaghetti in half, brush with some olive oil and bake for 20–30 minutes, skin side up. Remove from the oven and remove the core with a fork, creating the spaghetti.
3.Heat one tablespoon of olive oil in a skillet. Cook the bacon for about 1 minute until crispy.
4.Quickly wipe out the pan with paper towels.
5.Heat another tablespoon of oil and sauté the garlic, tomato, and chives for 2–3 minutes. Add the spaghetti and sauté for another 5 minutes, occasionally stirring to keep from burning.
6.Begin to add the cottage cheese, about two tablespoons at a time. If the sauce becomes thick, add about a cup of water. The sauce should be creamy but not too runny or thick. Allow cooking for another 3 minutes.
7.Serve immediately.



**Nutrition:**
Calories: 305
Total Fat: 21 g
Net Carbs: 8 g
Protein: 18 g

### 129.Spiced Sorghum and Berries

**Preparation Time**: 5 minutes
**Cooking Time:** 1 hour
**Servings:** 1
**Ingredients:**
•1/4 cup whole-grain sorghum
•1/4 teaspoon ground cinnamon
•1/4 teaspoon Chinese five-spice powder
•3/4 cups water
•1/4 cup unsweetened nondairy milk
•1/4 teaspoon vanilla extract
•1/2 tablespoons pure maple syrup
•1/2 tablespoon chia seed
•1/8 cup sliced almonds
•1/2 cups fresh raspberries, divided
**Directions:**
1.Using a large pot over medium-high heat, stir together the sorghum, cinnamon, five-spice powder, and water.
2.Wait for the water to a boil, cover it, and reduce the heat to medium-low.
3.Cook for one hour, or until the sorghum is soft and chewy. If the sorghum grains are still hard, add another cup of water and cook for 15 minutes more.
4.Using a glass measuring cup, whisk together the milk, vanilla, and maple syrup to blend.
5.Add the mixture to the sorghum and the chia seeds, almonds, and one cup of raspberries. Gently stir to combine.
6.When serving, top with the remaining one cup of fresh raspberries.
**Nutrition:**

Calories: 289

Fat: 8 g

Protein: 9 g

Carbohydrates: 52 g

Fiber: 10 g

## 130.Raw-Cinnamon-Apple Nut Bowl

**Preparation Time**: 15 minutes

**Cooking Time:** 1 hour to chill

**Servings:** 1

**Ingredients:**

•One green apple halved, seeded, and cored

•3/4 Honeycrisp apples, halved, seeded, and cored

•1/4 teaspoon freshly squeezed lemon juice

•One pitted Medrol dates

•1/8 teaspoon ground cinnamon

•Pinch ground nutmeg

•1/2 tablespoons chia seeds, plus more for serving (optional)

•1/4 tablespoon hemp seed

•1/8 cup chopped walnuts

•Nut butter, for serving (optional)

**Directions:**

1.Finely dice half the green apple and one Honey crisp apple. With the lemon juice, store it in an airtight container while you work on the next steps.

2.Coarsely chop the remaining apples and the dates. Transfer to a food processor and add the cinnamon and nutmeg.

3.Check it several times to see if it's mixing, then processes for 2 to 3 minutes to puree. Stir the puree into the reserved diced apples.

4.Stir in the chia seeds (if using), hemp seeds, and walnuts.

5.Chill for at least one hour.

6.                    Enjoy!

7.Serve as it is or top with additional chia seeds and nut butter (if using).

**Nutrition:**

Calories: 274

Fat: 8 g

Protein: 4 g

Carbohydrates: 52 g

Fiber: 9 g

## 131.Peanut Butter and Cacao Breakfast Quinoa

**Preparation Time**: 5 Minutes

**Cooking Time:** 10 Minutes

**Servings:** 1

**Ingredients:**

•1/3 cup quinoa flakes

•1/2 cup unsweetened nondairy milk,

•1/2 cup of water

•1/8 cup raw cacao powder

•One tablespoon natural creamy peanut butter

•1/8 teaspoon ground cinnamon

•One banana, mashed

•Fresh berries of choice, for serving

•Chopped nuts of choice, for serving

**Directions:**

1.Using an 8-quart pot over medium-high heat, stir together the quinoa flakes, milk, water, cacao powder, peanut butter, and cinnamon.

2.Cook and stir it until the mixture begins to simmer. Turn the heat to medium-low and cook for 3 to 5 minutes, stirring frequently.

3.Stir in the bananas and cook until hot.

4.Serve topped with fresh berries, nuts, and a splash of milk.

**Nutrition:**

Calories: 471

Fat: 16g

Protein: 18g

Carbohydrates: 69g

Fiber: 16g

### 132.Vanilla Buckwheat Porridge

**Preparation Time**: 5 minutes

**Cooking Time:** 25 minutes

**Servings:** 1

**Ingredients:**

•One cup of water

•1/4 cup raw buckwheat grouts

•1/4 teaspoon ground cinnamon

•1/4 banana, sliced

•1/16 cup golden raisins

•1/16 cup dried currants

•1/16 cup sunflower seeds

•1/2 tablespoons chia seeds

•1/4 tablespoon hemp seeds

•1/4 tablespoon sesame seeds, toasted

•1/8 cup unsweetened nondairy milk

•1/4 tablespoon pure maple syrup

•1/4 teaspoon vanilla extract

**Directions:**

1.Boil the water in a pot. Stir in the buckwheat, cinnamon, and banana.

2.Cook the mixture. Mix it and wait for it to boil, then reduce the heat to medium-low.

3.Cover the pot and cook for 15 minutes, or until the buckwheat is tender.

4.Remove from the heat.

5.Stir in the raisins, currants, sunflower seeds, chia seeds, hemp seeds, sesame seeds, milk, maple syrup, and vanilla. Cover the pot. Wait for 10 minutes before serving.

6.Serve as it is or top as desired.

**Nutrition:**

Calories: 353

Fat: 11 g

Protein: 10 g

Carbohydrates: 61 g

Fiber: 10 g

### 133.Polenta with Seared Pears

**Preparation Time**: 10 minutes

**Cooking Time:** 50 minutes

**Servings:** 1

**Ingredients:**

•One cup water, divided, plus more as needed

•1/2 cups coarse cornmeal

•One tablespoon pure maple syrup

•1/4 tablespoon molasses

•1/4 teaspoon ground cinnamon

•1/2 ripe pears, cored and diced

•1/4 cup fresh cranberries

•1/4 teaspoon chopped fresh rosemary leaves

**Directions:**

1.In a pan, cook 5 cups of water to a simmer.

2.While whisking continuously to avoid clumping, slowly pour in the cornmeal. Cook, often stirring with a heavy spoon, for 30 minutes. The polenta should be thick and creamy.

3.While the polenta cooks, in a saucepan over medium heat, stir together the maple syrup, molasses, the remaining 1/4 cup of water, and the cinnamon until combined.

4.Bring it to a simmer. Add the pears and cranberries. Cook for 10 minutes, occasionally stirring, until the pears are tender and start to brown.

5.Remove from the heat. Stir in the rosemary and let the mixture sit for 5 minutes. If it is too thick, add another 1/4 cup of water and return to the heat.

6.Top with the cranberry-pear mixture.

**Nutrition:**

Calories: 282

Fat: 2 g

Protein: 4 g

Carbohydrates: 65 g

Fiber: 12 g

### 134. Best Whole Wheat Pancakes

**Preparation Time**: 10 minutes
**Cooking Time:** 20 minutes
**Servings:** 1
**Ingredients:**
- 3/4 tablespoons ground flaxseed
- Two tablespoons warm water
- 1/2 cups whole wheat pastry flour
- 1/8 cup rye flour
- 1/2 tablespoons double-acting baking powder
- 1/4 teaspoon ground cinnamon
- 1/8 teaspoon ground ginger
- One cup unsweetened nondairy milk
- 3/4 tablespoons pure maple syrup
- 1/4 teaspoon vanilla extract

**Directions:**
1. Mix the warm water and flaxseed in a large bowl. Set aside for at least 5 minutes.
2. Whisk together the pastry and rye flours, baking powder, cinnamon, and ginger.
3. Whisk together the milk, maple syrup, and vanilla in a large bowl. Make use of a spatula, fold the wet ingredients into the dry ingredients. Fold in the soaked flaxseed until fully incorporated.
4. Heat a large skillet or nonstick griddle over medium-high heat.
5. Working in batches, three to four pancakes at a time, add 1/4-cup portions of batter to the hot skillet.
6. Until golden brown, cook for 3 to 4 minutes each side or no liquid batter is visible.

**Nutrition:**
Calories: 301
Fat: 4 g
Protein: 10 g

Carbohydrates: 57 g
Fiber: 10 g

### 135. Spiced Pumpkin Muffins

**Preparation Time**: 15 minutes
**Cooking Time:** 20 minutes
**Servings:** 1
**Ingredients:**
- 1/6 tablespoons ground flaxseed
- 1/24 cup of water
- 1/8 cups whole wheat flour
- 1/6 teaspoons baking powder
- 5/6 teaspoons ground cinnamon
- 1/12 teaspoon baking soda
- 1/12 teaspoon ground ginger
- 1/16 teaspoon ground nutmeg
- 1/32 teaspoon ground cloves
- 1/6 cup pumpkin puree
- 1/12 cup pure maple syrup
- 1/24 cup unsweetened applesauce
- 1/24 cup unsweetened nondairy milk
- 1/2 teaspoons vanilla extract

**Directions:**
1. Preheat the oven to 350°F. Line a 12-cup metal muffin pan with parchment paper liners or use a silicone muffin pan.
2. First, mix the flaxseed and water in a large bowl then keep it aside.
3. In a medium bowl, stir together the flour, baking powder, cinnamon, baking soda, ginger, nutmeg, and cloves.
4. In a medium bowl, stir up the maple syrup, pumpkin puree, applesauce, milk, and vanilla. Crease the wet ingredients into the dry ingredients making use of a spatula.
5. Fold the soaked flaxseed into the batter until evenly combined, but do not over mix the batter, or your muffins will become

dense. Spoon about 1/4 cup of batter per muffin into your prepared muffin pan.

6.Bake for 18 to 20 minutes, or until a toothpick inserted into the center of a muffin comes out clean. Remove the muffins from the pan.

7.Transfer to a wire rack for cooling.

8.Store in an airtight container that is at room temperature.

**Nutrition:**

Calories: 115

Fat: 1 g

Protein: 3 g

Carbohydrates: 25 g

Fiber: 3 g

### 136.Pesto Zucchini Noodles

**Preparation Time**: 10 minutes

**Cooking Time:** 30 minutes

**Servings:** 4

**Ingredients:**

•4 zucchinis, spiralized

•1 tbsp. avocado oil

•2 garlic cloves, chopped

•2/3 cup olive oil

•1/3 cup parmesan cheese, grated

•2 cups fresh basil

•1/3 cup almonds

•1/8 tsp. black pepper

•3/4 tsp. sea salt

**Directions:**

1.Add zucchini noodles into a colander and sprinkle with 1/4 teaspoon of salt.

2.Cover and let sit for 30 minutes.

3.Drain zucchini noodles well and pat dry.

4.Preheat the oven to 400 F.

5.Place almonds on a parchment-lined baking sheet and bake for 6-8 minutes.

6.Transfer toasted almonds into the food processor and process until coarse.

7.Add olive oil, cheese, basil, garlic, pepper, and remaining salt in a food processor with almonds and process until pesto texture.

8.Heat avocado oil in a large pan over medium-high heat.

9.Add zucchini noodles and cook for 4-5 minutes.

10.Pour pesto over zucchini noodles, mix well and cook for 1 minute.

11.Serve immediately with baked salmon.

**Nutrition:**

Calories: 525 Cal

Fat: 47.4 g

Carbohydrates: 9.3 g

Sugar: 3.8 g

Protein: 16.6 g

Cholesterol: 30 mg

### 137.Stewed Herbed Fruit

**Preparation Time**: 15 minutes

**Cooking Time:** 6 to 8 hours

**Servings:** 12

**Ingredients:**

•2 cups dried apricots

•2 cups prunes

•2 cups dried unsulphured pears

•2 cups dried apples

•1 cup dried cranberries

•1/4 cup honey

•6 cups water

•1 teaspoon dried thyme leaves

•1 teaspoon dried basil leaves

**Directions:**

1.In a 6-quart slow cooker, mix all of the ingredients.

2.Cover and cook on low for 6 to 8 hours, or until the fruits have absorbed the liquid and are tender.

3.Store in the refrigerator for up to 1 week.

4.You can freeze the fruit in 1-cup portions for more extended storage.

**Nutrition:**
Calories: 242 Cal
Carbohydrates: 61 g
Sugar: 43 g
Fiber: 9 g
Fat: 0 g
Saturated Fat: 0 g
Protein: 2 g
Sodium: 11 mg

# Dinner Recipes

### 138.Zucchini Salmon Salad

**Preparation Time:** 5 minutes
**Cooking Time:** 10 minutes
**Servings:** 3
**Ingredients:**

- 2 salmon fillets
- 2 tablespoons soy sauce
- 2 zucchinis, sliced
- Salt and pepper to taste
- 2 tablespoons extra virgin olive oil
- 2 tablespoons sesame seeds
- Salt and pepper to taste

**Directions:**

1.Drizzle the salmon with soy sauce.
2.Heat a grill pan over medium flame. Cook salmon on the grill on each side for 2-3 minutes.
3.Season the zucchini with salt and pepper and place it on the grill as well. Cook on each side until golden.
4.Place the zucchini, salmon and the rest of the ingredients in a bowl.
5.Serve the salad fresh.

**Nutrition:**
Calories: 224
Fat: 19g
Protein: 18g
Carbohydrates: 0g

### 139.Pan Fried Salmon

**Preparation Time:** 5 minutes
**Cooking Time:** 20 minutes
**Servings:** 4
**Ingredients:**

- 4 salmon fillets
- Salt and pepper to taste
- 1 teaspoon dried oregano
- 1 teaspoon dried basil
- 3 tablespoons extra virgin olive oil

**Directions:**

1.Season the fish with salt, pepper, oregano and basil.
2.Heat the oil in a pan and place the salmon in the hot oil, with the skin facing down.
3.Fry on each side for 2 minutes until golden brown and fragrant.
4.Serve the salmon warm and fresh.

**Nutrition:**
Calories: 327
Fat: 25g
Protein: 36g
Carbohydrates: 0.3g

### 140.Grilled Salmon with Pineapple Salsa

**Preparation Time:** 5 minutes
**Cooking Time:** 30 minutes
**Servings:** 4
**Ingredients:**

- 4 salmon fillets
- Salt and pepper to taste
- 2 tablespoons Cajun seasoning
- 1 fresh pineapple, peeled and diced
- 1 cup cherry tomatoes, quartered
- 2 tablespoons chopped cilantro
- 2 tablespoons chopped parsley
- 1 teaspoon dried mint
- 2 tablespoons lemon juice
- 2 tablespoons extra virgin olive oil
- 1 teaspoon honey
- Salt and pepper to taste

**Directions:**

1.Add salt, pepper and Cajun seasoning to the fish.
2.Heat a grill pan over medium flame. Cook fish on the grill on each side for 3-4 minutes.

3.For the salsa, mix the pineapple, tomatoes, cilantro, parsley, mint, lemon juice and honey in a bowl. Season with salt and pepper.
4.Serve the grilled salmon with the pineapple salsa.

**Nutrition:**
Calories: 332
Fat: 12g
Protein: 34g
Carbohydrates: 0g

## 141.Mediterranean Chickpea Salad

**Preparation Time:** 5 minutes
**Cooking Time:** 20 minutes
**Servings:** 6
**Ingredients:**
- 1 can chickpeas, drained
- 1 fennel bulb, sliced
- 1 red onion, sliced
- 1 teaspoon dried basil
- 1 teaspoon dried oregano
- 2 tablespoons chopped parsley
- 4 garlic cloves, minced
- 2 tablespoons lemon juice
- 2 tablespoons extra virgin olive oil
- Salt and pepper to taste

**Directions:**
1.Combine the chickpeas, fennel, red onion, herbs, garlic, lemon juice and oil in a salad bowl.
2.Add salt and pepper and serve the salad fresh.

**Nutrition:**
Calories: 200
Fat: 9g
Protein: 4g
Carbohydrates: 28g

## 142.Warm Chorizo Chickpea Salad

**Preparation Time:** 5 minutes
**Cooking Time:** 20 minutes
**Servings:** 6
**Ingredients:**
- 1 tablespoon extra virgin olive oil
- 4 chorizo links, sliced
- 1 red onion, sliced
- 4 roasted red bell peppers, chopped
- 1 can chickpeas, drained
- 2 cups cherry tomatoes
- 2 tablespoons balsamic vinegar
- Salt and pepper to taste

**Directions:**
1.Heat the oil in a skillet and add the chorizo. Cook briefly just until fragrant then add the onion, bell peppers and chickpeas and cook for 2 additional minutes.
2.Transfer the mixture in a salad bowl then add the tomatoes, vinegar, salt and pepper.
3.Mix well and serve the salad right away.

**Nutrition:**
Calories: 359
Fat: 18g
Protein: 15g
Carbohydrates: 21g

## 143.Greek Roasted Fish

**Preparation Time:** 5 minutes
**Cooking Time:** 30 minutes
**Servings:** 4
**Ingredients:**
- 4 salmon fillets
- 1 tablespoon chopped oregano
- 1 teaspoon dried basil
- 1 zucchini, sliced
- 1 red onion, sliced
- 1 carrot, sliced
- 1 lemon, sliced

•2 tablespoons extra virgin olive oil

•Salt and pepper to taste

**Directions:**

1.addall the ingredients in a deep dish baking pan.

2.Season with salt and pepper and cook in the preheated oven at 350F for 20 minutes.

3.Serve the fish and vegetables warm.

**Nutrition:**

Calories: 328

Fat: 13g

Protein: 38g

Carbohydrates: 8g

## 144.Tomato Fish Bake

**Preparation Time:** 5 minutes

**Cooking Time:** 30 minutes

**Servings:** 4

**Ingredients:**

•4 cod fillets

•4 tomatoes, sliced

•4 garlic cloves, minced

•1 shallot, sliced

•1 celery stalk, sliced

•1 teaspoon fennel seeds

•1 cup vegetable stock

•Salt and pepper to taste

**Directions:**

1.Layer the cod fillets and tomatoes in a deep dish baking pan.

2.Add the rest of the ingredients and add salt and pepper.

3.Cook in the preheated oven at 350F for 20 minutes.

4.Serve the dish warm or chilled.

**Nutrition:**

Calories: 299

Fat: 3g

Protein: 64g

Carbohydrates: 2g

## 145.Garlicky Tomato Chicken Casserole

**Preparation Time:** 5 minutes

**Cooking Time:** 50 minutes

**Servings:** 4

**Ingredients:**

•4 chicken breasts

•2 tomatoes, sliced

•1 can diced tomatoes

•2 garlic cloves, chopped

•1 shallot, chopped

•1 bay leaf

•1 thyme sprig

•½ cup dry white wine

•½ cup chicken stock

•Salt and pepper to taste

**Directions:**

1.Combine the chicken and the remaining ingredients in a deep dish baking pan.

2.Adjust the taste with salt and pepper and cover the pot with a lid or aluminum foil.

3.Cook in the preheated oven at 330F for 40 minutes.

4.Serve the casserole warm.

**Nutrition:**

Calories: 313

Fat: 8g

Protein: 47g

Carbohydrates: 6g

## 146.Chicken Cacciatore

**Preparation Time:** 5 minutes

**Cooking Time:** 45 minutes

**Servings:** 6

**Ingredients:**

•2 tablespoons extra virgin olive oil

•6 chicken thighs

•1 sweet onion, chopped

•2 garlic cloves, minced

•2 red bell peppers, cored and diced

•2 carrots, diced

•1 rosemary sprig

•1 thyme sprig

•4 tomatoes, peeled and diced

•½ cup tomato juice

•¼ cup dry white wine

•1 cup chicken stock

•1 bay leaf

•Salt and pepper to taste

**Directions:**

1.Heat the oil in a heavy saucepan.

2.Cook chicken on all sides until golden.

3.Stir in the onion and garlic and cook for 2 minutes.

4.Stir in the rest of the ingredients and season with salt and pepper.

5.Cook on low heat for 30 minutes.

6.Serve the chicken cacciatore warm and fresh.

**Nutrition:**

Calories: 363

Fat: 14g

Protein: 42g

Carbohydrates: 9g

## 147.Fennel Wild Rice Risotto

**Preparation Time:** 5 minutes

**Cooking Time:** 35 minutes

**Servings:** 6

**Ingredients:**

•2 tablespoons extra virgin olive oil

•1 shallot, chopped

•2 garlic cloves, minced

•1 fennel bulb, chopped

•1 cup wild rice

•¼ cup dry white wine

•2 cups chicken stock

•1 teaspoon grated orange zest

•Salt and pepper to taste

**Directions:**

1.Heat the oil in a heavy saucepan.

2.Add the garlic, shallot and fennel and cook for a few minutes until softened.

3.Stir in the rice and cook for 2 additional minutes then add the wine, stock and orange zest, with salt and pepper to taste.

4.Cook on low heat for 20 minutes.

5.Serve the risotto warm and fresh.

**Nutrition:**

Calories: 162

Fat: 2g

Protein: 8g

Carbohydrates: 20g

## 148.Wild Rice Prawn Salad

**Preparation Time:** 5 minutes

**Cooking Time:** 35 minutes

**Servings:** 6

**Ingredients:**

•¾ cup wild rice

•1¾ cups chicken stock

•1 pound prawns

•Salt and pepper to taste

•2 tablespoons lemon juice

•2 tablespoons extra virgin olive oil

•2 cups arugula

**Directions:**

1.Combine the rice and chicken stock in a saucepan and cook until the liquid has been absorbed entirely.

2.Transfer the rice in a salad bowl.

3.Season the prawns with salt and pepper and drizzle them with lemon juice and oil.

4.Heat a grill pan over medium flame.

5.Place the prawns on the hot pan and cook on each side for 2-3 minutes.

6.For the salad, combine the rice with arugula and prawns and mix well.

7.Serve the salad fresh.

**Nutrition:**
Calories: 207
Fat: 4g
Protein: 20.6g
Carbohydrates: 17g

### 149.Chickpea Sandwich Filling

**Preparation Time:** 5 minutes
**Cooking Time:** 0 minutes
**Servings:** 2
**Ingredients:**
○ounces chickpeas
•1 green onion, chopped
•½ teaspoon dried dill
•1 tablespoon mayonnaise
•1 tablespoon lime juice
•Extra:
•¼ teaspoon salt
•1/8 teaspoon ground black pepper
**Directions:**
1.Take a medium bowl, add chickpeas in it, and then add remaining ingredients.
**2.**Stir until well mixed and when ready, serve filling as a sandwich between two bread slices.
**Nutrition:**
356 Cal
7.5 g Fats
11.6 g Protein
60.6 g Carb
7 g Fiber

### 150.Chicken Broccoli Salad with Avocado Dressing

**Preparation Time:** 5 minutes
**Cooking Time:** 40 minutes
**Servings:** 6
**Ingredients:**
•2 chicken breasts
•1 pound broccoli, cut into florets
•1 avocado, peeled and pitted
•½ lemon, juiced
•2 garlic cloves
•¼ teaspoon chili powder
•¼ teaspoon cumin powder
•Salt and pepper to taste
**Directions:**
1.Cook the chicken in a large pot of salty water.
2.Drain and cut the chicken into small cubes. Place in a salad bowl.
3.Add the broccoli and mix well.
4.Combine the avocado, lemon juice, garlic, chili powder, cumin powder, salt and pepper in a blender. Pulse until smooth.
5.Spoon the dressing over the salad and mix well.
6.Serve the salad fresh.
**Nutrition:**
Calories: 195
Fat: 11g
Protein: 14g
Carbohydrates: 3g

### 151.Seafood Paella

**Preparation Time:** 5 minutes
**Cooking Time:** 45 minutes
**Servings:** 8
**Ingredients:**
•2 tablespoons extra virgin olive oil
•1 shallot, chopped
•2 garlic cloves, chopped
•1 red bell pepper, cored and diced
•1 carrot, diced
•2 tomatoes, peeled and diced
•1 cup wild rice
•1 cup tomato juice
•2 cups chicken stock
•1 chicken breast, cubed
•Salt and pepper to taste
•2 monkfish fillets, cubed

•½ pound fresh shrimps, peeled and deveined
•½ pound prawns
•1 thyme sprig
•1 rosemary sprig

**Directions:**

1.Heat the oil in a skillet and stir in the shallot, garlic, bell pepper, carrot and tomatoes. Cook for a few minutes until softened.

2.Stir in the rice, tomato juice, stock, chicken, salt and pepper and cook on low heat for 20 minutes.

3.Add the rest of the ingredients and cook for 10 additional minutes.

4.Serve the paella warm and fresh.

**Nutrition:**

Calories: 245

Fat: 8g

Protein: 27g

Carbohydrates: 20.6g

## 152.Broccoli Parmesan Pasta

**Preparation Time:** 10 minutes

**Cooking Time:** 10 minutes

**Servings:** 2

**Ingredients:**

•ounces broccoli florets
•tablespoons olive oil
•2 tablespoons grated parmesan cheese
•2 ounces rotini pasta, boiled
•ounces spaghetti, boiled
•Extra:
•1/3 teaspoon salt
•¼ teaspoon ground black pepper

**Directions:**

1Chop broccoli florets into small pieces, place in a heatproof bowl, cover with a plastic wrap, and then microwave for 3 to 5 minutes until tender.

2Drain broccoli well to remove all the moisture and then set aside until required.

3Meanwhile, take a medium pot half full with water, place it over medium-high heat, bring the water to a boil, then add pasta and spaghetti and cook for 5 to 8 minutes until tender.

4Drain the pasta, return it into the pot, add broccoli and cheese, and then stir in salt and black pepper until combined.

**Nutrition:**

353 Cal

g Fats

9.7 g Protein

34g Carb

5.4 g Fiber

## 153.Herbed Roasted Chicken Breasts

**Preparation Time:** 5 minutes

**Cooking Time:** 50 minutes

**Servings:** 4

**Ingredients:**

•2 tablespoons extra virgin olive oil
•2 tablespoons chopped parsley
•2 tablespoons chopped cilantro
•1 teaspoon dried oregano
•1 teaspoon dried basil
•2 tablespoons lemon juice
•Salt and pepper to taste
•4 chicken breasts

**Directions:**

1.Combine the oil, parsley, cilantro, oregano, basil, lemon juice, salt and pepper in a bowl.

2.Spread this mixture over the chicken and rub it well into the meat.

3.Place in a deep dish baking pan and cover with aluminum foil.

4.Cook in the preheated oven at 350F for 20 minutes then remove the foil and cook for 25 additional minutes.

5.Serve the chicken warm and fresh with your favorite side dish.

**Nutrition:**

Calories: 330

Fat: 15g

Protein: 40.7g

Carbohydrates: 1g

## 154.Peanut Butter Mocha Smoothie

**Preparation Time:** 5 minutes

**Cooking Time:** 0 minutes

**Servings:** 2

**Ingredients:**

- ounces sliced pear
- tablespoons instant coffee powder
- 1 ½ cup almond milk, unsweetened

**Directions:**

1. Place all the ingredients in the order into a food processor or blender, and then pulse for 1 to 2 minutes until smooth.

2. Distribute smoothie between two glasses and then serve.

**Nutrition:**

117 Cal

3.6 g Fats

1 g Protein

20.1 g Carb

2 g Fiber

## 155.Garlic Mashed Potatoes

**Preparation Time:** 5 minutes

**Cooking Time:** 10 minutes

**Servings:** 2

**Ingredients:**

- russet potatoes
- 1 clove of garlic
- 1 cup of water



- 1 tablespoon white miso paste
- 1/3 cup almond milk, unsweetened
- Extra:
- 1 1/3 teaspoon salt
- ¼ teaspoon black pepper

**Directions:**

1Peel the potatoes, cut them into ½-inch rounds, and then place them into a medium pot.

2Cover potatoes with water, add 1 teaspoon salt and garlic, place the pot over medium-high heat and bring to a boil.

3Then switch heat to medium level and then cook potatoes for 10 to 15 minutes until tender.

4When done, drain the potatoes, return them into the pot, then add milk and mash well until smooth.

5Stir in remaining salt and black pepper until mixed, add miso paste and whip the mixture by using an immersion blender until reach to desired consistency.

**Nutrition:**

274.5 Cal

0.6 g Fats

5.5 g Protein

61.8 g Carb

g Fiber

## 156.Marinated Chicken Breasts

**Preparation Time:** 5 minutes

**Cooking Time:** 2 hours

**Servings:** 4

**Ingredients:**

- 4 chicken breasts
- Salt and pepper to taste
- 1 lemon, juiced
- 1 rosemary sprig
- 1 thyme sprig
- 2 garlic cloves, crushed

•2 sage leaves
•3 tablespoons extra virgin olive oil
•½ cup buttermilk

**Directions:**

1.1. Boil the chicken with salt and pepper and place it in a resealable bag.

2.2. Add remaining ingredients and seal bag.

3.3. Refrigerate for at least 1 hour.

4.4. After 1 hour, heat a roasting pan over medium heat, then place the chicken on the grill.

5.5. Cook on each side for 8-10 minutes or until juices are gone.

6.Serve the chicken warm with your favorite side dish.

**Nutrition:**

Calories: 371

Fat: 21g

Protein: 46g

Carbohydrates: 2g

### 157.Seared Tofu in Soy Sauce and Black Pepper

**Preparation Time:** 35 minutes

**Cooking Time:** 8 minutes

**Servings:** 2

**Ingredients:**

•ounces tofu, ¼-inch thick sliced
•1 green onion, chopped
•tablespoons soy sauce
•¼ teaspoon ground black pepper
•1 teaspoon sesame seeds
•Extra:
•1 tablespoon olive oil

**Directions:**

1Cut tofu into ¼-inch pieces, place them into a medium bowl and then add soy sauce and black pepper.

2Stir until coated and then let the tofu marinate for a minimum of 30 minutes.

3Then take a medium skillet pan, place it over medium-high heat, add oil and when hot, add tofu pieces and cook for 2 to 3 minutes per side until golden brown and crisp.

4When done, garnish tofu pieces with sesame seeds and onion and then serve.

**Nutrition:**

154 Cal

11 g Fats

10 g Protein

3 g Carb

1 g Fiber

### 158.Herbed Brown Rice

**Preparation Time:** 10 minutes

**Cooking Time:** 25 minutes

**Servings:** 2

**Ingredients:**

2/3 cup brown rice

¼ teaspoon salt

1 teaspoon Italian seasoning

1 tablespoon unsalted butter

1 ½ cup vegetable broth

Extra:

1/8 teaspoon ground black pepper

**Directions:**

Take a medium saucepan, place it over medium heat, add butter and when it melts, add rice, stir well, and then cook for 3 minutes.

Pour in broth, season with salt, black pepper, and Italian seasoning, stir until combined, and then bring the mixture to a boil.

Switch heat to medium-low heat, simmer rice for 20 to 25 minutes until rice has absorbed all the liquid and turned tender.

**Nutrition:**

136 Cal

3 g Fats

3 g Protein

24 g Car

1g Fiber

## 159.Cauliflower Rice Stuffed Peppers

**Preparation Time:** 10 minutes

**Cooking Time:** 25 minutes

**Servings:** 2

**Ingredients:**

•1 red bell pepper

•1 green bell pepper

•ounces cauliflower florets

•1 green onion, chopped

•ounces white beans

•Extra:

•½ teaspoon salt

•¼ teaspoon ground black pepper

•½ teaspoon red chili powder

**Directions:**

1Switch on the oven, then set it to 375 degrees F and let it preheat.

2Meanwhile, place the cauliflower florets into a food processor and then pulse for 1 minute until the mixture resembles rice.

3Then take a medium skillet pan, place it over medium heat, add oil and when hot, add cauliflower rice, season with salt and black pepper, and then cook for 2 minutes, covering the pan.

4Remove pan from heat, then add remaining ingredients except for red pepper and stir until mixed.

5Prepare the pepper and for this, cut each pepper into half, remove the stem and seeds and then arrange them into a baking dish.

6Stuff each pepper with cauliflower and black bean mixture, cover with the foil, and then bake for 15 minutes.

7Uncover the baking dish, switch heat of the oven to 400 degrees F and then continue baking for 5 to 10 minutes until peppers have turned soft and the top has turned golden brown.

**Nutrition:**

207 Cal

5 g Fats

9.3 g Protein

35.1 g Carb

10.4 g Fiber

## 160.Black Bean and Brown Rice Bowl

**Preparation Time:** 5 minutes

**Cooking Time:** 10 minutes

**Servings:** 2

**Ingredients:**

•ounces black beans

•1 cup of brown rice

•1 tablespoon olive oil

•ounces tomato sauce

•1 cup vegetable broth

•Extra:

•1/3 teaspoon salt

•1 teaspoon red chili powder

**Directions:**

1Take a medium skillet pan, place it over medium-high heat, add oil and when hot, add rice and stir in red chili powder.

2Cook the rice for 2 minutes until nicely golden brown, add remaining ingredients and stir until combined.

3Switch heat to medium-low level and cook rice for 10 to 15 minutes until rice has turned tender.

4When done, remove the pan from heat, let the mixture for 5 minutes and then fluff with by using a fork.

**Nutrition:**

577 Cal

10.3 g Fats

14.4 g Protein
106.7 g Carb
g Fiber

### 161. Chai Cardamom Vanilla Smoothie

**Preparation Time:** 5 minutes
**Cooking Time:** 0 minutes
**Servings:** 2
**Ingredients:**
½ teaspoon ground ginger
½ teaspoon ground cinnamon
½ teaspoon ground cloves
½ teaspoon ground cardamom
2 cups almond milk, unsweetened
Extra:
½ teaspoon ground nutmeg
½ teaspoon ground allspice
**Directions:**
Place all the ingredients in the order into a food processor or blender, and then pulse for 1 to 2 minutes until smooth.
Distribute smoothie between two glasses and then serve.
**Nutrition:**
92 Cal
5.7 g Fats
2.3 g Protein
7.8 g Carb
0.5 g Fiber

### 162. Cilantro and Lime Broccoli Rice

**Preparation Time:** 5 minutes
**Cooking Time:** 8 minutes
**Servings:** 2
**Ingredients:**
•ounces broccoli florets, finely chopped
•green onions, white and green part separated
•tablespoons chopped cilantro
•½ teaspoon garlic powder
•1 teaspoon lime juice
•Extra:
•¼ teaspoon cayenne pepper
•1 tablespoon olive oil
**Directions:**
1Take a medium skillet pan, place it over medium heat, add oil and when hot, add white parts of green onion and then cook for 1 to 2 minutes until softened.
2Stir in garlic, add broccoli, stir until mixed, then cover the pan and cook for 4 to 5 minutes until broccoli has turned slightly soft.
3Add lime juice and cilantro, sprinkle with cayenne pepper, and then cook for 30 seconds.
4Taste to adjust seasoning and then serve.
**Nutrition:**
101 Cal
6.7 g Fats
2 g Protein
72 g Carb
2 g Fiber

### 163. Spicy Garlic Pasta

**Preparation Time:** 5 minutes
**Cooking Time:** 5 minutes
**Servings:** 2
**Ingredients:**
•ounces fettuccine pasta, boiled
•1 tablespoon minced garlic
•½ teaspoon red chili flakes
•1 teaspoon lime juice
•1 ½ tablespoon olive oil
**Directions:**
1Take a medium skillet pan, place it over medium heat, add oil and when hot, add garlic and then cook for 1 minute until golden.

**2**Stir in chili flakes, cook for 20 seconds, then add pasta and toss to coat.

**3**Drizzle lime juice over pasta, cook for 1 minute until hot, and then serve.

**Nutrition:**

490 Cal

11.4 g Fats

13.5 g Protein

83.3 g Carb

4 g Fiber

### 164.Simple Beef Roast

**Preparation Time:** 10 minutes

**Cooking Time:** 8 hours

**Servings:** 8

**Ingredients:**

- 5 pounds' beef roast
- 2 tablespoons Italian seasoning
- 1 cup beef stock
- 1 tablespoon sweet paprika
- 3 tablespoons olive oil

**Directions:**

1.In your slow cooker, mix all the ingredients, cover and cook on low for 8 hours.

2.Carve the roast, divide it between plates and serve.

**Nutrition:**

Calories 587,

Fat 24.1,

Fiber 0.3,

Carbs 0.9,

Protein 86.5

### 165.Honey Garlic Butter Roasted Carrots

**Preparation Time:** 5 minutes

**Cooking Time:** 20 minutes

**Servings:** 2

**Ingredients:**

- carrots
- ½ tablespoon minced garlic
- 1/8 teaspoon salt
- 2/3 tablespoon honey
- 1 tablespoon chopped cilantro
- Extra:
- 1/8 teaspoon ground black pepper
- 1 2/3 tablespoon butter, unsalted

**Directions:**

1Switch on the oven, then set it to 425 degrees F and let it preheat.

2Meanwhile, prepare the carrot, and for this, peel them and diagonally cut them into 2-inch pieces.

3Take a medium skillet pan, place it over medium heat, add butter and when it melts, add garlic and then cook for 1 minute until golden.

4Remove pan from heat, add honey into the pan and then stir until well combined.

5Add carrots into the pan, season with salt and black pepper and mix until well coated.

6Arrange carrots in a single layer on a baking sheet greased with oil and then bake for 15 to 18 minutes until carrots have become tender and golden brown.

**Nutrition:**

143 Cal

9.5 g Fats

0.7 g Protein

14 g Carb

21 g Fiber

### 166.Stuffed Bell Peppers with Quinoa

**Preparation Time:** 10 minutes

**Cooking Time:** 35 minutes

**Servings:** 2

**Ingredients:**

- 2 bell peppers
- 1/3 cup quinoa
- 3 oz. chicken stock

•¼ cup onion, diced

•½ teaspoon salt

•¼ teaspoon tomato paste

•½ teaspoon dried oregano

•1/3 cup sour cream

•1 teaspoon paprika

**Directions:**

1.Trim the bell peppers and remove the seeds.

2.Then combine together chicken stock and quinoa in the pan.

3.Add salt and boil the ingredients for 10 minutes or until quinoa will soak all liquid.

4.Then combine together cooked quinoa with dried oregano, tomato paste, and onion.

5.Fill the bell peppers with the quinoa mixture and arrange in the casserole mold.

6.Add sour cream and bake the peppers for 25 minutes at 365F.

7.Serve the cooked peppers with sour cream sauce from the casserole mold.

**Nutrition:**

Calories 237

Fat 10.3

Fiber 4.5

Carbs 31.3

Protein 6.9

## 167.Creamy Penne

**Preparation Time:** 10 minutes

**Cooking Time:** 25 minutes

**Servings:** 4

**Ingredients:**

•½ cup penne, dried

•9 oz. chicken fillet

•1 teaspoon Italian seasoning

•1 tablespoon olive oil

•1 tomato, chopped

•1 cup heavy cream

•1 tablespoon fresh basil, chopped

•½ teaspoon salt

•2 oz. Parmesan, grated

•1 cup water, for cooking

**Directions:**

1.Pour water in the pan, add penne, and boil it for 15 minutes. Then drain water.

2.Pour olive oil in the skillet and heat it up.

3.Slice the chicken fillet and put it in the hot oil.

4.Sprinkle chicken with Italian seasoning and roast for 2 minutes from each side.

5.Then add fresh basil, salt, tomato, and grated cheese.

6.Stir well.

7.Add heavy cream and cooked penne.

8.Cook the meal for 5 minutes more over the medium heat. Stir it from time to time.

**Nutrition:**

Calories 388

Fat 23.4

Fiber 0.2

Carbs 17.6

Protein 17.6

## 168.Pork and Peppers Chili

**Preparation Time:** 5 minutes

**Cooking Time:** 8 hours 5 minutes

**Servings:** 4

**Ingredients:**

•1 red onion, chopped

•2 pounds' pork, ground

•4 garlic cloves, minced

•2 red bell peppers, chopped

•1 celery stalk, chopped

•25 ounces' fresh tomatoes, peeled, crushed

•¼ cup green chilies, chopped

•2 tablespoons fresh oregano, chopped

•2 tablespoons chili powder

•A pinch of salt and black pepper

•A drizzle of olive oil

**Directions:**

1.Heat up a sauté pan with the oil over medium-high heat and add the onion, garlic and the meat. Mix and brown for 5 minutes then transfer to your slow cooker.

2.Add the rest of the ingredients, toss, cover and cook on low for 8 hours.

3.Divide everything into bowls and serve.

**Nutrition:**

Calories 448

Fat 13

Fiber 6.6

Carbs 20.2

Protein 63g

## 169.Chicken Breast Soup

**Preparation Time:** 5 minutes

**Cooking Time:** 4 hours

**Servings:** 4

**Ingredients:**

- 3 chicken breasts, skinless, boneless, cubed
- 2 celery stalks, chopped
- 2 carrots, chopped
- 2 tablespoons olive oil
- 1 red onion, chopped
- 3 garlic cloves, minced
- 4 cups chicken stock
- 1 tablespoon parsley, chopped

**Directions:**

1.In your slow cooker, mix all the ingredients except the parsley, cover and cook on High for 4 hours.

2.Add the parsley, stir, ladle the soup into bowls and serve.

**Nutrition:**

Calories 445,

Fat 21.1,

Fiber 1.6,

Carbs 7.4,

Protein 54,3

## 170.Oregano Pork Mix

**Preparation Time:** 5 minutes

**Cooking Time:** 7 hours and 6 minutes

**Servings:** 4

**Ingredients:**

- 2 pounds' pork roast
- 7 ounces' tomato paste
- 1 yellow onion, chopped
- 1 cup beef stock
- 2 tablespoons ground cumin
- 2 tablespoons olive oil
- 2 tablespoons fresh oregano, chopped
- 1 tablespoon garlic, minced
- ½ cup fresh thyme, chopped

**Directions:**

1.Heat up a sauté pan with the oil over medium-high heat, add the roast, brown it for 3 minutes on each side and then transfer to your slow cooker.

2.Add the rest of the ingredients, toss a bit, cover and cook on low for 7 hours.

3.Slice the roast, divide it between plates and serve.

**Nutrition:**

Calories 623,

Fat 30.1,

Fiber 6.2,

Carbs 19.3,

Protein 69,2

## 171.Light Paprika Moussaka

**Preparation Time:** 15 minutes

**Cooking Time:** 45 minutes

**Servings:** 3

**Ingredients:**

- 1 eggplant, trimmed
- 1 cup ground chicken
- 1/3 cup white onion, diced
- 3 oz. Cheddar cheese, shredded
- 1 potato, sliced

•1 teaspoon olive oil

•1 teaspoon salt

•½ cup milk

•1 tablespoon butter

•1 tablespoon ground paprika

•1 tablespoon Italian seasoning

•1 teaspoon tomato paste

**Directions:**

1.Slice the eggplant lengthwise and sprinkle with salt.

2.Pour olive oil in the skillet and add sliced potato.

3.Roast potato for 2 minutes from each side.

4.Then transfer it in the plate.

5.Put eggplant in the skillet and roast it for 2 minutes from each side too.

6.Pour milk in the pan and bring it to boil.

7.Add tomato paste, Italian seasoning, paprika, butter, and Cheddar cheese.

8.Then mix up together onion with ground chicken.

9.Arrange the sliced potato in the casserole in one layer.

10.Then add ½ part of all sliced eggplants.

11.Spread the eggplants with ½ part of chicken mixture.

12.Then add remaining eggplants.

13.Pour the milk mixture over the eggplants.

14.Bake moussaka for 30 minutes at 355F.

**Nutrition:**

Calories 387,

Fat 21.2,

Fiber 8.9,

Carbs 26.3,

Protein 25.4

## 172.Cauliflower Curry

**Preparation Time:** 5 minutes

**Cooking Time:** 5 hours

**Servings:** 4

**Ingredients:**

•1 cauliflower head, florets separated

•2 carrots, sliced

•1 red onion, chopped

•¾ cup coconut milk

•2 garlic cloves, minced

•2 tablespoons curry powder

•A pinch of salt and black pepper

•1 tablespoon red pepper flakes

•1 teaspoon garam masala

**Directions:**

1.In your slow cooker, mix all the ingredients.

2.Cover, cook on high for 5 hours, divide into bowls and serve.

**Nutrition:**

Calories 160,

Fat 11.5,

Fiber 5.4,

Carbs 14.7,

Protein 3,6

## 173.Balsamic Beef and Mushrooms Mix

**Preparation Time:** 5 minutes

**Cooking Time:** 8 hours

**Servings:** 4

**Ingredients:**

•2 pounds' beef, cut into strips

•¼ cup balsamic vinegar

•2 cups beef stock

•1 tablespoon ginger, grated

•Juice of ½ lemon

•1 cup brown mushrooms, sliced

•A pinch of salt and black pepper

•1 teaspoon ground cinnamon

**Directions:**

1.Mix all the ingredients In your slow cooker,, cover and cook on low for 8 hours.

2.Divide everything between plates and
serve.
**Nutrition:**
Calories 446,
Fat 14,
Fiber 0.6,
Carbs 2.9,
Protein 70,8

## 174.Cucumber Bowl with Spices and Greek Yogurt

**Preparation Time:** 10 minutes
**Cooking Time:** 20 minutes
**Servings:** 3
**Ingredients:**
•4 cucumbers
•½ teaspoon chili pepper
•¼ cup fresh parsley, chopped
•¾ cup fresh dill, chopped
•2 tablespoons lemon juice
•½ teaspoon salt
•½ teaspoon ground black pepper
•¼ teaspoon sage
•½ teaspoon dried oregano
•1/3 cup Greek yogurt
**Directions:**
1.Make the cucumber dressing: blend the dill
and parsley until you get green mash.
2.Then combine together green mash with
lemon juice, salt, ground black pepper, sage,
dried oregano, Greek yogurt, and chili
pepper.
3.Churn the mixture well.
4.Chop the cucumbers roughly and combine
them with cucumber dressing. Mix up well.
5.Refrigerate the cucumber for 20 minutes.
**Nutrition:**
Calories 114
Fat 1.6
Fiber 4.1

Carbs 23.2
Protein 7.6

## 175.Zucchini Omelet

**Preparation Time**: 10 minutes
**Cooking Time:** 10 minutes
**Servings:** 1
**Ingredients:**
•1/2 teaspoon butter
•1/2 zucchini, julienned
•One egg
•1/8 teaspoon fresh basil, chopped
•1/8 teaspoon red pepper flakes, crushed
•Salted and newly ground black pepper, to
taste
**Directions:**
1.Preheat the Instant Crisp Air Fryer to 355
degrees F.
2.Melt butter on a medium heat using a
skillet.
3.Add zucchini and cook for about 3-4
minutes.
4.In a bowl, add the eggs, basil, red pepper
flakes, salt, and black pepper and beat well.
5.Add cooked zucchini and gently stir to
combine.
6.Transfer the mixture into the Instant Crisp
Air Fryer pan. Lock the air fryer lid.
7.Cook for about 10 minutes. Also, you may
opt to wait until it is done thoroughly.
**Nutrition:**
Calories: 285
Fat: 20.5 g
Protein: 8.6 g

## 176.Prosciutto Wrapped Mozzarella Balls

**Preparation Time:** 10 minutes
**Cooking Time:** 10 minutes

**Servings:** 4
**Ingredients:**
- 8 Mozzarella balls, cherry size
- 4 oz. bacon, sliced
- ¼ teaspoon ground black pepper
- ¾ teaspoon dried rosemary
- 1 teaspoon butter

**Directions:**
1. Sprinkle the sliced bacon with ground black pepper and dried rosemary.
2. Wrap every Mozzarella ball in the sliced bacon and secure them with toothpicks.
3. Melt butter.
4. Brush wrapped Mozzarella balls with butter.
5. Line the tray with the baking paper and arrange Mozzarella balls in it.
6. Bake the meal for 10 minutes at 365F.

**Nutrition:**
Calories 323
Fat 26.8
Fiber 0.1
Carbs 0.6
Protein 20.6

### 177.Cauliflower Rice

**Preparation Time**: 5 minutes
**Cooking Time:** 20 minutes
**Servings:** 1
**Ingredients:**
Round 1:
- 1/2 tsp. turmeric
- 1/2 cup of diced carrot
- 1/8 cup of diced onion
- 1/2 tbsp. low-sodium soy sauce
- 1/8 block of extra firm tofu
Round 2:
- 1/2 cup of frozen peas
- 1/4 minced garlic cloves
- 1/2 cup of chopped broccoli
- 1/2 tbsp. minced ginger

- 1/4 tbsp. rice vinegar
- 1/4 tsp. toasted sesame oil
- 1/2 tbsp. reduced-sodium soy sauce
- 1/2 cup of riced cauliflower

**Directions:**
1. Crush tofu in a large bowl and toss with all the Round one ingredient.
2. Lock the air fryer lid — preheat the Instant Crisp Air Fryer to 370 degrees. Also, set the temperature to 370°F, set time to 10 minutes, and cook 10 minutes, making sure to shake once.
3. In another bowl, toss ingredients from Round 2 together.
4. Add Round 2 mixture to Instant Crisp Air Fryer and cook another 10 minutes to shake 5 minutes.
5. Enjoy!

**Nutrition:**
Calories: 67
Fat: 8 g
Protein: 3 g
Sugar: 0 g

### 178.Air Fryer Asparagus

**Preparation Time**: 5 minutes
**Cooking Time:** 8 minutes
**Servings:** 1
**Ingredients:**
- Nutritional yeast
- Olive oil non-stick spray
- One bunch of asparagus

**Directions:**
1. Wash the asparagus. Do not forget to trim off thick, woody ends.
2. Spray with olive oil spray and sprinkle with yeast.
3. In your Instant Crisp Air Fryer, lay the asparagus in a singular layer. Set the

temperature to 360°F. Limit the time to eight minutes.
**Nutrition:**
Calories: 17
Fat: 4 g
Protein: 9 g

### 179.Bell-Pepper Corn Wrapped in Tortilla

**Preparation Time**: 5 minutes
**Cooking Time:** 15 minutes
**Servings:** 1
**Ingredients:**
•1/4 small red bell pepper, chopped
•1/4 small yellow onion, diced
•1/4 tablespoon water
•1/2 cobs grilled corn kernels
•One large tortilla
•One-piece commercial vegan nuggets, chopped
•Mixed greens for garnish
**Directions:**
1.Preheat the Instant Crisp Air Fryer to 400°F.
2.In a skillet heated over medium heat, sauté the vegan nuggets and the onions, bell peppers, and corn kernels. Set aside.
3.Place filling inside the corn tortillas.
4.Lock the air fryer lid. Fold the tortillas and place inside the Instant Crisp Air Fryer, cook for 15 minutes until the tortilla wraps are crispy.
5.Serve with mixed greens on top.
**Nutrition:**
Calories: 548
Fat: 20.7g
Protein: 46g

### 180.Mediterranean Burrito

**Preparation Time:** 10 minutes
**Cooking Time:** 0 minutes
**Servings:** 2
**Ingredients:**
•2 wheat tortillas
•2 oz. red kidney beans, canned, drained
•2 tablespoons hummus
•2 teaspoons tahini sauce
•1 cucumber
•2 lettuce leaves
•1 tablespoon lime juice
•1 teaspoon olive oil
•½ teaspoon dried oregano
**Directions:**
1.Mash the red kidney beans until you get a puree.
2.Then spread the wheat tortillas with beans mash from one side.
3.Add hummus and tahini sauce.
4.Cut the cucumber into the wedges and place them over tahini sauce.
5.Then add lettuce leaves.
6.Make the dressing: mix up together olive oil, dried oregano, and lime juice.
7.Drizzle the lettuce leaves with the dressing and wrap the wheat tortillas in the shape of burritos.
**Nutrition:**
Calories 288
Fat 10.2
Fiber 14.6
Carbs 38.2
Protein 12.5

### 181.Sweet Potato Bacon Mash

**Preparation Time:** 10 minutes
**Cooking Time:** 20 minutes
**Servings:** 4
**Ingredients:**
•3 sweet potatoes, peeled
•4 oz. bacon, chopped

•1 cup chicken stock

•1 tablespoon butter

•1 teaspoon salt

•2 oz. Parmesan, grated

**Directions:**

1.Chop sweet potato and put it in the pan.

2.Add chicken stock and close the lid.

3.Boil the vegetables for 15 minutes or until they are soft.

4.After this, drain the chicken stock.

5.Mash the sweet potato with the help of the potato masher. Add grated cheese and butter.

6.Mix up together salt and chopped bacon. Fry the mixture until it is crunchy (10-15 minutes).

7.Add cooked bacon in the mashed sweet potato and mix up with the help of the spoon.

8.It is recommended to serve the meal warm or hot.

**Nutrition:**

Calories 304

Fat 18.1

Fiber 2.9

Carbs 18.8

Protein 17

## 182.Mixed Fruit Parfait

**Preparation Time:** 5 minutes

**Cooking Time:** 0 minutes

**Servings:** 2

**Ingredients:**

•ounces of cherries mixed fruit

•tablespoons chia seeds

•½ tablespoons shredded coconut, unsweetened

•tablespoons maple syrup

•ounces almond milk, unsweetened

•Extra:

•½ teaspoon vanilla extract, unsweetened

**Directions:**

1Take a medium bowl, place chia and coconut in it, add maple syrup and vanilla, pour in the milk and whisk until well combined.

2Let the mixture rest for 30 minutes, then stir it and refrigerate for a minimum of 3 hours or overnight.

3Assemble parfait and for this, divide half of the chia mixture into the bottom of serving glass, and then top evenly with three-fourth of mixed fruit.

4Cover berries with remaining chia seed mixture and then place remaining mixed fruit on top.

**Nutrition:**

235 Cal

9.2 g Fats

2.9 g Protein

35.3 g Carb

g Fiber

## 183.Avocado Fries

**Preparation Time**: 10 minutes

**Cooking Time:** 7 minutes

**Servings:** 1

**Ingredients:**

•One avocado

•1/8 tsp. salt

•1/4 cup of panko breadcrumbs

•Bean liquid (aquafaba) from a 15-ounce can of white or garbanzo beans

**Directions:**

1.Peel, pit, and slice up avocado.

2.Toss salt and breadcrumbs together in a bowl. Place the aquafaba into another bowl.

3.Dredge slices of avocado first in the aquafaba and then in panko, making sure you are evenly coating.

4.Place coated avocado slices into a single layer in the Instant Crisp Air Fryer. Set temperature to 390°F and set time to 5 minutes.

5.Serve with your favorite Keto dipping sauce!

**Nutrition:**

Calories: 102

Fat: 22g

Protein: 9g

Sugar: 1g

### 184.Garlic Chicken Balls

**Preparation Time:** 15 minutes

**Cooking Time:** 10 minutes

**Servings:** 4

**Ingredients:**

•2 cups ground chicken

•1 teaspoon minced garlic

•1 teaspoon dried dill

•1/3 carrot, grated

•1 egg, beaten

•1 tablespoon olive oil

•¼ cup coconut flakes

•½ teaspoon salt

**Directions:**

1.In the mixing bowl mix up together ground chicken, minced garlic, dried dill, carrot, egg, and salt.

2.Stir the chicken mixture with the help of the fingertips until homogenous.

3.Then make medium balls from the mixture.

4.Coat every chicken ball in coconut flakes.

5.Heat up olive oil in the skillet.

6.Add chicken balls and cook them for 3 minutes from each side. The cooked chicken balls will have a golden-brown color.

**Nutrition:**

Calories 200

Fat 11.5

Fiber 0.6

Carbs 1.7

Protein 21.9



### 185.Vietnamese Turmeric Fish with Mango and Herbs Sauce

**Preparation Time:** 15 minutes

**Cooking Time:** 30 minutes

**Servings:** 4

**Ingredients:**

For the Fish:

•Coconut oil to fry the fish, 2 tablespoons

•Fresh codfish, skinless and boneless, 1 ¼ lbs. (cut into 2-inch piece wide)

•Pinch of sea salt, to taste

Fish Marinade:

•Chinese cooking wine, 1 tablespoon

•Turmeric powder, 1 tablespoon

•Sea salt, 1 teaspoon

•Olive oil, 2 tablespoons

•Minced ginger, 2 teaspoons

Mango Dipping Sauce:

•Juice of ½ lime

•Medium-sized ripe mango, 1

•Rice vinegar, 2 tablespoons

•Dry red chili pepper, 1 teaspoon (stir in before serving)

•Garlic clove, 1

•Infused scallion and dill oil

•Fresh dill, 2 cups

•Scallions, 2 cups (slice into long thin shape)

•A pinch of sea salt, to taste.

Toppings

•Nuts (pine or cashew nuts)

•Lime juice (as much as you like)

•Fresh cilantro (as much as you like)

**Directions:**

1.Add all the ingredients under "Mango Dipping Sauce" into your food processor. Blend until you get your preferred consistency.

2.Add two tablespoons of coconut oil in a large non-stick frying pan and heat over high heat. Once hot, add the pre-marinated fish.

Add the slices of the fish into the pan individually. Divide into batches for easy frying, if necessary.

3.Once you hear a loud sizzle, reduce the heat to medium-high.

4.Do not move or turn the fish until it turns golden brown on one side; then turn it to the other side to fry, about 5 minutes on each side. Add more coconut oil to the pan if needed. Season with the sea salt.

5.Transfer the fish to a large plate. You will have some oil left in the frypan, which you will use to make your scallion and dill infused oil.

6.Using the remaining oil in the frypan, set to medium-high heat, add 2 cups of dill, and 2 cups of scallions.

7.Put off the heat after you have added the dill and scallions. Toss them gently for about 15 seconds, until the dill and scallions have wilted. Add a dash of sea salt to season.

8.Pour the dill, scallion, and infused oil over the fish. Serve with mango dipping sauce, nuts, lime, and fresh cilantro.

**Nutrition:**

Calories: 234

Fat: 23 g

Protein: 76 g

Sugar: 5 g

### 186.Mediterranean Baked Penne

**Preparation Time**: 25 minutes

**Cooking Time:** 1 hour 20 minutes

**Servings:** 8

**Ingredients:**

•Extra-virgin olive oil, 1 tablespoon

•Fine dry breadcrumbs, ½ cup

•Small zucchini, 2 (chopped)

•Medium eggplant, 1 (chopped)

•Medium onion, 1 (chopped)

•Red bell pepper, 1 (seeded and chopped)

•Celery, 1 stalk (sliced)

•Garlic, 1 clove (minced)

•Salt and freshly ground pepper to taste

•Dry white wine, ¼ cup

•Plum tomatoes, 28-ounces (drained and coarsely chopped, juice reserved)

•Freshly grated Parmesan cheese, 2 tablespoons

•Large eggs, 2 (lightly beaten)

•Coarsely grated part-skim mozzarella cheese, 1 ½ cups

•Dried penne rig ate or rigatoni, 1 pound

**Directions:**

1.Preheat your oven to 375 degrees F. Apply nonstick spray on a 3-quart baking dish. Then coat the dish with ¼ cup of breadcrumbs, tapping out the excess.

2.Heat the oil in a large non-stick skillet over medium-high heat. Then add the onion, celery, bell pepper, eggplant, and zucchini.

3.Cook for about 10 minutes, occasionally stirring, until smooth. Then add the garlic and cook for another minute. Add the wine, stir and cook for about 2 minutes, long enough for the wine to almost evaporate.

4.Then add the juice and tomatoes. Bring to a simmer, then cook for about 10 to 15 minutes, until thickened, season with pepper and salt.

5.Transfer to a large bowl and allow to cool.

6.Pour water into a pot, add some salt, and then allow to boil. Add the penne into the boiling salted water to cook for about 10 minutes, until al dente.

7.Drain and rinse the pasta under running water. Toss the pasta with the vegetable mixture, then stir in the mozzarella.

8.Scoop the pasta mixture and place into the prepared baking dish. Drizzle the broken eggs evenly over the top.

9.Mix the Parmesan and ¼ cups of breadcrumbs in a small bowl, then sprinkle evenly over the top of the dish.

10.Place the dish into the oven to bake for about 40 to 50 minutes, until bubbly and golden.

11.Allow to rest for 10 min before you serve.

**Nutrition:**
Calories: 372
Protein: 45 g
Fat: 8 g
Sugar: 2 g

### 187.Prawn Arrabbiata

**Preparation Time**: 35 minutes
**Cooking Time:** 30 minutes
**Servings:** 1
**Ingredients:**
•Raw or cooked prawns, 1 cup
•Extra virgin olive oil, 1 tablespoon
•Buckwheat pasta, ½ cup
•Chopped parsley, 1 tablespoon
•Celery, ¼ cup (finely chopped)
•Tinned chopped tomatoes, 2 cups
•Red onion, 1/3 cup (finely chopped)
•Garlic clove, 1 (finely chopped)
•Extra virgin olive oil, 1 teaspoon
•Dried mixed herbs, 1 teaspoon
•Bird's eye chili, 1 (finely chopped)
•White wine, 2 tablespoons (optional)
**Directions:**
1.Add the olive oil into your fry-pan and fry the dried herbs, celery, and onions over medium-low heat for about two minutes.

2.Increase heat to medium, add the wine and cook for another min.

3.Add the tomatoes to the pan and allow to simmer for about 30 minutes, over medium-low heat, until you get a nice creamy consistency.

4.Add a little water if the sauce gets too thick.

5.While the sauce is cooking, cook the pasta following the instruction on the packet. Drain the water once the pasta is done cooking, toss with the olive oil, and set aside until needed.

6.If using raw prawns, add them to your sauce and cook for another four minutes, until the prawns turn opaque and pink, then add the parsley. If using cooked prawns, add them at the same time with the parsley and allow the sauce to boil.

7.Add the already cooked pasta to the sauce, mix them, and serve.

**Nutrition:**
Calories: 321
Protein: 19 g
Fat: 2 g
Carbohydrate: 23 g

### 188.Brown Basmati Rice Pilaf

**Preparation Time**: 10 minutes
**Cooking Time:** 3 minutes
**Servings:** 2
**Ingredients:**
•½ tablespoon vegan butter
•½ cup mushrooms, chopped
•½ cup brown basmati rice
•2-3 tablespoons water
•1/8 teaspoon dried thyme
•Ground pepper to taste
•½ tablespoon olive oil
•¼ cup green onion, chopped
•1 cup vegetable broth
•¼ teaspoon salt
•¼ cup chopped, toasted pecans

**Directions:**
1.Place a saucepan over medium-low heat. Add butter and oil.
2.When it melts, add mushrooms and cook until slightly tender.
3.Stir in the green onion and brown rice. Cook for 3 minutes. Stir constantly.
4.Stir in the broth, water, salt, and thyme.
5.When it begins to boil, lower the heat and cover with a lid. Simmer until rice is cooked. Add more water or broth if required.
6.Stir in the pecans and pepper.
7.Serve.
**Nutrition:**
Calories 189
Fats 11 g
Carbohydrates 19 g
Proteins 4 g

90.      Shakshuka
**Preparation Time**: 10 minutes
**Cooking Time:** 30 minutes
**Servings:** 1
**Ingredients:**
•Chopped parsley, 1 tablespoon
•Extra virgin olive oil, 1 teaspoon
•Paprika, 1 teaspoon
•Red onion, ½ cup (finely chopped)
•Kale, 30g (stems removed and roughly chopped)
•Garlic clove, 1 (finely chopped)
•Celery, 30g (finely chopped)
•Bird's eye chili, 1 (finely chopped)
•Ground turmeric, 1 teaspoon
•Ground cumin, 1 teaspoon
•Tinned chopped tomatoes, 2 cups
•Medium eggs, 2
**Directions:**

1.Place a small, deep-sided frying pan over medium-low heat. Add the oil once hot, then add the chili, spices, celery, garlic, and onions. Fry for about 2 minutes.
2.Add the tomatoes, then allow the sauce to simmer gently for approx. 20 min while stirring frequently.
3.Add the kale to the pot and cook for another five minutes. Add a little water if the sauce gets too thick. Stir in the parsley once the sauce becomes nicely creamy.
4.Create two little wells in the sauce, then break each egg into the wells. Reduce your heat to the lowest and cover the pan with a foil or with its lid.
5.Allow the eggs to cook for about 10 minutes, or until the whites are firm and the yolks remain runny. Cook for another four minutes if you want the yolks to be firm.
6.Serve immediately.
**Nutrition:**
Calories: 657
Protein: 87 g
Fat: 4 g
Sugar: 6 g

### 189.Chicken & Cauliflower Rice Bowls
**Preparation Time**: 10 minutes
**Cooking Time:** 20 minutes
**Servings:** 4
**Ingredients:**
•1/3 cup of salsa
•1 quantity of 14.5 oz. of can fire-roasted diced tomatoes
•1 canned chipotle pepper + 1 teaspoon sauce
•½ teaspoon of dried oregano
•1 teaspoon of cumin
•1 ½ lb. of boneless, skinless chicken breast

•¼ teaspoon of salt
•1 cup of reduced-fat shredded Mexican cheese blend
•4 cups of frozen riced cauliflower
•½ medium-sized avocado, sliced
**Directions:**
1.Combine the first ingredients in a blender and blend until they become smooth
2.Place chicken inside your instant pot, and pour the sauce over it. Cover the lid and close the pressure valve.
3.Set it to 20 minutes at high temperature. Let the pressure release on its own before opening.
4.Remove the piece and the chicken and then add it back to the sauce.
5.Microwave the riced cauliflower according to the directions on the package.
6.Before you serve, divide the riced cauliflower, cheese, avocado, and chicken equally among the four bowls.
**Nutrition:**
Calories: 287
Protein: 35 g
Carbohydrate: 19 g
Fat: 12 g

## 190.Chicken and Kale Curry

**Preparation Time**: 20 min
**Cooking Time:** 1 hour
**Servings:** 3
**Ingredients:**
•Boiling water, 250 ml
•Skinless and boneless chicken thighs, 7 oz.
•Ground turmeric, 2 tablespoons
•Olive oil, 1 tablespoon
•Red onions, 1 (diced)
•Bird's eye chili, 1 (finely chopped)
•Freshly chopped ginger, ½ tablespoon
•Curry powder, ½ tablespoon

•Garlic, 1 ½ cloves (crushed)
•Cardamom pods, 1
•Tinned coconut milk, light, 100 ml
•Chicken stock, 2 cups
•Tinned chopped tomatoes, 1 cup
Direction:
1.Place the chicken thighs in a non-metallic bowl, add one tablespoon of turmeric and one teaspoon of olive oil. Mix together and keep aside to marinate for approx. 30 minutes.
2.Fry the chicken thighs over medium heat for about 5 minutes until well cooked and brown on all sides. Remove from the pan and set aside.
3.Add the remaining oil into a frypan on medium heat. Then add the onion, ginger, garlic, and chili. Fry for about 10 minutes until soft.
4.Add one tablespoon of the turmeric and half a tablespoon of curry powder to the pan and cook for another 2 minutes.
5.Then add the cardamom pods, coconut milk, tomatoes, and chicken stock. Allow simmering for thirty minutes.
6.Add the chicken once the sauce has reduced a little into the pan, followed by the kale. Cook until the kale is tender and the chicken is warm enough.
7.Serve with buckwheat.
8.Garnish with the chopped coriander.
**Nutrition:**
Calories: 313 g
Protein: 13 g
Fat: 6 g
Carbohydrate: 23 g

## 191.Zucchini Risotto

**Preparation Time**: 10 minutes
**Cooking Time:** 5 minutes

**Servings:** 8
**Ingredients:**
- 2 tablespoons olive oil
- 4 cloves garlic, finely chopped
- 1.5 pounds Arborio rice
- 6 tomatoes, chopped
- 2 teaspoons chopped rosemary
- 6 zucchini, finely diced
- 1 ¼ cups peas, fresh or frozen
- 12 cups hot vegetable stock
- Salt to taste
- Freshly ground pepper

**Directions:**
1. Place a large, heavy-bottomed pan over medium heat. Add oil. When the oil is heated, add onion and sauté until translucent.
2. Stir in the tomatoes and cook until soft.
3. Stir in the rice and rosemary. Mix well.
4. Add half the stock and cook until dry. Stir frequently.
5. Add remaining stock and cook for 3-4 minutes.
6. Add courgette and peas and cook until rice is tender. Add salt and pepper to taste.
7. Stir in the basil. Let it sit for 5 minutes.

**Nutrition:**
Calories 406
Fats 5 g
Carbohydrates 82 g
Proteins 14 g

### 192. Walnut and Date Porridge

**Preparation Time:** 10 minutes
**Cooking Time:** 0 minutes
**Servings:** 1
**Ingredients:**
- Strawberries, ½ cup (hulled)
- Milk or dairy-free alternative, 200 ml
- Buckwheat flakes, ½ cup
- Medjool date, 1 (chopped)
- Walnut butter, 1 teaspoon, or chopped walnut halves

**Directions:**
1. Place the date and the milk in a pan, heat gently before adding the buckwheat flakes. Then cook until the porridge gets to your desired consistency.
2. Add the walnuts, stir, then top with the strawberries.
3. Serve.

**Nutrition:**
Calories: 254
Protein: 65 g
Fat: 4 g
Vitamin B

# Snacks and Appetizers

### 193.Healthy Cookies
**Preparation Time:** 4 minutes
**Cooking Time:** 15 minutes
**Servings:** 1
**Ingredients:**
- 1 ¾ cup of quick oats
- 2 large ripe bananas
- 4 tsp peanut butter
- 1/3 cup crushed nuts of your choice
- ½ tsp pure vanilla extract
- ¼ cup shredded coconut

**Directions:**
1.Preheat your oven to 350 degrees Fahrenheit.
2.Mash the bananas in a bowl and add the oats and mix them well to combine. Fold any optional add ins such as ¼ cup chocolate chips. You can add honey to taste.
3.Line your baking tray with parchment paper and drop one tsp of cookie dough per cookie into your tray. Press down with a metal spoon into the shape of the cookies.
4.Bake for 20 minutes depending on your oven or cook them until they are golden brown on top.
5.Remove and allow to cool before serving.
**Nutrition:**
Calories 24
Carbohydrates 5g
Proteins 1g
Calcium: 4mg
Potassium: 29mg.

### 194.Eggplant Dip
**Preparation Time: 10 minutes**
**Cooking Time: 40 minutes**
 **Servings: 4**
**Ingredients:**
- 1 eggplant, poked with a fork
- 2 tablespoons tahini paste
- 2 tablespoons lemon juice
- 2 garlic cloves, minced
- 1 tablespoon olive oil
- Salt and black pepper to the taste
- 1 tablespoon parsley, chopped

**Directions:**
1.Put the eggplant in a roasting pan, bake at 400° F for 40 minutes, cool down, peel and transfer to your food processor.
2.Add the rest of the ingredients except the parsley, pulse well, divide into small bowls and serve as an appetizer with the parsley sprinkled on top.
**Nutrition:**
Calories 121;
Fat 4.3 g;
Fiber 1 g;
Carbs 1.4 g;
Protein 4.3 g

### 195.Veggie Fritters
**Preparation Time: 10 minutes**
**Cooking Time: 10 minutes**
**Servings: 4**
**Ingredients:**
- 2 garlic cloves, minced
- 2 yellow onions, chopped
- 4 scallions, chopped
- 2 carrots, grated
- 2 teaspoons cumin, ground
- ½ teaspoon turmeric powder
- Salt and black pepper to the taste
- ¼ teaspoon coriander, ground
- 2 tablespoons parsley, chopped
- ¼ teaspoon lemon juice
- ½ cup almond flour
- 2 beets, peeled and grated

•2 eggs, whisked
•¼ cup tapioca flour
•3 tablespoons olive oil
**Directions:**
1.In a bowl, combine the garlic with the onions, scallions and the rest of the ingredients except the oil, stir well and shape medium fritters out of this mix.
2.Heat up a pan with the oil over medium-high heat, add the fritters, cook for 5 minutes on each side, arrange on a platter and serve.
**Nutrition:**
Calories 209;
Fat 11.2 g;
Fiber 3 g;
Carbs 4.4 g;
Protein 4.8 g

## 196.White Bean Dip

**Preparation Time: 10 minutes**
**Cooking Time: 0 minute**
**Servings: 4**
**Ingredients:**
•15 ounces canned white beans, drained and rinsed
•6 ounces canned artichoke hearts, drained and quartered
•4 garlic cloves, minced
•1 tablespoon basil, chopped
•2 tablespoons olive oil
•Juice of ½ lemon
•Zest of ½ lemon, grated
•Salt and black pepper to the taste
**Directions:**
1.In your food processor, combine the beans with the artichokes and the rest of the ingredients except the oil and pulse well.
2.Add the oil gradually, pulse the mix again, divide into cups and serve as a party dip.

**Nutrition:**
Calories 274;
Fat 11.7 g;
Fiber 6.5 g;
Carbs 18.5 g;
Protein 16.5 g

## 197.Grilled Avocado Caprese Crostini

**Preparation Time:** 10 minutes
**Cooking Time:** 20 minutes
**Servings:** 2
**Ingredients:**
•1 avocado thinly sliced
•9 ounces ripened cherry tomatoes
•ounces fresh bocconcini in water
•2 tsp balsamic glaze
•8 pieces Italian baguette
•½ a cup basil leaves
**Directions:**
1.Preheat your oven to 375 degrees Fahrenheit
2.Arrange your baking sheet properly before spraying them on top with olive oil.
3.Bake your item of choice until they are well done or golden brown. Rub your crostini with the cut side of garlic while they are still warm and you can season them with pepper and salt.
4.Divide the basil leaves on each side of bread and top up with tomato halves, avocado slices and bocconcini. Season it with pepper and salt.
5.Broil it for 4 minutes and when the cheese starts to melt through remove and drizzle balsamic glaze before serving.
**Nutrition:**
Calories 278
Fat 10g
Carbohydrates 37g

Proteins 10g
Sodium: 342 Mg
Potassium: 277mg

### 198.Mushroom Caprese Stuffed Garlic Butter

**Preparation Time:** 5 minutes
**Cooking Time:** 10 minutes
**Servings:** 6
**Ingredients:**
•For Garlic butter
•2 tsp of butter
•2 cloves garlic 1 tsp parsley finely chopped
•For the mushrooms
•6 large portobello mushrooms, washed and dried well with paper towel.
•6 mozzarella cheese balls thinly sliced
•1 cup grape tomatoes thinly sliced
•Fresh basil for garnishing
•For balsamic glaze
•2 tsp brown sugar
•¼ cup balsamic vinegar
**Directions:**
1.Preheat the oven to broil setting on high heat. Arrange the oven shelf and place it in the right direction.
2.Combine the garlic butter ingredients in a small pan and melt until the garlic begins to be fragrant. Brush the bottoms of the mushroom and place them on the buttered section of the baking tray.
3.Flip and brush the remaining garlic over each cap. Fill each mushroom with tomatoes and mozzarella slices and grill until the cheese has melted. Drizzle the balsamic glaze and sprinkle some salt to taste.
4.If you are making the balsamic glaze from scratch, combine the sugar and vinegar in a small pan and reduce the heat to low. Allow it to simmer for 6 minutes or until the mixture has thickened well.
**Nutrition:**
Calories 101
Fat 5g
Carbohydrates 12g
Proteins 2g
Sodium: 58mg
Potassium: 377 Mg

### 199.Cheesy Mashed Sweet Potato Cakes

**Preparation Time:** 10 minutes
**Cooking Time:** 30 minutes
**Servings:** 4
**Ingredients:**
•¾ cup bread crumbs
•4 cups mashed potatoes
•½ cup onions
•2 cup of grated mozzarella cheese
•¼ cup fresh grated parmesan cheese
•2 large cloves finely chopped
•1 egg
•2 tsp finely chopped parsley
•Salt and pepper to taste
**Directions:**
1.Line your baking sheet with foil. Wash, peel and cut the sweet potatoes into 6 pieces. Arrange them inside the baking sheet and drizzle a small amount of oil on top before seasoning with salt and pepper.
2.Cover with a baking sheet and bake it for 45 minutes. once cooked transfer them into a mixing bowl and mash them well with a potato masher.
3.To the sweet potatoes in a bowl add green onions, parmesan, mozzarella, garlic, egg, parsley and bread crumbs. Mash and combine the mixture together using the masher.

4.Put the remaining ¼ cup of the breadcrumbs in a place. Scoop a tsp of mixture into your palm and form round patties around ½ and inch thick. Dredge your patties in the breadcrumbs to cover both sides and set them aside.

5.Heat a tablespoon of oil in a medium nonstick pan. when the oil is hot begin to cook the patties in batches 4 or 5 per session and cook each side for 6 minutes until they turn golden brown. Using a spoon or spatula flip them. Add oil to prevent burning.

**Nutrition:**
Calories 126
Fat 6g
Carbs 15g
Proteins 3g
Sodium: 400mg

## 200.Cheesy Garlic Sweet Potatoes

**Preparation Time:** 10 minutes
**Cooking Time:** 25 minutes
**Servings:** 4
**Ingredients:**
•Sea salt
•¼ cup garlic butter melt
•¾ cup shredded mozzarella cheese
•½ cup of parmesan cheese freshly grated
•4 medium sized sweet potatoes
•2 tsp freshly chopped parsley
**Directions:**
1.Heat the oven to 400 degrees Fahrenheit and brush the potatoes with garlic butter and season each with pepper and salt. Arrange the cut side down on a greased baking sheet until the flesh is tender or they turn golden brown.

2.Remove them from the oven, flip the cut side up and top up with parsley and parmesan cheese.

3.Change the settings of your instant fryer oven to broil and on medium heat add the cheese and melt it. sprinkle salt and pepper to taste. Serve them warm

**Nutrition:**
Calories 356
Fat 9g
Carbohydrates 13g
Proteins 5g
Potassium: 232mg
Sodium: 252mg

## 201.Crispy Garlic Baked Potato Wedges

**Preparation Time:** 5 minutes
**Cooking Time:** 10 minutes
**Servings:** 3
**Ingredients:**
•3 tsp salt
•1 tsp minced garlic
•6 large russet
•¼ cup olive oil
•1 tsp paprika
•2/3 finely grated parmesan cheese
•2 tsp freshly chopped parsley
**Directions:**
1.Preheat the oven into 350 degrees Fahrenheit and line the baking sheet with a parchment pepper.

2.Cut the potatoes into halfway length and cut each half in half lengthways again. Make 8 wedges.

3.In a small jug combine garlic, oil, paprika and salt and place your wedges in the baking sheets. Pour the oil mixture over the potatoes and toss them to ensure that they are evenly coated.

4.Arrange the potato wedges in a single layer on the baking tray and sprinkle salt and parmesan cheese if needed. Bake for 35 minutes turning the wedges once half side is cooked.

5.Flip the other side until they are both golden brown.

6.Sprinkle parsley and the remaining parmesan before serving.

**Nutrition:**

Calories 324

Fat 6g

Carbs 8g

Proteins 2g

Sodium: 51mg

Potassium: 120mg

## 202.Sticky Chicken Thai Wings

**Preparation Time:** 10 minutes

**Cooking Time:** 30 minutes

**Servings:** 6

**Ingredients:**

•3 pounds chicken wings removed

•1 tsp sea salt to taste

For the glaze:

•¾ cup Thai sweet chili sauce

•¼ cup soy sauce

•4 tsp brown sugar

•4 tsp rice wine vinegar

•3 tsp fish sauce

•2 tsp lime juice

•1 tsp lemon grass minced

•2 tsp sesame oil

•1 tsp garlic minced

1.**Directions:**

2.Preheat the oven to 350 degrees Fahrenheit. Lightly spray your baking tray with cooking tray and set it aside. To prepare the glaze combine the ingredients in a small bowl and whisk them until they are well combined. Pour half of the mixture into a pan and reserve the rest.

3.Trim any excess skin off the wing edges and season it with pepper and salt. Add the wings to a baking tray and pour the sauce over the wings tossing them for the sauce to evenly coat. Arrange them in a single layer and bake them for 15 minutes.

4.While the wings are in the oven, bring your glaze to simmer in medium heat until there are visible bubbles.

5.Once the wings are cooled on one side rotate each piece and bake for an extra 10 minutes. Baste them and return them into the oven to allow for more cooking until they are golden brown. Garnish with onion slices, cilantro, chili flakes and sprinkle the remain salt. Serving with glaze of your choice.

**Nutrition:**

Calories: 256

Fat :16g

Carbohydrates 19g

Proteins: 20g

Potassium: 213mg

Sodium: 561mg

## 203.Coconut Shrimp

**Preparation Time:** 15 minutes

**Cooking Time:** 15 minutes

**Servings:** 6

**Ingredients:**

•Salt and pepper

•1-pound jumbo shrimp peeled and deveined

•½ cup all-purpose flour

For batter:

•½ cup beer

•1 tsp baking powder

•½ cup all-purpose flour

•1 egg

For coating:

•1 cup panko bread crumbs

•1 cup shredded coconut

**Directions:**
1.Line the baking tray with parchment paper.
2.In a shallow bowl add ½ cup flour for dredging and in another bowl whisk the batter ingredients. The batter should resemble a pancake consistency. If it is too thick add a little mineral or beer whisking in between. In another bowl mix together the shredded coconut and bread crumbs.
3.Dredge the shrimp in flour shaking off any excess before dipping in the batter and coat it with bread crumb mixture. Lightly press the coconut into the shrimp.
4.Place them into the baking sheet and repeat the process until you have several.
5.In a Dutch oven skillet heat vegetable oil until it is nice and hot fry the frozen shrimp batches for 3 minutes per side. Drain them on a paper towel lined plate.
6.Serve immediately with sweet chili sauce.

**Nutrition:**
Calories: 409
Fat 11g
Carbohydrates 46g
Proteins 30g
Sodium: 767mg
Potassium: 345mg

## 204.Spicy Korean Cauliflower Bites

**Preparation Time:** 15 minutes
**Cooking Time:** 30 minutes
**Servings:** 4
**Ingredients:**
•2 eggs
•1 lb. cauliflower
•2/3 cups of corn starch
•2 tsp smoked paprika
•1 tsp garlic grated
•1 tsp ginger grated
•1 lb. panko
•1 tsp sea salt
For the Korean barbecue sauce:
•1 cup ketchup
•½ cup Korea chili flakes
•½ cup minced garlic
•½ cup red pepper

**Directions:**
1.Cut the cauliflower into small sizes based on your taste and preference.
2.In a small bowl add cornstarch and eggs and mix them until they are smooth.
3.Add onions, garlic, ginger, smoked paprika and coat them with panko.
4.Apply some pressure so that the panko can stick and repeat this with all the cauliflower.

**Nutrition:**
Calories: 141
Fat: 12 g
Carbs: 23 g
Protein: 27 g

## 205. Grilled Salmon Burger

**Preparation Time:** 15 minutes
**Cooking Time:** 10 minutes
**Servings:** 4
**Ingredients:**
•16 ounces (450 g) pink salmon fillet, minced
•1 cup (250 g) prepared mashed potatoes
•1 shallot (about 40 g), chopped
•1 large egg (about 60 g), lightly beaten
•2 tablespoons (7 g) fresh coriander, chopped
•4 Hamburger buns (about 60 g each), split
•1 large tomato (about 150 g), sliced
•8 (15 g) Romaine lettuce leaves
•1/4 cup (60 g) mayonnaise
•Salt and freshly ground black pepper
•Cooking oil spray
**Directions:**

1.Combine the salmon, mashed potatoes, shallot, egg, and coriander in a mixing bowl. Season with salt and pepper.

2.Spoon about 2 tablespoons of mixture and form into patties.

3.Preheat your grill or griddle on high. Grease with cooking oil spray.

4.Grill the salmon patties for 4-5 minutes on each side or until cooked through. Transfer to a clean plate and cover to keep warm.

5.Spread some mayonnaise on the bottom half of buns. Top with lettuce, salmon patty, and tomato. Cover with bun tops.

6.Serve and enjoy.

**Nutrition:**

Calories: 395

Fat - 18.0 g

Carbohydrates - 38.8 g

Protein - 21.8 g

Sodium - 383 mg

## 206.Salmon Burger

**Preparation Time:** 15 minutes

**Cooking Time:** 15 minutes

**Servings:** 6

**Ingredients:**

•16 ounces (450 g) pink salmon, minced

•1 cup (250 g) prepared mashed potatoes

•1 medium (110 g) onion, chopped

•1 stalk celery (about 60 g), finely chopped

•1 large egg (about 60 g), lightly beaten

•2 tablespoons (7 g) fresh cilantro, chopped

•1 cup (100 g) breadcrumbs

•Vegetable oil, for deep frying

•Salt and freshly ground black pepper

**Directions:**

1.Combine the salmon, mashed potatoes, onion, celery, egg, and cilantro in a mixing bowl. Season to taste and mix thoroughly. Spoon about 2 Tablespoon mixture, roll in

114

breadcrumbs, and then form into small patties.

2.Heat oil in non-stick frying pan. Cook your salmon patties for 5 minutes on each side or until golden brown and crispy.

3.Serve in burger buns and with coleslaw on the side if desired.

4.Enjoy.

**Nutrition:**

Calories 230

Fat 7.9 g

Carbs 20.9 g

Protein 18.9 g

Sodium 298 mg

## 207.Salmon Sandwich with Avocado and Egg

**Preparation Time:** 15 minutes

**Cooking Time:** 10 minutes

**Servings:** 4

**Ingredients:**

•8 ounces (250 g) smoked salmon, thinly sliced

•1 medium (200 g) ripe avocado, thinly sliced

•4 large poached eggs (about 60 g each)

•4 slices whole wheat bread (about 30 g each)

•2 cups (60 g) arugula or baby rocket

•Salt and freshly ground black pepper

**Directions:**

1.Place 1 bread slice on a plate top with arugula, avocado, salmon, and poached egg. Season with salt and pepper. Repeat procedure for the remaining ingredients.

2.Serve and enjoy.

**Nutrition:**

Calories: 310

Fat: 18.2 g

Carbohydrates: 16.4 g

Protein: 21.3 g

Sodium: 383 mg

## 208. Onion and Cauliflower Dip

**Preparation Time**: 20 minutes
**Cooking Time:** 30 minutes
**Servings:** 24
**Ingredients:**
- 1 and ½ cups chicken stock
- 1 cauliflower head, florets separated
- ¼ cup mayonnaise
- ½ cup yellow onion, chopped
- ¾ cup cream cheese
- ½ teaspoon chili powder
- ½ teaspoon cumin, ground
- ½ teaspoon garlic powder
- Salt and black pepper to the taste

**Directions:**
1. Put the stock in a pot, add cauliflower and onion, heat up over medium heat, and cook for 30 minutes.
2. Add chili powder, salt, pepper, cumin, and garlic powder and stir.
3. Also, add cream cheese and stir a bit until it melts.
4. Blend using an immersion blender and mix with the mayo.
5. Transfer to a bowl and keep in the fridge for 2 hours before you serve it.
6. Enjoy!

**Nutrition:**
Calories: 40 kcal
Protein: 1.23 g
Fat: 3.31 g
Carbohydrates: 1.66 g
Sodium: 72 mg

## 209. Chicken Enchilada Bake

**Preparation Time**: 20 minutes
**Cooking Time:** 50 minutes
**Servings:** 5

**Ingredients:**
- 5 oz. Shredded chicken breast (boil and shred ahead) or 99 percent fat-free white chicken can be used in a pan.
- 1 can tomato paste
- 1 low sodium chicken broth can be fat-free
- 1/4 cup cheese with low fat mozzarella
- 1 tablespoon oil
- 1 tbsp. of salt
- Ground cumin, chili powder, garlic powder, oregano, and onion powder (all to taste)
- 1 to 2 zucchinis sliced longways (similar to lasagna noodles) into thin lines
- Sliced (optional) olives

**Directions:**
1. Add olive oil in sauce pan over medium/high heat, stir in tomato paste and seasonings, and heat in chicken broth for 2-3 min.
2. Stirring regularly to boil, turn heat to low for 15 min.
3. Set aside and cool to ambient temperature.
4. Pull-strip of zucchini through enchilada sauce and lay flat on the pan's bottom in a small baking pan.
5. Next, add the chicken a little less than 1/4 cup of enchilada sauce and mix it.
6. Attach chicken to the cover ends to end of the baking tray.
7. Sprinkle some bacon over the chicken.
8. Add another layer of the pulled zucchini via enchilada sauce (similar to lasagna making).
9. When needed, cover with the remaining cheese and olives on top. Bake for 35 to 40 minutes.
10. Keep an eye on them.
11. When the cheese starts getting golden, cover with foil.
12. Serve and enjoy!

**Nutrition:**
Calories: 312 Cal
Carbohydrates: 21.3 g
Protein: 27 g
Fat: 10.2 g

### 210.Marinated Eggs

**Preparation Time**: 2 hours and 10 minutes
**Cooking Time:** 7 minutes
**Servings:** 4
**Ingredients:**
•6 eggs
•1 and ¼ cups water
•¼ cup unsweetened rice vinegar
•2 tablespoons coconut aminos
•Salt and black pepper to the taste
•2 garlic cloves, minced
•1 teaspoon stevia 4 ounces cream cheese
•1 tablespoon chives, chopped
**Directions:**
1.Put the eggs in a pot, add water to cover, bring to a boil over medium heat, cover and cook for 7 minutes.
2.Rinse eggs with cold water and leave them aside to cool down.
3.In a bowl, mix one cup water with coconut aminos, vinegar, stevia, and garlic and whisk well.
4.Put the eggs in this mix, cover with a kitchen towel, and leave them aside for 2 hours, rotating from time to time.
5.Peel eggs, cut in halves, and put egg yolks in a bowl.
6.Add ¼ cup water, cream cheese, salt, pepper, and chives and stir well.
7.Stuff egg whites with this mix and serve them.
8.Enjoy!
**Nutrition:**
Calories: 289 kcal
Protein: 15.86 g



Fat: 22.62 g
Carbohydrates: 4.52 g
Sodium: 288 mg

### 211.Sausage and Cheese Dip

**Preparation Time**: 10 minutes
**Cooking Time:** 130 minutes
**Servings:** 28
**Ingredients:**
•8 ounces cream cheese
•A pinch of salt and black pepper
•16 ounces sour cream
•8 ounces pepper jack cheese, chopped
•15 ounces canned tomatoes mixed with habaneros
•1-pound Italian sausage, ground
•¼ cup green onions, chopped
**Directions:**
1.Heat up a pan over medium heat, add sausage, stir and cook until it browns.
2.Add tomatoes mix, stir and cook for 4 minutes more.
3.Add a pinch of salt, pepper, and the green onions, stir and cook for 4 minutes.
4.Spread pepper jack cheese on the bottom of your slow cooker.
5.Add cream cheese, sausage mix, and sour cream, cover and cook on High for 2 hours.
6.Uncover your slow cooker, stir dip, transfer to a bowl, and serve.
7.Enjoy!
**Nutrition:**
Calories: 132 kcal
Protein: 6.79 g
Fat: 9.58 g
Carbohydrates: 6.22 g
Sodium: 362 mg

## 212.Pumpkin Muffins

**Preparation Time**: 10 minutes
**Cooking Time:** 15 minutes
**Servings:** 18
**Ingredients:**
•¼ cup sunflower seed butter
•¾ cup pumpkin puree
•2 tablespoons flaxseed meal
•¼ cup coconut flour
•½ cup erythritol
•½ teaspoon nutmeg, ground
•1 teaspoon cinnamon, ground
•½ teaspoon baking soda
•1 egg ½ teaspoon baking powder
•A pinch of salt
**Directions:**
1.In a bowl, mix butter with pumpkin puree and egg and blend well.
2.Add flaxseed meal, coconut flour, erythritol, baking soda, baking powder, nutmeg, cinnamon, and a pinch of salt and stir well.
3.Spoon this into a greased muffin pan, introduce in the oven at 350 degrees F and bake for 15 minutes.
4.Leave muffins to cool down and serve them as a snack.
5.Enjoy!
**Nutrition:**
Calories: 65 kcal
Protein: 2.82 g
Fat: 5.42 g
Carbohydrates: 2.27 g
Sodium: 57 mg

## 213.Personal Pizza Biscuit

**Preparation Time**: 5 minutes
**Cooking Time:** 15 minutes
**Servings:** 1
**Ingredients:**
•1 sachet  select
•Buttermilk Cheddar Herb Biscuit.
•2 tbsp. cold water
•Cooking spray
•2 tbsp. no-sugar-added tomato sauce
•1/4 cup reduced-fat shredded cheese
**Directions:**
1.Preheat oven to 350°F.
2.Mix biscuit and water, and spread mixture into a small, circular crust shape onto a greased, foil-lined baking sheet.
3.Bake for 10 minutes.
4.Top with tomato sauce and cheese, and cook till cheese is melted about 5 minutes.
**Nutrition:**
Fats: 3.2 g
Cholesterol: 9.8 mg
Sodium: 10.5 mg
Protein: 3.6 g

## 214.Salmon Spinach and Cottage Cheese Sandwich

**Preparation Time:** 15 minutes
**Cooking Time:** 10 minutes
**Servings:** 4
**Ingredients:**
•4 ounces (125 g) cottage cheese
•1/4 cup (15 g) chives, chopped
•1 teaspoon (5 g) capers
•1/2 teaspoon (2.5 g) grated lemon rind
•4 (2 oz. or 60 g) smoked salmon
•2 cups (60 g) loose baby spinach
•1 medium (110 g) red onion, sliced thinly
•8 slices rye bread (about 30 g each)
•Kosher salt and freshly ground black pepper
**Directions:**
1.Preheat your griddle or Panini press.
2.Mix together cottage cheese, chives, capers, and lemon rind in a small bowl.

3.Spread and divide the cheese mixture on 4 bread slices. Top with spinach, onion slices, and smoked salmon.

4.Cover with remaining bread slices.

5.Grill the sandwiches until golden and grill marks form on both sides.

6.Transfer to a serving dish.

7.Serve and enjoy.

**Nutrition:**

Calories: 261

Fat 9.9 g

Carbohydrates 22.9 g

Protein 19.9 g

Sodium - 1226 mg

### 215.Pesto Crackers

**Preparation Time**: 10 minutes

**Cooking Time:** 17 minutes

**Servings:** 6

**Ingredients:**

•½ teaspoon baking powder

•Salt and black pepper to the taste

•1 and ¼ cups almond flour

•¼ teaspoon basil, dried 1 garlic clove, minced

•2 tablespoons basil pesto

•A pinch of cayenne pepper

•3 tablespoons ghee

**Directions:**

1.In a bowl, mix salt, pepper, baking powder, and almond flour.

2.Add garlic, cayenne, and basil and stir.

3.Add pesto and whisk.

4.Also, add ghee and mix your dough with your finger.

5.Spread this dough on a lined baking sheet, introduce in the oven at 325 degrees F and bake for 17 minutes.

6.Leave aside to cool down, cut your crackers, and serve them as a snack.

7.Enjoy!



**Nutrition:**

Calories: 9 kcal

Protein: 0.41 g

Fat: 0.14 g

Carbohydrates: 1.86 g

Sodium: 2 mg

### 216.Bacon Cheeseburger

**Preparation Time**: 10 minutes

**Cooking Time:** 30 minutes

**Servings:** 4

**Ingredients:**

•1 lb. lean ground beef

•1/4 cup chopped yellow onion

•1 clove garlic, minced

•1 tbsp. yellow mustard

•1 tbsp. Worcestershire sauce

•1/2 tsp. salt

•Cooking spray

•4 ultra-thin slices cheddar cheese, cut into 6 equal-sized rectangular pieces

•3 pieces of turkey bacon, each cut into 8 evenly-sized rectangular pieces

•24 dill pickle chips

•4-6 green leaf

•Lettuce leaves, torn into 24 small square-shaped pieces

•12 cherry tomatoes, sliced in half

**Directions:**

1.Pre-heat oven to 400°F.

2.Combine the garlic, salt, onion, Worcestershire sauce, and beef in a medium-sized bowl, and mix well.

3.Form mixture into 24 small meatballs.

4.Put meatballs onto a foil-lined baking sheet and cook for 12-15 minutes.

5.Leave oven on.

6.Top every meatball with a piece of cheese, then go back to the oven until cheese melts for about 2 to 3 minutes.

7.Let meatballs cool.

8.To assemble bites: on a toothpick layer a cheese-covered meatball, piece of bacon, piece of lettuce, pickle chip, and a tomato half.

**Nutrition:**
Fat: 14 g
Cholesterol: 41 mg
Carbohydrates: 30 g
Protein: 15 g

## 217.Chicken and Mushrooms

**Preparation Time**: 10 minutes
**Cooking Time:** 15 minutes
**Servings:** 6
**Ingredients:**
•2 chicken breasts
•1 cup of sliced white champignons
•1 cup of sliced green chilies
•1/2 cup scallions hacked
•1 teaspoon of chopped garlic
•1 cup of low-fat cheddar shredded cheese (1-1,5 lb. grams fat / ounce)
•1 tablespoon of olive oil
•1 tablespoon of butter
**Directions:**
1.Fry the chicken breasts with olive oil.
2.When needed, salt and pepper.
3.Grill breasts of chicken in a plate with grill.
4.For every serving, weigh 4 ounces of chicken. (Make two servings, save leftovers for another meal).
5.In a butter pan, stir in mushrooms, green peppers, scallions, and garlic until smooth, and a little dark.
6.Place the chicken in a baking platter.

7.Cover with mushroom combination.
8.Top on ham.
9.Place the cheese in a 350 oven until it melts.
**Nutrition:**
Carbohydrates: 2 g
Protein: 23 g
Fat: 11 g
Cholesterol: 112 mg
Sodium: 198 mg
Potassium: 261 mg

## 218.Cheeseburger Pie

**Preparation Time**: 20 minutes
**Cooking Time:** 90 minutes
**Servings:** 4
**Ingredients:**
•1 large spaghetti squash
•1 lb. lean ground beef
•1/4 cup diced onion
•2 eggs
•1/3 cup low-fat, plain Greek yogurt
•2 tbsp. tomato sauce
•1/2 tsp. Worcestershire sauce
•2/3 cup reduced-fat, shredded cheddar cheese
•2 oz. dill pickle slices
•Cooking spray
**Directions:**
1.Preheat oven to 400°F. Slice spaghetti squash in half lengthwise; dismiss pulp and seeds.
2.Spray insides with cooking spray.
3.Place squash halves cut-side- down onto a foil-lined baking sheet, and bake for 30 minutes.
4.Once cooked, let cool to before scraping squash flesh with a fork to remove spaghetti-like strands; set aside.

5.Push squash strands in the bottom and up sides of the greased pie pan, creating an even layer.

6.Meanwhile, set up pie filling.

7.In a lightly greased, medium-sized skillet, cook beef and onion over medium heat 8 to 10 minutes, sometimes stirring, until meat is brown.

8.Drain and remove from heat.

9.In a medium-sized bowl, whisk together eggs, tomato paste, Greek yogurt, and Worcestershire sauce. Stir in ground beef mixture.

10. Pour pie filling over squash crust.

11. Sprinkle meat filling with cheese, and then top with dill pickle slices.

12. Bake for 40 minutes.

**Nutrition:**

Calories: 409 Cal

Fat: 24.49 g

Carbohydrates: 15.06 g

Protein: 30.69 g

## 219.Salmon Feta and Pesto Wrap

**Preparation Time:** 15 minutes

**Cooking Time:** 10 minutes

**Servings:** 4

**Ingredients:**

•8 ounces (250 g) smoked salmon fillet, thinly sliced

•1 cup (150 g) feta cheese

•8 (15 g) Romaine lettuce leaves

•4 (6-inch) pita bread

•1/4 cup (60 g) basil pesto sauce

**Directions:**

1.Place 1 pita bread on a plate. Top with lettuce, salmon, feta cheese, and pesto sauce. Fold or roll to enclose filling. Repeat procedure for the remaining ingredients.

2.Serve and enjoy.



**Nutrition:**

Calories: 379

Fat 17.7 g

Carbohydrates: 36.6 g

Protein: 18.4 g

Sodium: 554 mg

## 220.Salmon Cream Cheese and Onion on Bagel

**Preparation Time:** 15 minutes

**Cooking Time:** 10 minutes

**Servings:** 4

**Ingredients:**

•8 ounces (250 g) smoked salmon fillet, thinly sliced

•1/2 cup (125 g) cream cheese

•1 medium (110 g) onion, thinly sliced

•4 bagels (about 80g each), split

•2 tablespoons (7 g) fresh parsley, chopped

•Freshly ground black pepper, to taste

**Directions:**

1.Spread the cream cheese on each bottom's half of bagels. Top with salmon and onion, season with pepper, sprinkle with parsley and then cover with bagel tops.

2.Serve and enjoy.

**Nutrition:**

Calories: 309

 Fat 14.1 g

Carbohydrates 32.0 g

Protein 14.7 g

Sodium 571 mg

## 221.Greek Baklava

**Preparation Time:** 20 minutes

**Cooking Time:** 20 minutes

**Servings:** 18

**Ingredients:**

•1 (16 oz.) package phyllo dough

•1 lb. chopped nuts

•1 cup butter

•1 teaspoon ground cinnamon
•1 cup water
•1 teaspoon. vanilla extract
•1/2 cup honey

**Directions:**

1.Preheat the oven to 175°C or 350°Fahrenheit. Spread butter on the sides and bottom of a 9-in by 13-in pan.

2.Chop the nuts then mix with cinnamon; set it aside. Unfurl the phyllo dough then halve the whole stack to fit the pan. Use a damp cloth to cover the phyllo to prevent drying as you proceed. Put two phyllo sheets in the pan then butter well. Repeat to make eight layered phyllo sheets. Scatter 2-3 tablespoons. nut mixture over the sheets then place two more phyllo sheets on top, butter then sprinkle with nuts. Layer as you go. The final layer should be six to eight phyllo sheets deep.

3.Make square or diamond shapes with a sharp knife up to the bottom of pan. You can slice into four long rows for diagonal shapes. Bake until crisp and golden for 50 minutes.

4.Meanwhile, boil water and melts to make the sauce; mix in honey and vanilla. Let it simmer for 20 minutes.

5.Take the baklava out of the oven then drizzle with sauce right away; cool. Serve the baklava in cupcake papers. You can also freeze them without cover. The baklava will turn soggy when wrapped.

**Nutrition:**

Calories: 393
Total Carbohydrate: 37.5 g
Cholesterol: 27 mg
Total Fat: 25.9 g
Protein: 6.1 g
Sodium: 196 mg

## 222.Glazed Bananas in Phyllo Nut Cups

**Preparation Time:** 30 minutes
**Cooking Time:** 45 minutes
**Servings:** 6 servings.

**Ingredients:**

•3/4 cup shelled pistachios
•1 teaspoon. ground cinnamon
•4 sheets phyllo dough, (14 inches x 9 inches)
•1/4 cup butter, melted
Sauce:
•3/4 cup butter, cubed
•3 medium firm bananas, sliced
•1/4 teaspoon. ground cinnamon
•3 to 4 cups vanilla ice cream

**Directions:**

1.Finely chop pistachios in a food processor; move to a bowl then mix in cinnamon. Slice each phyllo sheet to 6 four-inch squares, get rid of the trimmings. Pile the squares then use plastic wrap to cover.

2.Slather melted butter on each square one at a time then scatter a heaping tablespoonful of pistachio mixture. Pile 3 squares, flip each at an angle to misalign the corners. Force each stack on the sides and bottom of an oiled eight-oz. custard cup. Bake for 15-20 minutes in a 350 degrees F oven until golden; cool for 5 minutes. Move to a wire rack to completely cool.

3.Melt and boil butter in a saucepan to make the sauce; lower heat. Mix in cinnamon and bananas gently; heat completely. Put ice cream in the phyllo cups until full then put banana sauce on top. Serve right away.

**Nutrition:**

Calories: 735
Total Carbohydrate: 82 g
Cholesterol: 111 mg

Total Fat: 45 g
Fiber: 3 g
Protein: 7 g
Sodium: 468 mg

### 223.Salmon Apple Salad Sandwich

**Preparation Time:** 15 minutes
**Cooking Time:** 10 minutes
**Servings:** 4
**Ingredients:**

•4 ounces (125 g) canned pink salmon, drained and flaked
•1 medium (180 g) red apple, cored and diced
•1 celery stalk (about 60 g), chopped
•1 shallot (about 40 g), finely chopped
•1/3 cup (85 g) light mayonnaise
•8 slices whole grain bread (about 30 g each), toasted
•8 (15 g) Romaine lettuce leaves
•Salt and freshly ground black pepper

**Directions:**

1.Combine the salmon, apple, celery, shallot, and mayonnaise in a mixing bowl. Season with salt and pepper.
2.Place 1 slices bread on a plate, top with lettuce and salmon salad, and then covers with another slice of bread. Repeat procedure for the remaining ingredients.
3.Serve and enjoy.

**Nutrition:**

Calories: 315
Fat - 11.3 g
Carbohydrates - 40.4 g
Protein - 15.1 g
Sodium - 469 mg

### 224.Smoked Salmon and Cheese on Rye Bread

**Preparation Time:** 15 minutes
**Cooking Time:** 10 minutes
**Servings:** 4

**Ingredients:**

•8 ounces (250 g) smoked salmon, thinly sliced
•1/3 cup (85 g) mayonnaise
•2 tablespoons (30 ml) lemon juice
•1 tablespoon (15 g) Dijon mustard
•1 teaspoon (3 g) garlic, minced
•4 slices cheddar cheese (about 2 oz. or 30 g each)
•8 slices rye bread (about 2 oz. or 30 g each)
•8 (15 g) Romaine lettuce leaves
•Salt and freshly ground black pepper

**Directions:**

1.Mix together the mayonnaise, lemon juice, mustard, and garlic in a small bowl. Flavor with salt and pepper and set aside.
2.Spread dressing on 4 bread slices. Top with lettuce, salmon, and cheese. Cover with remaining rye bread slices.
3.Serve and enjoy.

**Nutrition:**

Calories: 365
Fat: 16.6 g
Carbohydrates: 31.6 g
Protein: 18.8 g
Sodium: 951 mg

### 225.Pan-Fried Trout

**Preparation Time:** 15 minutes
**Cooking Time:** 10 minutes
**Servings:** 4
**Ingredients:**

•1 ¼ pounds trout fillets
•1/3 cup white, or yellow, cornmeal
•¼ teaspoon anise seeds
•¼ teaspoon black pepper
•½ cup minced cilantro, or parsley
•Vegetable cooking spray
•Lemon wedges

**Directions:**

1.Coat fish with combined cornmeal, spices, and cilantro, pressing it gently into fish. Spray large skillet with cooking spray; heat over medium heat until hot.

2.Add fish and cook until fish is tender and flakes with fork, about 5 minutes on each side. Serve with lemon wedges.

**Nutrition:**

Calories: 207

Total Carbohydrate: 19 g

Cholesterol: 27 mg

Total Fat: 16 g

Fiber: 4 g

Protein: 18g

# Drinks

### 226.Avocado Blueberry Smoothie

**Preparation Time**: 5 minutes
**Cooking Time:** 5 minutes
**Servings:** 1
**Ingredients:**

- 1 tsp chia seeds
- ½ cup unsweetened coconut milk
- 1 avocado
- ½ cup blueberries

**Directions:**

1.Add all the listed ingredients to the blender and blend until smooth and creamy.
2.Serve immediately and enjoy.

**Nutrition:**

Calories: 389
Fat: 34.6g
Carbs: 20.7g
Protein: 4.8g
Fiber: 0g

### 227.Vegan Blueberry Smoothie

**Preparation Time**: 5 minutes
**Cooking Time:** 5 minutes
**Servings:** 2
**Ingredients:**

- 2 cups blueberries
- 1 tbsp hemp seeds
- 1 tbsp chia seeds
- 1 tbsp flax meal
- 1/8 tsp orange zest, grated
- 1 cup fresh orange juice
- 1 cup unsweetened coconut milk

**Directions:**

1.Toss all your ingredients into your blender then process till smooth and creamy.
2.Serve immediately and enjoy.

**Nutrition:** Calories: 212 Fat: 6.6g Carbs: 36.9g Protein: 5.2g Fiber: 0g

### 228.Berry Peach Smoothie

**Preparation Time**: 5 minutes
**Cooking Time:** 5 minutes
**Servings:** 2
**Ingredients:**

- 1 cup coconut water
- 1 tbsp hemp seeds
- 1 tbsp agave
- ½ cup strawberries
- ½ cup blueberries
- ½ cup cherries
- ½ cup peaches

**Directions:**

1.Toss all your ingredients into your blender then process till smooth and creamy.
2.Serve immediately and enjoy.

**Nutrition:** Calories: 117 Fat: 2.5g Carbs: 22.5g Protein: 3.5g Fiber: 0g

### 229.Cantaloupe Blackberry Smoothie

**Preparation Time**: 5 minutes
**Cooking Time:** 5 minutes
**Servings:** 2
**Ingredients:**

- 1 cup coconut milk yogurt
- ½ cup blackberries
- 2 cups fresh cantaloupe
- 1 banana

**Directions:**

1.Toss all your ingredients into your blender then process till smooth.
2.Serve and enjoy.

**Nutrition:** Calories: 160 Fat: 4.5g Carbs: 33.7g Protein: 1.8g Fiber: 0g

### 230.Cantaloupe Kale Smoothie

**Preparation Time**: 5 minutes

**Cooking Time:** 5 minutes
**Servings:** 2
**Ingredients:**
•8 oz. water
•1 orange, peeled
•3 cups kale, chopped
•1 banana, peeled
•2 cups cantaloupe, chopped
•1 zucchini, chopped
**Directions:**
1.Toss all your ingredients into your blender then process till smooth and creamy.
2.Serve immediately and enjoy.
**Nutrition:** Calories: 203 Fat: 0.5g Carbs: 49.2g Protein: 5.6g Fiber: 0g

### 231.Mix Berry Cantaloupe Smoothie

**Preparation Time**: 5 minutes
**Cooking Time:** 5 minutes
**Servings:** 2
**Ingredients:**
•1 cup alkaline water
•2 fresh Seville orange juices
•¼ cup fresh mint leaves
•1 ½ cups mixed berries
•2 cups cantaloupe
Directions
1.Toss all your ingredients into your blender then process till smooth.
2.Serve immediately and enjoy.
**Nutrition:** Calories: 122 Fat: 1g Carbs: 26.1g Protein: 2.4g Fiber: 0g

### 232.Avocado Kale Smoothie

**Preparation Time**: 5 minutes
**Cooking Time:** 5 minutes
**Servings:** 3
**Ingredients:**
•1 cup water
•½ Seville orange, peeled
•1 avocado
•1 cucumber, peeled
•1 cup kale
•1 cup ice cubes
**Directions:**
1.Toss all your ingredients into your blender then process till smooth and creamy.
2.Serve immediately and enjoy.
**Nutrition:** Calories: 160 Fat: 13.3g Carbs: 11.6g Protein: 2.4g Fiber: 0g

### 233.Apple Kale Cucumber Smoothie

**Preparation Time**: 5 minutes
**Cooking Time:** 5 minutes
**Servings:** 1
**Ingredients:**
•¾ cup water
•½ green apple, diced
•¾ cup kale
•½ cucumber
**Directions:**
1.Toss all your ingredients into your blender then process till smooth and creamy.
2.Serve immediately and enjoy.
**Nutrition:** Calories: 86 Fat: 0.5g Carbs: 21.7g Protein: 1.9g Fiber: 0g

### 234.Refreshing Cucumber Smoothie

**Preparation Time**: 5 minutes
**Cooking Time:** 5 minutes
**Servings:** 2
**Ingredients:**
•1 cup ice cubes
•20 drops liquid stevia
•2 fresh lime, peeled and halved
•1 tsp lime zest, grated
•1 cucumber, chopped

•1 avocado, pitted and peeled
•2 cups kale
•1 tbsp creamed coconut
•¾ cup coconut water
**Directions:**
1.Toss all your ingredients into your blender then process till smooth and creamy.
2.Serve immediately and enjoy.
**Nutrition:** Calories: 313 Fat: 25.1g Carbs: 24.7g Protein: 4.9g Fiber: 0g

### 235.Cauliflower Veggie Smoothie
**Preparation Time**: 5 minutes
**Cooking Time:** 5 minutes
**Servings:** 4
**Ingredients:**
•1 zucchini, peeled and chopped
•1 Seville orange, peeled
•1 apple, diced
•1 banana
•1 cup kale
•½ cup cauliflower
**Directions:**
1.Toss all your ingredients into your blender then process till smooth and creamy.
2.Serve immediately and enjoy.
**Nutrition:** Calories: 71 Fat: 0.3g Carbs: 18.3g Protein: 1.3g Fiber: 0g

### 236.Soursop Smoothie
**Preparation Time**: 5 minutes
**Cooking Time:** 5 Minutes
**Servings:** 2
**Ingredients:**
•3 quartered frozen Burro Bananas
•1-1/2 cups of Homemade Coconut Milk
•1/4 cup of Walnuts
•1 teaspoon of Sea Moss Gel
•1 teaspoon of Ground Ginger
•1 teaspoon of Soursop Leaf Powder
•1 handful of Kale



**Directions:**
1.Prepare and put all ingredients in a blender or a food processor.
2.Blend it well until you reach a smooth consistency.
3.Serve and enjoy your Soursop Smoothie!
4.Useful Tips:
5.If you don't have frozen Bananas, you can use fresh ones.
**Nutrition:** Calories: 213 Fat: 3.1g  Carbs: 6g Protein: 8g Fiber: 4.3g

### 237.Cucumber-Ginger Water
**Preparation Time**: 5 minutes
**Cooking Time:** 5 Minutes
**Servings:** 2
**Ingredients:**
•1 sliced Cucumber
•1 smashed thumb of Ginger Root
•2 cups of Spring Water
**Directions:**
1.Prepare and put all ingredients in a jar with a lid.
2.Let the water infuse overnight. Store it in the refrigerator.
3.Serve and enjoy your Cucumber-Ginger Water throughout the day!
**Nutrition:** Calories: 117 Fat: 2g Carbs: 6g Protein: 9.7g Fiber: 2g

### 238.Strawberry Milkshake
**Preparation Time**: 5 minutes
**Cooking Time:** 5 Minutes
**Servings:** 2
**Ingredients:**
•2 cups of Homemade Hempseed Milk
•1 cup of frozen Strawberries
•Agave Syrup, to taste
**Directions:**
1.Prepare and put all ingredients in a blender or a food processor.

2.Blend it well until you reach a smooth consistency.

3.Serve and enjoy your Strawberry Milkshake!

4.Useful Tips

5.If you don't have Homemade Hempseed Milk, you can add Homemade Walnut Milk instead.

6.If you don't have frozen Strawberries, you can use fresh ones.

**Nutrition:** Calories: 222 Fat: 4g Carbs: 3g Protein: 6g Fiber: 1g

### 239.Cactus Smoothie

**Preparation Time**: 5 minutes

**Cooking Time:** 10 Minutes

**Servings:** 2

**Ingredients:**

•1 medium Cactus

•2 cups of Homemade Coconut Milk

•2 frozen Baby Bananas

•1/2 cup of Walnuts

•1 Date

•2 teaspoons of Hemp Seeds

**Directions:**

1.Take the Cactus, remove all pricks, wash it, and cut into medium pieces.

2.Put all the listed ingredients in a blender or a food processor.

3.Blend it well until you reach a smooth consistency.

4.Serve and enjoy your Cactus Smoothie!

5.Useful Tips

6.If you don't have Homemade Coconut Milk, you can add Homemade Walnut Milk or Homemade Hempseed Milk instead.

7.If you don't have frozen Bananas, you can use fresh ones.

8.If you don't have Baby Bananas, add 1 Burro Banana instead.

**Nutrition:** Calories: 123 Fat: 3g Carbs: 6g Protein: 2.5g Fiber: 0g

### 240.Prickly Pear Juice

**Preparation Time**: 5 minutes

**Cooking Time:** 10 Minutes

**Servings:** 2

**Ingredients:**

•6 Prickly Pears

•1/3 cup of Lime Juice

•1/3 cup of Agave

•1-1/2 cups of Spring Water*

**Directions:**

1.Take Prickly Pear, cut off the ends, slice off the skin, and put in a blender. Do the same with the other pears.

2.Add Lime Juice with Agave to the blender and blend well for 30–40 seconds.

3.Strain the prepared mixture through a nut milk bag or cheesecloth and pour it back into the blender.

4.Pour Spring Water in and blend it repeatedly.

5.Serve and enjoy your Prickly Pear Juice!

6.Useful Tips:

7.If you want a cold drink, add a tray of ice cubes instead.

8.like and serve it on top of the braised greens.

**Nutrition:** Calories: 312 Fat: 6g Carbs: 11g Protein: 8g Fiber: 2g

# Vegetable Recipes

### 241.Baby Corn in Chili-Turmeric Spice

**Preparation Time:** 5 minutes

 **Cooking Time:**  8 minutes

**Servings:** 5

**Ingredients:**

- ¼ cup water
- ¼ teaspoon baking soda
- ¼ teaspoon salt
- ¼ teaspoon turmeric powder
- ½ teaspoon curry powder
- ½ teaspoon red chili powder
- 1 cup chickpea flour or besan
- 10 pieces' baby corn, blanched

**Directions:**

1.Preheat the air fryer to 4000F.

2.Line the air fryer basket with aluminum foil and brush with oil.

3.In a mixing bowl, mix all ingredients except for the corn.

4.Whisk until well combined.

5.Dip the corn in the batter and place inside the air fryer. Cook for 8 minutes until golden brown.

**Nutrition:**

Calories: 89

Carbohydrates: 14.35g

Protein: 4.75g

Fat: 1.54g

### 242.Creamy Cauliflower and Broccoli

**Preparation Time:** 4 minutes

**Cooking Time:** 16 minutes

**Servings:** 6

**Ingredients:**

- 1-pound cauliflower florets
- 1-pound broccoli florets
- 2 ½ tablespoons sesame oil
- 1/2 teaspoon smoked cayenne pepper
- 3/4 teaspoon sea salt flakes
- 1 tablespoon lemon zest, grated
- 1/2 cup Colby cheese, shredded

**Directions:**

1.Prepare the cauliflower and broccoli using your favorite steaming method. Then, drain them well; add the sesame oil, cayenne pepper, and salt flakes.

2.Air-fry at 390 degrees F for approximately 16 minutes; make sure to check the vegetables halfway through the cooking time.

3.Afterwards, stir in the lemon zest and Colby cheese; toss to coat well and serve immediately!

**Nutrition:**

Calories: 133

Fat: 9.0g

Carbs: 9.5g

Protein:  5.9g

Sugars: 3.2g

Fiber: 3.6g

### 243.Buttered Carrot-Zucchini with Mayo

**Preparation Time:** 15 minutes

**Cooking Time:**  25 minutes

**Servings:** 4

**Ingredients:**

- 1 tablespoon grated onion
- 2 tablespoons butter, melted
- 1/2-pound carrots, sliced
- 1-1/2 zucchinis, sliced
- 1/4 cup water
- 1/4 cup mayonnaise
- 1/4 teaspoon prepared horseradish
- 1/4 teaspoon salt
- 1/4 teaspoon ground black pepper

•1/4 cup Italian bread crumbs

**Directions:**

1.Lighten skillet with cooking spray. Add the carrots. Cook for 360 minutes at 360oF. Add the zucchini and continue cooking for another 5 minutes.

2.Meanwhile, in a bowl, whisk together the pepper, salt, horseradish, onion, mayonnaise, and water. Pour into a vegetable skillet. Pull well over the coat.

3.In a small bowl, combine the melted butter and breadcrumbs. Sprinkle over the vegetables.

4.Cook for 10 minutes at 390oF until tops are lightly browned.

5.Serve and enjoy.

**Nutrition:**

Calories: 223

Carbs: 13.8g

Protein: 2.7g

Fat: 17.4g

## 244.Baked Portobello, Pasta 'n Cheese

**Preparation Time:** 10 minutes

**Cooking Time:** 30 minutes

**Servings:** 4

**Ingredients:**

•1 cup milk

•1 cup shredded mozzarella cheese

•1 large clove garlic, minced

•1 tablespoon vegetable oil

•1/4 cup margarine

•1/4 teaspoon dried basil

•1/4-pound Portobello mushrooms, thinly sliced

•2 tablespoons all-purpose flour

•2 tablespoons soy sauce

•4-ounce penne pasta, cooked according to manufacturer's Directions for Cooking

•5-ounce frozen chopped spinach, thawed

**Directions:**

1.Lightly grease baking pan of air fryer with oil. For 2 minutes, heat on 360oF. Add mushrooms and cook for a minute. Transfer to a plate.

2.In same pan, melt margarine for a minute. Stir in basil, garlic, and flour. Cook for 3 minutes. Stir and cook for another 2 minutes. Stir in half of milk slowly while whisking continuously. Cook for another 2 minutes. Mix well. Cook for another 2 minutes. Stir in remaining milk and cook for another 3 minutes.

3.Add cheese and mix well.

4.Stir in soy sauce, spinach, mushrooms, and pasta. Mix well. Top with remaining cheese.

5.Cook for 15 minutes at 390oF until tops are lightly browned.

6.Serve and enjoy.

**Nutrition:**

Calories: 482

Carbs: 32.1g

Protein: 16.0g

Fat: 32.1g

## 245.Simple Green Beans with Butter

**Preparation Time:** 2 minutes

**Cooking Time:** 10 minutes

**Servings:** 4

**Ingredients:**

•3/4 pound green beans, cleaned

•1 tablespoon balsamic vinegar

•1/4 teaspoon kosher salt

•1/2 teaspoon mixed peppercorns, freshly cracked

•1 tablespoon butter

•2 tablespoons toasted sesame seeds, to serve

**Directions:**
1.Set your Air Fryer to cook at 390 degrees F.
2.Mix the green beans with all of the above ingredients, apart from the sesame seeds. Set the timer for 10 minutes.
3.Meanwhile, toast the sesame seeds in a small-sized nonstick skillet; make sure to stir continuously.
4.Serve sautéed green beans on a nice serving platter sprinkled with toasted sesame seeds. Bon appétit!
**Nutrition:**
Calories: 73
Fat: 3.0g
Carbs: 6.1g
Protein: 1.6g
Sugars: 1.2g
Fiber: 2.1g

## 246.Brown Rice, Spinach 'n Tofu Frittata

**Preparation Time:** 20 minutes
**Cooking Time:** 55 minutes
**Servings:** 4
**Ingredients:**
•½ cup baby spinach, chopped
•½ cup kale, chopped
•½ onion, chopped
•½ teaspoon turmeric
•1 ¾ cups brown rice, cooked
•1 flax egg (1 tablespoon flaxseed meal + 3 tablespoon cold water)
•1 package firm tofu
•1 tablespoon olive oil
•1 yellow pepper, chopped
•2 tablespoons soy sauce
•2 teaspoons arrowroot powder
•2 teaspoons Dijon mustard
•2/3 cup almond milk
•3 big mushrooms, chopped

•3 tablespoons nutritional yeast
•4 cloves garlic, crushed
•4 spring onions, chopped
•a handful of basil leaves, chopped
**Directions:**
1.Preheat the air fryer to 3750F. Grease a pan that will fit inside the air fryer.
2.Prepare the frittata crust by mixing the brown rice and flax egg. Press the rice onto the baking dish until you form a crust. Brush with a little oil and cook for 10 minutes.
3.Meanwhile, heat olive oil in a skillet over medium flame and sauté the garlic and onions for 2 minutes.
4.Add the pepper and mushroom and continue stirring for 3 minutes.
5.Stir in the kale, spinach, spring onions, and basil. Remove from the pan and set aside.
6.In a food processor, pulse together the tofu, mustard, turmeric, soy sauce, nutritional yeast, vegan milk and arrowroot powder. Pour in a mixing bowl and stir in the sautéed vegetables.
7.Pour the vegan frittata mixture over the rice crust and cook in the air fryer for 40 minutes.
**Nutrition:**
Calories: 226
Carbohydrates: 30.44g
Protein: 10.69g
Fat: 8.05g

## 247.Baked Zucchini Recipe from Mexico

**Preparation Time:** 10 minutes
**Cooking Time:** 30 minutes
**Servings:** 4
**Ingredients:**
•1 tablespoon olive oil
•1-1/2 pounds' zucchini, cubed
•1/2 cup chopped onion

•1/2 teaspoon garlic salt
•1/2 teaspoon paprika
•1/2 teaspoon dried oregano
•1/2 teaspoon cayenne pepper, or to taste
•1/2 cup cooked long-grain rice
•1/2 cup cooked pinto beans
•1-1/4 cups salsa
•3/4 cup shredded Cheddar cheese
**Directions:**
1.Lightly grease baking pan of air fryer with olive oil. Add onions and zucchini and for 10 minutes, cook on 360oF. Halfway through cooking time, stir.
2.Season with cayenne, oregano, paprika, and garlic salt. Mix well.
3.Stir in salsa, beans, and rice. Cook for 5 minutes.
4.Stir in cheddar cheese and mix well.
5.Cover pan with foil.
6.Cook for 15 minutes at 390oF until bubbly.
7.Serve and enjoy.
**Nutrition:**
Calories: 263
Carbs: 24.6g
Protein: 12.5g
Fat: 12.7g

### 248.Banana Pepper Stuffed with Tofu 'n Spices

**Preparation Time:** 5 minutes
**Cooking Time:** 10 minutes
**Servings:** 8
**Ingredients:**
•½ teaspoon red chili powder
•½ teaspoon turmeric powder
•1 onion, finely chopped
•1 package firm tofu, crumbled
•1 teaspoon coriander powder
•3 tablespoons coconut oil
•8 banana peppers, top end sliced and seeded
•Salt to taste
**Directions:**
1.Preheat the air fryer for 5 minutes.
2.In a mixing bowl, combine the tofu, onion, coconut oil, turmeric powder, red chili powder, coriander power, and salt. Mix until well-combined.
3.Scoop the tofu mixture into the hollows of the banana peppers.
4.Place the stuffed peppers in the air fryer.
5.Close and cook for 10 minutes at 3250F.
**Nutrition:**
Calories: 72
Carbohydrates: 4.1g
Protein: 1.2g
Fat: 5.6

### 249.Baked Potato Topped with Cream cheese 'n Olives

**Preparation Time:** 15 minutes
**Cooking Time:** 40 minutes
**Servings:** 1
**Ingredients:**
•¼ teaspoon onion powder
•1 medium russet potato, scrubbed and peeled
•1 tablespoon chives, chopped
•1 tablespoon Kalamata olives
•1 teaspoon olive oil
•1/8 teaspoon salt
•a dollop of vegan butter
•a dollop of vegan cream cheese
**Directions:**
1.Place inside the air fryer basket and cook for 40 minutes. Be sure to turn the potatoes once halfway.

2.Place the potatoes in a mixing bowl and pour in olive oil, onion powder, salt, and vegan butter.

3.Preheat the air fryer to 4000F.

4.Serve the potatoes with vegan cream cheese, Kalamata olives, chives, and other vegan toppings that you want.

**Nutrition:**

Calories: 504

Carbohydrates: 68.34g

Protein: 9.31g

Fat: 21.53g

### 250.Brussels Sprouts with Balsamic Oil

**Preparation Time:** 5 minutes

**Cooking Time:** 15 minutes

**Servings:** 4

**Ingredients:**

•¼ teaspoon salt

•1 tablespoon balsamic vinegar

•2 cups Brussels sprouts, halved

•2 tablespoons olive oil

**Directions:**

1.Preheat the air fryer for 5 minutes.

2.Mix all ingredients in a bowl until the zucchini fries are well coated.

3.Place in the air fryer basket.

4.Close and cook for 15 minutes for 3500F.

**Nutrition:**

Calories: 82

Carbohydrates: 4.6g

Protein: 1.5g

Fat: 6.8g

### 251.Bell Pepper-Corn Wrapped in Tortilla

**Preparation Time:** 5 minutes

**Cooking Time:** 15 minutes

**Servings:** 4

**Ingredients:**

•1 small red bell pepper, chopped

•1 small yellow onion, diced

•1 tablespoon water

•2 cobs grilled corn kernels

•4 large tortillas

•4 pieces' commercial vegan nuggets, chopped

•mixed greens for garnish

**Directions:**

1.Preheat the air fryer to 4000F.

2.In a skillet heated over medium heat, water sauté the vegan nuggets together with the onions, bell peppers, and corn kernels. Set aside.

3.Place filling inside the corn tortillas.

4.Fold the tortillas and place inside the air fryer and cook for 15 minutes until the tortilla wraps are crispy.

5.Serve with mix greens on top.

6.**Nutrition:**

Calories: 548

Carbohydrates: 43.54g

Protein: 46.73g

Fat: 20.76g

### 252.Black Bean Burger with Garlic-Chipotle

**Preparation Time:** 10 minutes

**Cooking Time:** 20 minutes

**Servings:** 3

**Ingredients:**

•½ cup corn kernels

•½ teaspoon chipotle powder

•½ teaspoon garlic powder

•¾ cup salsa

•1 ¼ teaspoon chili powder

•1 ½ cup rolled oats

•1 can black beans, rinsed and drained

•1 tablespoon soy sauce

**Directions:**

1.In a mixing bowl, combine all Ingredients and mix using your hands.
2.Form small patties using your hands and set aside.
3.Brush patties with oil if desired.
4.Place the grill pan in the air fryer and place the patties on the grill pan accessory.
5.Close the lid and cook for 20 minutes on each side at 3300F.
**Nutrition:**
Calories: 395
Carbs: 52.2g
Protein: 24.3g
Fat: 5.8g

# Vegan Recipes

### 253. Vegan Edamame Quinoa Collard Wraps

**Preparation Time**: 5 minutes
**Cooking Time:** 15 minutes
**Servings:** 4
**Ingredients:**
For the wrap:
•Collard leaves; 2 to 3
•Grated carrot; 1/4 cup
•Sliced cucumber; 1/4 cup
•Red bell pepper; 1/4; thin strips
•Orange bell pepper; 1/4; thin strips
•Cooked quinoa; 1/3 cup
•Shelled defrosted edamame; 1/3 cup
For the dressing:
•Fresh ginger root; 3 tablespoons; peeled and chopped
•Cooked chickpeas; 1 cup
•Clove of garlic; 1
•Rice vinegar; 4 tablespoons
•Low sodium tamari/coconut aminos; 2 tablespoons
•Lime juice; 2 tablespoons
•Water; 1/4 cup
•Few pinches of chili flakes
•Stevia; 1 pack
**Directions:**
1.For the dressing, combine all the ingredients and purée in a food processor until smooth.
2.Load into a little jar or tub, and set aside.
3.Place the collar leaves on a flat surface, covering one another to create a tighter tie.
4.Take one tablespoon of ginger dressing and blend it up with the prepared quinoa.
5.Spoon the prepared quinoa onto the leaves and shape a simple horizontal line at the closest end.

6.Supplement the edamame with all the veggie fillings left over.
7.Drizzle around one tablespoon of the ginger dressing on top, then fold the cover's sides inwards.
8.Pullover the fillings, the side of the cover closest to you, then turn the whole body away to seal it up.
**Nutrition:**
Calories: 295 Cal
Sugar: 3 g
Sodium: 200 mg
Fat: 13 g

### 254. Baked Eggplant with Marinara

**Preparation Time:** 20 minutes
**Cooking Time:**  45 minutes
**Servings:** 3
**Ingredients:**
•1 clove garlic, sliced
•1 large eggplants
•1 tablespoon olive oil
•1 tablespoon olive oil
•1/2 pinch salt, or as needed
•1/4 cup and 2 tablespoons dry bread crumbs
•1/4 cup and 2 tablespoons ricotta cheese
•1/4 cup grated Parmesan cheese
•1/4 cup grated Parmesan cheese
•1/4 cup water, plus more as needed
•1/4 teaspoon red pepper flakes
•1-1/2 cups prepared marinara sauce
•1-1/2 teaspoons olive oil
•2 tablespoons shredded pepper jack cheese
•salt and freshly ground black pepper to taste
**Directions:**
1.Cut the eggplant crosswise into 5 pieces. Peel a pumpkin, grate it and cut it into two cubes.

2.Lightly turn skillet with 1 Tbsp. olive oil.
Heat the oil at 390 ° F for 5 minutes. Add half
of the aubergines and cook 2 minutes on each
side. Transfer to a plate.

3.Add 1 tablespoon of olive oil and add garlic.
Cook for one minute. Add the chopped
aubergines. Season with pepper flakes and
salt. Cook for 4 minutes. Lower the heat to
330oF and continue cooking the eggplants
until soft, about 8 more minutes.

4.Stir in water and marinara sauce. Cook for 7
minutes until heated through. Stirring every
now and then. Transfer to a bowl.

5.In a bowl, whisk well pepper, salt, pepper
jack cheese, Parmesan cheese, and ricotta.
Evenly spread cheeses over eggplant strips
and then fold in half.

6.Lay folded eggplant in baking pan. Pour
marinara sauce on top.

7.In a small bowl whisk well olive oil, and
bread crumbs. Sprinkle all over sauce.

8.Cook for 15 minutes at 390oF until tops are
lightly browned.

9.Serve and enjoy.

**Nutrition:**
Calories: 405
Carbs: 41.1g
Protein: 12.7g
Fat: 21.4g

### 255.Crispy-Topped Baked Vegetables

**Preparation Time**: 10 minutes
**Cooking Time**: 40 minutes
**Servings**: 4
**Ingredients:**
•2 tbsp. olive oil
•1 onion, chopped
•1 celery stalk, chopped
•2 carrots, grated
•1/2-pound turnips, sliced
•1 cup vegetable broth
•1 tsp. turmeric
•Sea salt and black pepper, to taste
•1/2 tsp. liquid smoke
•1 cup Parmesan cheese, shredded
•2 tbsp fresh chives, chopped

**Directions:**
1.Set oven to 360ºF and grease a baking dish
with olive oil.

2.Set a skillet over medium heat and warm
olive oil.

3.Sweat the onion until soft, and place in the
turnips, carrots, and celery; and cook for 4
minutes.

4.Remove the vegetable mixture to the
baking dish.

5.Combine vegetable broth with turmeric,
pepper, liquid smoke, and salt.

6.Spread this mixture over the vegetables.

7.Sprinkle with Parmesan cheese and bake for
about 30 minutes.

8.Garnish with chives to serve.

**Nutrition:**
Calories: 242 Cal
Fats: 16.3 g
Carbohydrates: 8.6 g
Protein: 16.3 g

### 256.Creamy Spinach and Mushroom Lasagna

**Preparation Time**: 60 minutes
**Cooking Time**: 20 minutes
**Servings**: 6
**Ingredients:**
•10 lasagna noodles
•1 package whole milk ricotta
•2 packages of frozen chopped spinach.

•4 cups mozzarella cheese (divided and shredded)
•3/4 cup grated fresh Parmesan
•3 tablespoons chopped fresh parsley leaves (optional)
For the Sauce:
•1/4 cup of butter (unsalted)
•2 cloves garlic
•1 pound of thinly sliced cremini mushroom
•1 diced onion
•1/4 cup flour
•4 cups milk, kept at room temperature
•1 teaspoon basil (dried)
•Pinch of nutmeg
•Salt and freshly ground black pepper, to taste

**Directions:**
1.Preheat oven to 352 degrees F.
2.To make the sauce, over a medium heat, melt your butter. Add garlic, mushrooms, and onion. Cook and stir at intervals until it becomes tender at about 3-4 minutes.
3.Whisk in flour until lightly browned, it takes about 1 minute for it to become brown.
4.Next, whisk in the milk gradually, and cook, constantly whisking, about 2-3 minutes till it becomes thickened. Stir in basil, oregano, and nutmeg, season with salt and pepper for taste.
5.Then set aside.
6.In another pot of boiling salted water, cook lasagna noodles according to the package instructions.
7.Spread one cup mushroom sauce onto the bottom of a baking dish; top it with four lasagna noodles, 1/2 of the spinach, one cup mozzarella cheese, and 1/4 cup Parmesan.
8.Repeat this process with remaining noodles, mushroom sauce, and cheeses.

9.Place into oven and bake for 35-45 minutes, or until it starts bubbling. Then boil for 2-3 minutes until it becomes brown and translucent.
10.          Let cool for 15 minutes.
11.          Serve it with garnished parsley (optional)

**Nutrition:**
Calories: 488.3 Cal
Fats: 19.3 g
Cholesterol: 88.4 mg
Sodium: 451.9 mg
Carbohydrates: 51.0 g
Dietary Fiber: 7.0 g
Protein: 25.0 g

### 257.Zucchini Parmesan Chips

**Difficulty:** Hard
**Preparation Time:** 5 minutes
**Cooking Time:** 8 minutes
**Servings:** 10
**Ingredients:**
•½ tsp. paprika
•½ C. grated parmesan cheese
•½ C. Italian breadcrumbs
•1 lightly beaten egg
•thinly sliced zucchinis

**Directions:**
1Use a very sharp knife or mandolin slicer to slice zucchini as thinly as you can. Pat off extra moisture.
2Beat egg with a pinch of pepper and salt and a bit of water.
3Combine paprika, cheese, and breadcrumbs in a bowl.
4Dip slices of zucchini into the egg mixture and then into breadcrumb mixture. Press gently to coat.

5With olive oil cooking spray, mist coated zucchini slices. Place into your air fryer in a single layer.

6Cook 8 minutes at 350 degrees.

7Sprinkle with salt and serve with salsa.

**Nutrition:**

Calories: 211

Fat: 16g

Protein: 8g

Sugar: 0g

### 258.Roasted Squash Puree

**Preparation Time**: 20 minutes

**Cooking Time:** 6 to 7 hours

**Servings:** 8

**Ingredients:**

•1 (3-pound) butternut squash, peeled, seeded, and cut into 1-inch pieces

•3 (1-pound) acorn squash, peeled, seeded, and cut into 1-inch pieces

•2 onions, chopped

•3 garlic cloves, minced

•2 tablespoons olive oil

•1 teaspoon dried marjoram leaves

•1/2 teaspoon salt

•1/8 teaspoon freshly ground black pepper

**Directions:**

1.In a 6-quart slow cooker, mix all of the ingredients.

2.Cover and cook on low for 6 to 7 hours, or until the squash is tender when pierced with a fork.

3.Use a potato masher to mash the squash right in the slow cooker.

**Nutrition:**

Calories: 175 Cal

Carbohydrates: 38 g

Sugar: 1 g

Fiber: 3 g

Fat: 4 g

Saturated Fat: 1 g

Protein: 3 g

Sodium: 149 mg

### 259.Roasted Root Vegetables

**Preparation Time**: 20 minutes

**Cooking Time:** 6 to 8 hours

**Servings:** 8

**Ingredients:**

•6 carrots, cut into 1-inch chunks

•2 yellow onions, each cut into 8 wedges

•2 sweet potatoes, peeled and cut into chunks

•6 Yukon Gold potatoes, cut into chunks

•8 whole garlic cloves, peeled

•4 parsnips, peeled and cut into chunks

•3 tablespoons olive oil

•1 teaspoon dried thyme leaves

•1/2 teaspoon salt

•1/8 teaspoon freshly ground black pepper

**Directions:**

1.In a 6-quart slow cooker, mix all of the ingredients.

2.Cover and cook on low for 6 to 8 hours, or until the vegetables are tender.

3.Serve and enjoy!

**Nutrition:**

Calories: 214 Cal

Carbohydrates: 40 g

Sugar: 7 g

Fiber: 6 g

Fat: 5 g

Saturated Fat: 1 g

Protein: 4 g

Sodium: 201 mg

### 260. Hummus

**Preparation Time**: 10 minutes
**Cooking Time:** 10 minutes
**Servings:** 32
**Ingredients:**
- 4 cups of cooked garbanzo beans
- 1 cup of water
- 11/2 tablespoons of lemon juice
- 2 teaspoons of ground cumin
- 11/2 teaspoon of ground coriander.
- 1 teaspoon of finely chopped garlic
- 1/2 teaspoon of salt
- 1/4 teaspoon of fresh ground pepper
- Paprika for garnish

**Directions:**
1. On a food processor, place together the garbanzo beans, lemon juice, water, garlic, salt, and pepper and process it until it becomes smooth and creamy.
2. To achieve your desired consistency, add more water.
3. Then spoon out the hummus in a serving bowl
4. Sprinkle your paprika and serve.

**Nutrition:**
Protein: 0.7 g
Carbohydrates: 2.5 g
Dietary Fiber: 0.6 g
Sugars: 0 g
Fat: 1.7 g

### 261. Thai Roasted Veggies

**Preparation Time**: 20 minutes
**Cooking Time:** 6 to 8 hours
**Servings:** 8
**Ingredients:**
- 4 large carrots, peeled and cut into chunks
- 2 onions, peeled and sliced
- 6 garlic cloves, peeled and sliced
- 2 parsnips, peeled and sliced
- 2 jalapeño peppers, minced
- 1/2 cup Roasted Vegetable Broth
- 1/3 cup canned coconut milk
- 3 tablespoons lime juice
- 2 tablespoons grated fresh ginger root
- 2 teaspoons curry powder

**Directions:**
1. In a 6-quart slow cooker, mix the carrots, onions, garlic, parsnips, and jalapeño peppers.
2. In a small bowl, mix the vegetable broth, coconut milk, lime juice, ginger root, and curry powder until well blended. Pour this mixture into the slow cooker.
3. Cover and cook on low for 6 to 8 hours, do it until the vegetables are tender when pierced with a fork.

**Nutrition:**
Calories: 69 Cal
Carbohydrates: 13 g
Sugar: 6 g
Fiber: 3 g
Fat: 3g
Saturated Fat: 3g
Protein: 1g
Sodium: 95mg

### 262. Cheesy Cauliflower Fritters

**Difficulty:** Medium
**Preparation Time:** 5 minutes
**Cooking Time:** 14 minutes
**Servings:** 8
**Ingredients:**
- ½ C. chopped parsley
- 1 C. Italian breadcrumbs
- 1/3 C. shredded mozzarella cheese
- 1/3 C. shredded sharp cheddar cheese
- 1 egg
- minced garlic cloves

•chopped scallions
•1 head of cauliflower
**Directions:**
1Cut cauliflower up into florets. Wash well and pat dry. Place into a food processor and pulse 20-30 seconds till it looks like rice.
2Place cauliflower rice in a bowl and mix with pepper, salt, egg, cheeses, breadcrumbs, garlic, and scallions.
3With hands, form 15 patties of the mixture. Add more breadcrumbs if needed.
4With olive oil, spritz patties, and place into your air fryer in a single layer.
5Cook 14 minutes at 390 degrees, flipping after 7 minutes.
**Nutrition:**
Calories: 209
Fat: 17g
Protein: 6g
Sugar: 0.5g

## 263.Crispy Jalapeno Coins
**Difficulty:** Hard
**Preparation Time:** 10 minutes
**Cooking Time:** 10 minutes
**Servings:** 8 to 10
**Ingredients:**
•1 egg
•2-3 tbsp. coconut flour
•1 sliced and seeded jalapeno
•Pinch of garlic powder
•Pinch of onion powder
•Pinch of Cajun seasoning (optional)
•Pinch of pepper and salt
**Directions:**
1Ensure your air fryer is preheated to 400 degrees.
2Mix together all dry ingredients.

3Pat jalapeno slices dry. Dip coins into egg wash and then into dry mixture. Toss to coat thoroughly.
4Add coated jalapeno slices to air fryer in a singular layer. Spray with olive oil.
5Cook just till crispy.
**Nutrition:**
Calories: 128
Fat: 8g
Protein: 7g
Sugar: 0g

## 264.Jicama Fries
**Difficulty:** Hard
**Preparation Time:** 10 minutes
**Cooking Time:** 20 minutes
**Servings:** 8
**Ingredients:**
•1 tbsp. dried thyme
•¾ C. arrowroot flour
•½ large Jicama
•eggs
**Directions:**
1Sliced jicama into fries.
2Whisk eggs together and pour over fries. Toss to coat.
3Mix a pinch of salt, thyme, and arrowroot flour together. Toss egg-coated jicama into dry mixture, tossing to coat well.
4Spray air fryer basket with olive oil and add fries. Cook 20 minutes on CHIPS setting. Toss halfway into the cooking process.
**Nutrition:**
Calories: 211
Fat: 19g
Protein: 9g
Sugar: 1g

## 265.Air Fryer Brussels Sprouts

**Difficulty:** Hard
**Preparation Time:** 5 minutes
**Cooking Time:** 10 minutes
**Servings:** 5
**Ingredients:**

- ¼ tsp. salt
- 1 tbsp. balsamic vinegar
- 1 tbsp. olive oil
- C. Brussels sprouts

**Directions:**

1Cut Brussels sprouts in half lengthwise. Toss with salt, vinegar, and olive oil till coated thoroughly.

2Add coated sprouts to air fryer, cooking 8-10 minutes at 400 degrees. Shake after 5 minutes of cooking.

3Brussels sprouts are ready to devour when brown and crisp!

**Nutrition:**

Calories: 118
Fat: 9g
Protein: 11g
Sugar: 1g

## 266.Spaghetti Squash Tots

**Difficulty:** Hard
**Preparation Time:** 5 minutes
**Cooking Time:** 15 minutes
**Servings:** 8 to 10
**Ingredients:**

- ¼ tsp. pepper
- ½ tsp. salt
- 1 thinly sliced scallion
- 1 spaghetti squash

**Directions:**

1Wash and cut the squash in half lengthwise. Scrape out the seeds.

2With a fork, remove spaghetti meat by strands and throw out skins.

3In a clean towel, toss in squash and wring out as much moisture as possible. Place in a bowl and with a knife slice through meat a few times to cut up smaller.

4Add pepper, salt, and scallions to squash and mix well.

5Create "tot" shapes with your hands and place in air fryer. Spray with olive oil.

6Cook 15 minutes at 350 degrees until golden and crispy!

**Nutrition:**

Calories: 231
Fat: 18g
Protein: 5g
Sugar: 0g

## 267.Cinnamon Butternut Squash Fries

**Difficulty:** Very Hard
**Preparation Time:** 10 minutes
**Cooking Time:** 10 minutes
**Servings:** 2
**Ingredients:**

- 1 pinch of salt
- 1 tbsp. Stevia
- ½ tsp. nutmeg
- tsp. cinnamon
- 1 tbsp. coconut oil
- ounces pre-cut butternut squash fries

**Directions:**

1In a plastic bag, pour in all ingredients. Coat fries with other components till coated and Stevia is dissolved.

2Spread coated fries into a single layer in the air fryer. Cook 10 minutes at 390 degrees until crispy.

**Nutrition:**

Calories: 175
Fat: 8g
Protein: 1g
Sugar: 5g

## 268.Carrot & Zucchini Muffins

**Difficulty:** Very Hard
**Preparation Time: 5 minutes**
**Cooking Time:  14 minutes**
**Servings:  4**
**Ingredients:**

- tablespoons butter, melted
- ¼ cup carrots, shredded
- ½ cup zucchini, shredded
- 1 ½ cups almond flour
- 1 tablespoon liquid Stevia
- teaspoons baking powder
- Pinch of salt
- eggs
- 1 tablespoon yogurt
- 1 cup milk

*Directions:*

1Preheat your air fryer to 350 degree Fahrenheit.
2Beat the eggs, yogurt, milk, salt, pepper, baking soda, and Stevia.
3Whisk in the flour gradually.
4Add zucchini and carrots.
5Grease muffin tins with butter and pour muffin batter into tins.  Cook for 14-minutes and serve.

*Nutrition:*
Calories:  224,
Total Fats:  12.3g,
 Carbs: 11.2g,
Protein:  14.2g

## 269.Curried Cauliflower Florets

**Difficulty:** Very Hard
**Preparation Time:** 5 minutes
**Cooking Time:**  10 minutes
**Servings:**  4
**Ingredients:**

- 1/4 cup sultanas or golden raisins
- ¼ teaspoon salt
- 1 tablespoon curry powder
- 1 head cauliflower, broken into small florets
- ¼ cup pine nuts
- ½ cup olive oil

**Directions:**

1.In a cup of boiling water, soak your sultanas to plump.  Preheat your air fryer to 350 degree Fahrenheit.
2.Add oil and pine nuts to air fryer and toast for a minute or so.
3. In a bowl toss the cauliflower and curry powder as well as salt, then add the mix to air fryer mixing well.
4.Cook for 10-minutes.  Drain the sultanas, toss with cauliflower, and serve.

**Nutrition:**
Calories:  275,
Total Fat:  11.3g,
Carbs:  8.6g,
Protein:  9.5g

## 270.Oat and Chia Porridge

**Difficulty:** Very Hard
**Preparation Time: 5 minutes**
**Cooking Time:  5 minutes**
**Servings:  4**
**Ingredients:**

- tablespoons peanut butter
- teaspoons liquid Stevia
- 1 tablespoon butter, melted
- cups milk
- cups oats
- 1 cup chia seeds

*Directions:*

1Preheat your air fryer to 390 degree Fahrenheit.
2Whisk the peanut butter, butter, milk and Stevia in a bowl.
3Stir in the oats and chia seeds.

4Pour the mixture into an oven-proof bowl and place in the air fryer and cook for 5-minutes.

***Nutrition:***

Calories:  228,

Total Fats:  11.4g,

Carbs:  10.2g,

Protein:  14.5g

## 271.Feta & Mushroom Frittata

**Difficulty:** Very Hard

**Preparation Time: 15 minutes**

**Cooking Time:  30 minutes**

**Servings:  4**

**Ingredients:**

- 1 red onion, thinly sliced
- cups button mushrooms, thinly sliced
- Salt to taste
- tablespoons feta cheese, crumbled
- medium eggs
- Non-stick cooking spray
- tablespoons olive oil

***Directions:***

1Saute the onion and mushrooms in olive oil over medium heat until the vegetables are tender.

2 Remove the vegetables from pan and drain on a paper towel-lined plate.

3 In a mixing bowl, whisk eggs and salt.  Coat all sides of baking dish with cooking spray.

4 Preheat your air fryer to 325 degree Fahrenheit.  Pour the beaten eggs into prepared baking dish and scatter the sautéed vegetables and crumble feta on top.  Bake in the air fryer for 30-minutes.  Allow to cool slightly and serve!

***Nutrition:***

Calories:  226,

Total Fat:  9.3g,

Carbs:  8.7g,

Protein:  12.6g

142

## 272.Butter Glazed Carrots

**Difficulty:** Very Hard

**Preparation Time:** 20 Minutes

**Cooking Time:** 15 minutes

**Servings:** 4

**Ingredients:**

- Baby carrots-2 cups
- Stevia-1 tbsps.
- Butter; melted-1/2 tbsps.
- Salt and black pepper- a pinch

**Directions:**

1Take a baking dish suitable to fit in your air fryer.

2Toss carrots with stevia, butter, salt and black peppers in that baking dish.

3Place this dish in the air fryer basket and seal the fryer.

4Cook the carrots for 10 minutes at 3500 F on Air fryer mode.

5Enjoy.

**Nutrition:**

Calories 151,

Fat 2,

Fiber 4,

Carbs 14,

Protein 4

# Low-Cost Recipes

### 273.Creamed Coconut Curry Spinach

**Preparation Time:** 30 minutes
**Cooking Time:** 30 seconds
**Servings:** 6
**Ingredients:**
•1-pound frozen spinach, thawed and drained of moisture
•1 small can whole fat coconut milk
•2 teaspoon yellow curry paste
•1 teaspoon lemon zest
•Cashews for garnish
**Directions:**
1.Heat a medium sized pan to medium high heat, then add the curry paste and cook for 30 seconds. Add a small amount of the coconut milk and stir to combine, and then cook until the paste is aromatic.
2.Add the spinach, and then season. Separate the rest of the ingredients, from the cashews, and allow the sauce to reduce slightly.
3.Keep the sauce creamy, but reduce it to coat the spinach well. Serve with chopped cashews.
**Nutrition:**
Calories: 191
Total Carbohydrate: 9 g
Cholesterol: 2 mg
Total Fat: 14 g
Fiber: 1 g
Protein: 4 g

### 274.Shrimp Salad Cocktails

**Preparation Time:** 35 minutes
**Cooking Time:** 35 minutes
**Servings:** 8 servings
**Ingredients:**
•2 cups mayonnaise
•1/4 cup ketchup
•1/4 cup lemon juice
•1 tablespoon. Worcestershire sauce
•2 lbs. peeled and deveined cooked large shrimp
•2 celery ribs, finely chopped
•3 tablespoons. minced fresh tarragon or 3 teaspoon dried tarragon
•1/4 teaspoon. salt 1/4 teaspoon pepper
•2 cups shredded romaine
•2 cups seedless red and/or green grapes, halved
•6 plum tomatoes, seeded and finely chopped
•1/2 cup chopped peeled mango or papaya
•Minced chives or parsley
**Directions:**
1.Combine Worcestershire sauce, lemon juice, ketchup and mayonnaise together in a small bowl. Combine pepper, salt, tarragon, celery and shrimp together in a large bowl. Put in 1 cup of dressing toss well to coat.
2.Scoop 1 tablespoon. of the dressing into 8 cocktail glasses. Layer each glass with 1/4 cup of lettuce, followed by 1/2 cup of the shrimp mixture, 1/4 cup of grapes, 1/3 cup of tomatoes and finally 1 tablespoon. of mango. Spread the remaining dressing over top; sprinkle chives on top. Serve immediately.
**Nutrition:**
Calories: 580
Total Carbohydrate: 16 g
Cholesterol: 192 mg
Total Fat: 46 g
Fiber: 2 g
Protein: 24 g

### 275.Garlic Chive Cauliflower Mash

**Preparation Time:** 20 minutes

**Cooking Time:** 18 minutes
**Servings:** 5
**Ingredients:**
•4 cups cauliflower
•1/3 cup vegetarian mayonnaise
•1 garlic clove
•1/2 teaspoon. kosher salt
•1 tablespoon. water
•1/8 teaspoon. pepper
•1/4 teaspoon. lemon juice
•1/2 teaspoon lemon zest
•1 tablespoons. Chives, minced
**Directions:**
1.In a bowl that is save to microwave, add the cauliflower, mayo, garlic, water, and salt/pepper and mix until the cauliflower is well coated. Cook on high for 15-18 minutes, until the cauliflower is almost mushy.
2.Blend the mixture in a strong blender until completely smooth, adding a little more water if the mixture is too chunky. Season with the remaining ingredients and serve.
**Nutrition:**
Calories: 178
Total Carbohydrate: 14 g
Cholesterol: 18 mg
Total Fat: 18 g
Fiber: 4 g
Protein: 2 g

## 276.Beet Greens with Pine Nuts Goat Cheese

**Preparation Time:** 25 minutes
**Cooking Time:** 15 minutes
**Servings:** 3
**Ingredients:**
•4 cups beet tops, washed and chopped roughly
•1 teaspoon. EVOO
•1 tablespoon. no stevia added balsamic vinegar
•2 oz. crumbled dry goat cheese
•2 tablespoons. Toasted pine nuts
**Directions:**
1.Warm the oil in a large pan, then cook the beet greens on medium high heat until they release their moisture. Let it cook until almost tender. Flavor with salt and pepper and remove from heat.
2.Toss the greens in a mixture of balsamic vinegar and olive oil, then top with the nuts and cheese. Serve warm.
**Nutrition:**
Calories: 215
Total Carbohydrate: 4 g
Cholesterol: 12 mg
Total Fat: 18 g
Fiber: 2 g
Protein: 10 g

## 277.Shrimp with Dipping Sauce

**Preparation Time:** 5 minutes
**Cooking Time:** 15 minutes
**Servings**: 6
**Ingredients:**
•1 tablespoon. reduced-sodium soy sauce
•2 teaspoons. Hot pepper sauce
•1 teaspoon. canola oil
•1/4 teaspoon. garlic powder
•1/8 to 1/4 teaspoon. cayenne pepper
•1 lb. uncooked medium shrimp, peeled and deveined
•2 tablespoons. Chopped green onions
Dipping Sauce:
•3 tablespoon. Reduced-sodium soy sauce
•1 teaspoon. rice vinegar
•1 tablespoon. orange juice
•2 teaspoons. Sesame oil
•2 teaspoons. Honey

•1 garlic clove, minced

•1-1/2 teaspoons. Minced fresh gingerroot

**Directions:**

1.Heat the initial 5 ingredients in a big nonstick frying pan for 30 seconds, then mix continuously.

2.Add onions and shrimp and stir fry for 4-5 minutes or until the shrimp turns pink. Mix together the sauce ingredients and serve it with the shrimp.

**Nutrition:**

Calories: 97

Total Carbohydrate: 4 g

Cholesterol: 112 mg

Total Fat: 3 g

Fiber: 0 g

Protein: 13 g

## 278.Celeriac Cauliflower Mash

**Preparation Time:** 20 minutes

**Cooking Time:** 12 minutes

**Servings:** 6

**Ingredients:**

•1 head cauliflower

•1 small celery root

•1/4 cup butter

•1 tablespoon. chopped rosemary

•1 tablespoon. chopped thyme

•1 cup cream cheese

**Directions:**

1.Skin the celery root and cut into small pieces. Cut the cauliflower into similar sized pieces and combine.

2.Toast the herbs in the butter in a large pan, until they become fragrant. Add the cauliflower and celery root and stir to combine. Season and cook at medium high until whatever moisture is in the vegetables releases itself, then covers and cook on low for 10-12 minutes.

3.Once the vegetables are soft, remove from the heat and place them in the blender. Make it smooth, then put the cream cheese and puree again. Season and serve.

**Nutrition:**

Calories: 225

Total Carbohydrate: 4 g

Cholesterol: 1 mg

Total Fat: 20 g

Fiber: 0 g

Protein: 5 g

## 279.Cheddar Drop Biscuits

**Preparation Time:** 30 minutes

**Cooking Time:** 15 minutes

**Servings:** 8

**Ingredients:**

•1/4 cup coconut oil

•4 eggs

•2 teaspoon. apple cider vinegar

•1 1/2 cup coarse almond meal

•1/2 teaspoon. baking powder, gluten free

•1/2 teaspoon. onion powder

•1/4 teaspoon. salt

•3/4 cup cheddar cheese

•2 tablespoons. Chopped jalapenos

**Directions:**

1.Line a sheet tray with parchment paper, and then preheat the oven to 400F

2.Mix the wet ingredients in a bowl until combined, then reserve. Mix the dry ingredients in a separate bowl until combined, and then add them to the wet ingredients, stirring until incorporated. Fold in the cheddar cheese and jalapenos.

3.Drop the dough onto the parchment paper into eight roughly equal pieces, and then shape as desired once they are on the tray.

4.Bake until golden brown, 12-15 minutes. Rotate the tray halfway through baking so browning is even.

5.Cool slightly and serve.

**Nutrition:**

Calories: 260

Total Carbohydrate: 4 g

Cholesterol: 8 mg

Total Fat: 22 g

Fiber: 1 g

Protein: 4 g

## 280.Roasted Radish with Fresh Herbs

**Preparation Time:** 15 minutes

**Cooking Time:** 10 minutes

**Servings:** 4

**Ingredients:**

- 1 tablespoon. coconut oil
- 1 bunch radishes
- 2 tablespoons. Minced chives
- 1 tablespoon. minced rosemary
- 1 tablespoon. minced thyme

**Directions:**

1.Wash the radishes, and then remove the tops and stems. Cut them into quarters and reserve.

2.Add the oil to a cast iron pan, then heat to medium. Add the radishes, and then season with salt and pepper. Cook on medium heat for 6-8 minutes, until almost tender, then add the herbs and cook through.

3.The radishes can be served warm with meats or chilled with salads.

**Nutrition:**

Calories: 123

Total Carbohydrate: 6 g

Cholesterol: 8 mg

Total Fat: 13 g

Fiber: 2 g

Protein: 6 g



## 281.Summer Bruschetta

**Preparation Time:** 15 minutes

**Cooking Time:** 3 hours

**Servings:** 4

**Ingredients:**

- Basil leaves (chopped) – 6
- Artichoke hearts (quartered) – ½ cup
- Kalamata olives (halved) – ¼ cup
- Capers – ¼ cup
- Roma tomatoes (diced) – 4
- Balsamic vinegar – 3 tablespoon
- Avocado oil – 3 tablespoon
- Onion powder – ¾ teaspoon
- Sea salt – ¾ teaspoon
- Black pepper – ½ teaspoon
- Garlic (minced) – 2 tablespoon

**Directions:**

1.Combine all the ingredients in the slow cooker and stir mix.

2.Cook for 3 hours on high, stirring the mix after every hour.

**Nutrition:**

Calories: 152

Total Carbohydrate: 4 g

Cholesterol: 1 mg

Total Fat: 13 g

Fiber: 4 g

Protein: 1 g

Sodium: 140 mg

## 282.Tomato Cheddar Fondue

**Preparation Time:** 20 minutes

**Cooking Time:** 30 minutes

**Servings:** 3-1/2 cups

**Ingredients:**

- 1 garlic clove, halved
- 6 medium tomatoes, seeded and diced
- 2/3 cup dry white wine
- 6 tablespoons. butter, cubed
- 1-1/2 teaspoons. dried basil

- Dash cayenne pepper
- 2 cups shredded cheddar cheese
- 1 tablespoon. all-purpose flour
- Cubed French bread and cooked shrimp

**Directions:**

1. Rub the bottom and sides of a fondue pot with a garlic clove. Set aside and discard the garlic.
2. Combine wine, butter, basil, cayenne and tomatoes in a large saucepan. On a medium low heat, bring mixture to a simmer, then decrease heat to low. Mix cheese with flour. Add to tomato mixture gradually while stirring after each addition until cheese is melted.
3. Pour into the Preparation timeared fondue pot and keep warm. Enjoy with shrimp and bread cubes.

**Nutrition:**

Calories: 118

Total Carbohydrate: 4 g

Cholesterol: 30 mg

Total Fat: 10 g

Fiber: 1 g

Protein: 4 g

### 283.Swiss Seafood Canapés

**Preparation Time:** 20 minutes

**Cooking Time:** 25 minutes

**Servings:** 4

**Ingredients:**

- 1 can (6 oz.) small shrimp, rinsed and drained
- 1 package (6 oz.) frozen crabmeat, thawed
- 1 cup shredded Swiss cheese
- 2 hard-boiled large eggs, chopped
- 1/4 cup finely chopped celery
- 1/4 cup mayonnaise
- 1/4 cup French salad dressing or seafood cocktail sauce
- 2 green onions, chopped
- Dash salt
- 1 loaf (16 oz.) snack rye bread

**Directions:**

1. Mix the first nine ingredients in a large bowl. Put bread on ungreased baking sheets.
2. Broil for 1 to 2 minutes, 4 to 6-inches from the heat or until lightly browned. Flip slices over; spread 1 rounded tablespoonful of seafood mixture on each. Broil for 4 to 5 more minutes or until heated through.

**Nutrition:**

Calories: 57

Total Carbohydrate: 5 g

Cholesterol: 22 mg

Total Fat: 3 g

Fiber: 1 g

Protein: 3 g

### 284.Squash & Zucchini

**Preparation Time:** 5 min

**Cooking Time:** 4-6 hours

**Servings:** 6

**Ingredients:**

- Zucchini (sliced and quartered) – 2 cups
- Yellow squash (sliced and quartered) – 2 cups
- Pepper – ¼ teaspoon
- Italian seasoning – 1 teaspoon
- Garlic powder – 1 teaspoon
- Sea salt – ½ teaspoon
- Butter (cubed) – ¼ cup
- Parmesan cheese (grated) – ¼ cup

**Directions:**

1. Combine all the ingredients in the slow cooker.
2. Cook covered for 4-6 hours on low.

**Nutrition:**

Calories: 122

Total Carbohydrate: 4 g

Cholesterol: 18 mg
Total Fat: 9.9 g
Fiber: 4 g
Protein: 14 g

### 285.Tasty Shrimp Spread

**Preparation Time:** 15 minutes
**Cooking Time:** 20 minutes
**Servings:** 2-1/2 cups
**Ingredients:**
- 1 package (8 oz.) cream cheese, softened
- 1/4 cup butter, softened
- 1/4 cup mayonnaise
- 1/2 lb. peeled and deveined cooked shrimp, finely chopped
- 1 medium onion, chopped
- Assorted crackers and/or fresh vegetables

**Directions:**
1. Combine mayonnaise, butter and cream cheese together in a small bowl.
2. Mix in onion and shrimp.
3. Refrigerate with a cover till serving. Serve with crackers and/or vegetables if you want.

**Nutrition:**
Calories: 189
Cholesterol: 73 mg
Total Fat: 17 g
Fiber: 0 g
Protein: 7 g

### 286.Creamy Coconut Spinach

**Preparation Time:** 10 minutes
**Cooking Time:** 25 minutes
**Servings:** 2
**Ingredients:**
- Baby spinach – 4 cups
- Coconut milk – ¼ cup
- Nutmeg – 1/8 teaspoon
- Granulated sugar substitute – 2 teaspoon
- Cayenne pepper - 1/8 teaspoon
- Salt – to taste

**Directions:**
1. Heat a saucepan and warm the coconut milk in it for 2 minutes.
2. Mix in the spinach, cooking until bright green and wilted.
3. Mix in the rest of the ingredients.

**Nutrition:**
Calories: 73
Total Carbohydrate: 4 g
Cholesterol: 0 mg
Total Fat: 7 g
Fiber: 4 g
Protein: 4 g

### 287.Smoothie bowl with berries, poppy seeds, nuts and seeds

**Preparation Time:** 15 minutes
**Cooking Time:** 0 minutes
**Servings:** 2
**Ingredients:**
- 5 chopped almonds
- 2 chopped walnuts
- 1 apple
- ¼ banana
- 300 g yogurt
- 60 g raspberries
- 20 g blueberries
- 20 g rolled oats, roasted in a pan
- 10 g poppy seeds
- 1 teaspoon pumpkin seeds
- Agave syrup

**Directions:**
1. Clean the fruit and let it drain.
2. Take some berries and set them aside.
3. Place the remaining berries in a tall mixing vessel.
4. Cut the banana into slices. Put a few aside.
5. Add the rest of the banana to the berries.
6. Remove the core of the apple and cut it into quarters.

7.Cut the quarters into thin wedges and set a few aside.

8.Add the remaining wedges to the berries.

9.Add the yogurt to the fruits and mix everything into a puree.

10.Sweeten the smoothie with the agave syrup.

11.Divide it into two bowls.

12.Serve it with the remaining fruit, poppy seeds, oatmeal, nuts and seeds.

**Nutrition:**

kcal: 284

Carbohydrates: 21 g

Protein: 11 g

Fat: 19 g

## 288.Whole grain bread and avocado

**Preparation Time:** 5 minutes

**Cooking Time:** 0 minutes

Serving: 1

**Ingredients:**

•2 slices of wholemeal bread

•60 g of cottage cheese

•1 stick of thyme

•½ avocado

•½ lime

•Chili flakes

•salt

•pepper

**Directions:**

1.Cut the avocado in half.

2.Remove the pulp and cut it into slices.

3.Pour the lime juice over it.

4.Wash the thyme and shake it dry.

5.Remove the leaves from the stem.

6.Brush the whole wheat bread with the cottage cheese.

7.Place the avocado slices on top.

8.Top with the chili flakes and thyme.

9.Add salt and pepper and serve.

**Nutrition:**

kcal: 490

Carbohydrates: 31 g

Protein: 19 g

Fat: 21 g

# Lean and Tasty Recipes

### 289.Aloo Gobi

**Preparation Time:** 15 Minutes
**Cooking Time:** 4 To 5 Hours
**Servings:** 4
**Ingredients:**
•1 large cauliflower, cut into 1-inch pieces
•1 large russet potato, peeled and diced
•1 medium yellow onion, peeled and diced
•1 cup canned diced tomatoes, with juice
•1 cup frozen peas
•¼ cup water
•1 (2-inch) piece fresh ginger, peeled and finely chopped
•1½ teaspoons minced garlic (3 cloves)
•1 jalapeño pepper, stemmed and sliced
•1 tablespoon cumin seeds
•1 tablespoon garam masala
•1 teaspoon ground turmeric
•1 heaping tablespoon fresh cilantro
•Cooked rice, for serving (optional)
**Directions:**
1.Combine the cauliflower, potato, onion, diced tomatoes, peas, water, ginger, garlic, jalapeño, cumin seeds, garam masala, and turmeric in a slow cooker; mix until well combined.
2.Cover and cook on low for 4 to 5 hours.
3.Garnish with the cilantro, and serve over cooked rice (if using).
**Nutrition:**
Calories: 115
Total fat: 1g
Protein: 6g
Sodium: 62mg
Fiber: 6g

### 290.Jackfruit Carnitas

**Preparation Time:** 15 Minutes
**Cooking Time:** 8 Hours
**Servings:** 4
**Ingredients:**
•2 (20-ounce) cans jackfruit, drained, hard pieces discarded
•¾ cup Very Easy Vegetable Broth (here) or store bought
•1 tablespoon ground cumin
•1 tablespoon dried oregano
•1½ teaspoons ground coriander
•1 teaspoon minced garlic (2 cloves)
•½ teaspoon ground cinnamon
•2 bay leaves
•Tortillas, for serving
•Optional toppings: diced onions, sliced radishes, fresh cilantro, lime wedges, Nacho Cheese (here)
**Directions:**
1.Combine the jackfruit, vegetable broth, cumin, oregano, coriander, garlic, cinnamon, and bay leaves in a slow cooker. Stir to combine.
2.Cover and cook on low for 8 hours or on high for 4 hours.
3.Use two forks to pull the jackfruit apart into shreds.
4.Remove the bay leaves. Serve in warmed tortillas with your favorite taco fixings.
**Nutrition:**
Calories: 286
Total fat: 2g
Protein: 6g
Sodium: 155mg
Fiber: 5g

### 291.Baked Beans

**Preparation Time:** 15 Minutes
**Cooking Time:** 6 Hours

**Servings:** 4
**Ingredients:**

- 2 (15-ounce) cans white beans, drained and rinsed
- 1 (15-ounce) can tomato sauce
- 1 medium yellow onion, finely diced
- 1½ teaspoons minced garlic (3 cloves)
- 3 tablespoons stevia
- 2 tablespoons molasses
- 1 tablespoon prepared yellow mustard
- 1 tablespoon chili powder
- 1 teaspoon soy sauce
- Pinch salt
- Freshly ground black pepper

**Directions:**

1. Place the beans, tomato sauce, onion, garlic, stevia, molasses, mustard, chili powder, and soy sauce into a slow cooker; mix well.
2. Cover and cook on low for 6 hours. Season with salt and pepper before serving.

**Nutrition:**

Calories: 468
Total fat: 2g
Protein: 28g
Sodium: 714mg
Fiber: 20g

## 292.Sweet Potato Pecan Muffins

**Difficulty:** Average
**Preparation Time:** 10 minutes
**Cooking Time:** 20 minutes
**Servings:** 2
**Ingredients:**

- Select Honey Sweet Potatoes – 2 sachets (1/2 condiment)
- Essential Spiced Gingerbread – 2 sachets (1/2 condiment)
- Water – 1 cup (1/2 condiment)
- Liquid egg substitute – 6 tbsp (3 healthy fat)
- Cashew milk, unsweetened - ¼ cup (1/2 healthy fat)
- Pumpkin pie spice - ½ tsp (1/4 condiment)
- Vanilla extract - ½ tsp (1/4 condiment)
- Baking powder - ½ tsp (1/4 condiment)
- Pecans, chopped - 1½ oz (2 healthy fats)

**Directions:**

1. Preheat the air fryer to 180°C.
2. Do the directions on the packet to make the Honey Sweet Potatoes.
3. Allow it to cool for some time.
4. Mix the prepared honey sweet potatoes and all the other ingredients, except the pecans.
5. Lightly spray the muffin pan and transfer the mix to the slots evenly.
6. Top it with chopped pecans.
7. Situate it in the air fryer tray and bake for 20 minutes.
8. Serve hot.

**Nutrition:**

- 383 Calories
- 21g Fat
- 15g Protein

## 293.Brussels Sprouts Curry

**Preparation Time:** 15 Minutes
**Cooking Time:** 7 To 8 Hours
**Servings:** 4
**Ingredients:**

- ¾ pound Brussels sprouts, bottoms cut off and sliced in half
- 1 can full-fat coconut milk
- 1 cup Very Easy Vegetable Broth (here) or store bought
- 1 medium onion, diced
- 1 medium carrot, thinly sliced

•1 medium red or Yukon potato, diced

•1½ teaspoons minced garlic (3 cloves)

•1 (1-inch) piece fresh ginger, peeled and minced

•1 small serrano chile, seeded and finely chopped

•2 tablespoons peanut butter

•1 tablespoon rice vinegar or other vinegar

•1 tablespoon cane sugar or agave nectar

•1 tablespoon soy sauce

•1 teaspoon curry powder

•1 teaspoon ground turmeric

•Pinch salt

•Freshly ground black pepper

•Cooked rice, for serving (optional)

**Directions:**

Place the Brussels sprouts, coconut milk, vegetable broth, onion, carrot, potato, garlic, ginger, serrano chile, peanut butter, vinegar, cane sugar, soy sauce, curry powder, and turmeric in a slow cooker. Mix well.

Cover and cook on low for 7 to 8 hours or on high for 4 to 5 hours.

Season with salt and pepper. Serve over rice (if using).

**Nutrition:**

Calories: 404

Total fat: 29g

Protein: 10g

Sodium: 544mg

Fiber: 8g

### 294.Jambalaya

**Preparation Time:** 15 Minutes

**Cooking Time:** 6 To 8 Hours

**Servings:** 4

**Ingredients:**

•2 cups Very Easy Vegetable Broth (here) or store bought

•1 large yellow onion, diced

•1 green bell pepper, seeded and chopped

•2 celery stalks, chopped

•1½ teaspoons minced garlic (3 cloves)

•1 (15-ounce) can dark red kidney beans, drained and rinsed

•1 (15-ounce) can black-eyed peas, drained and rinsed

•1 (15-ounce) can diced tomatoes, drained

•2 tablespoons Cajun seasoning

•2 teaspoons dried oregano

•2 teaspoons dried parsley

•1 teaspoon cayenne pepper

•1 teaspoon smoked paprika

•½ teaspoon dried thyme

•Cooked rice, for serving (optional)

**Directions:**

1.Combine the vegetable broth, onion, bell pepper, celery, garlic, kidney beans, black-eyed peas, diced tomatoes, Cajun seasoning, oregano, parsley, cayenne pepper, smoked paprika, and dried thyme in a slow cooker; mix well.

2.Cover and cook on low for 6 to 8 hours.

3.Serve over rice (if using).

**Nutrition:**

Calories: 428

Total fat: 2g

Protein: 28g

Sodium: 484mg

Fiber: 19g

### 295.Mushroom-Kale Stroganoff

**Preparation Time:** 15 Minutes

**Cooking Time:** 6 To 8 Hours

**Servings:** 4

**Ingredients:**

•1 pound mushrooms, sliced

•1½ cups Very Easy Vegetable Broth (here) or store bought

- 1 cup stemmed and chopped kale
- 1 small yellow onion, diced
- 2 garlic cloves, minced
- 2 tablespoons all-purpose flour
- 2 tablespoons ketchup or tomato paste
- 2 teaspoons paprika
- ½ cup vegan sour cream
- ¼ cup chopped fresh parsley
- Cooked rice, pasta, or quinoa, for serving

**Directions:**
1. Combine the mushrooms, vegetable broth, kale, onion, garlic, flour, ketchup or tomato paste, and paprika in a slow cooker. Mix thoroughly.
2. Cover and cook on low for 6 to 8 hours.
3. Stir in the sour cream and parsley just before serving.
4. Serve over rice, pasta, or quinoa.

**Nutrition:**
Calories: 146
Total fat: 7g
Protein: 8g
Sodium: 417mg
Fiber: 3g

## 296. Sloppy Joe Filling

**Preparation Time:** 15 Minutes
**Cooking Time:** 6 To 8 Hours
**Servings:** 4
**Ingredients:**
- 3 cups textured vegetable protein
- 3 cups water
- 2 (6-ounce) cans tomato paste, or 1 cup ketchup
- 1 medium yellow onion, diced
- ½ medium green bell pepper, finely diced
- 2 teaspoons minced garlic (4 cloves)
- 4 tablespoons vegan Worcestershire sauce

- 3 tablespoons stevia
- 3 tablespoons apple cider vinegar
- 3 tablespoons prepared yellow mustard
- 2 tablespoons hot sauce (optional)
- 1 tablespoon salt
- 1 teaspoon chili powder
- Sliced, toasted buns or cooked rice, for serving

**Directions:**
1. Combine the textured vegetable protein, water, tomato paste, onion, bell pepper, garlic, Worcestershire sauce, stevia, vinegar, mustard, hot sauce (if using), salt, and chili powder in a slow cooker. Mix well.
2. Cover and cook on low for 6 to 8 hours or on high for 4 to 5 hours.
3. Serve on sliced, toasted buns or over rice.

**Nutrition:**
Calories: 452
Total fat: 4g
Protein: 75g
Sodium: 2,242mg
Fiber: 11g

## 297. Breakfast Scones with Blueberry Almond

**Difficulty:** Difficult
**Preparation Time:** 10 minutes
**Cooking Time:** 20 minutes
**Servings:** 2
**Ingredients:**
- Blueberry Almond Hot Cereal – 2 sachets (1/2 healthy fat)
- Flaxseed ground - ¼ cup (1/4 condiment)
- Sugar substitute, zero-calorie – 1 pkt (1/4 condiment)
- Baking powder - ½ tsp (1/4 condiment)
- Solid butter, unsalted, cut into ½" thickness – 1 tbsp. (1/2 healthy fat)

- Liquid egg white - 1½ tbsp (1 healthy fat)
- Greek yogurt, plain, low fat - 1½ tbsp (1 lean)
- Cinnamon ground – 1/8 tsp (1/4 condiment)

**Directions:**

1. Combine Blueberry Almond Hot Cereal, baking powder, and sugar substitute in a food processor.
2. Put butter cubes and blitz to form a rough, coarse meal. Let there be rice-sized butter pieces to get the scone structure.
3. Now add Greek yogurt, egg white, almond extract, cashew milk, and process until it turns to a dough form.
4. Line a baking paper in the air fryer baking tray.
5. Make 4 flat circles of dough and place them on the baking paper.
6. Drizzle some cinnamon powder on top.
7. Bake it at 205°C for 20 minutes, until it turns to a golden brown.
8. Allow it to cool and cut into half to make 8 wedges.
9. Serve and enjoy.

**Nutrition:**

- 277 Calories
- 13.6g Fat
- 7g Protein

### 298.Mini Pepper Nachos

**Difficulty:** Average
**Preparation Time:** 10 minutes
**Cooking Time:** 13 minutes
**Servings:** 2
**Ingredients:**

- Jalapeno pepper, diced - ¼ cup (1/2 green)
- Bell pepper, halved, cored – 12 nos. (2 greens)
- Chicken breast, canned in low sodium water – 6 oz (3 lean)

- Avocado, mashed – 3 oz (2 healthy fats)
- Greek yogurt, plain, low fat - ¼ cup (1/2 healthy fat)
- Cheddar cheese, low fat, divided – 1 cup (1/2 healthy fat)
- Chili powder - ½ tsp (1/2 condiment)
- Scallions, chopped - ¼ cup. (1/2 green)

**Directions:**

1. Drain the chicken thoroughly.
2. Put the diced jalapeno pepper in the air fryer tray and spray some cooking spray oil.
3. Air fry it at 200°C for 2-3 minutes until they become tender.
4. Transfer them to a large bowl, add chicken, yogurt, avocado, half portion of cheese, jalapeno, chili powder, and combine to mix.
5. In the air fryer tray, arrange the bell pepper and fill the chicken mixture.
6. Top them with the remaining cheese.
7. Bake it for 10 minutes until the cheese starts to melt.
8. Serve with garnished scallion.

Nutrition

- 457 Calories
- 18.5g Fat
- 40g Protein

### 299.Rice With Vegetables

**Preparation Time:** 15 Minutes
**Cooking Time:** 4 To 6 Hours
**Servings:** 4
**Ingredients:**

- 3 (15-ounce) cans black-eyed peas, drained and rinsed
- 1 (14.5-ounce) can Cajun-style stewed tomatoes, with juice
- 2 cups hot water
- 1 cup stemmed and chopped kale
- ¾ cup finely diced red bell pepper

•½ cup sliced scallions
•1 medium jalapeño pepper, seeded and minced
•1 teaspoon minced garlic (2 cloves)
•1½ teaspoons hot sauce
•1 vegetable bouillon cube
•Cooked rice, for serving

**Directions:**

1.Combine the black-eyed peas, tomatoes, hot water, kale, bell pepper, scallions, jalapeño, garlic, hot sauce, and bouillon cube in a slow cooker. Stir to combine.

2.Cover and cook on low for 4 to 6 hours.

3.Serve over cooked rice.

**Nutrition:**

Calories: 164

Total fat: 2g

Protein: 10g

Sodium: 250mg

Fiber: 8g

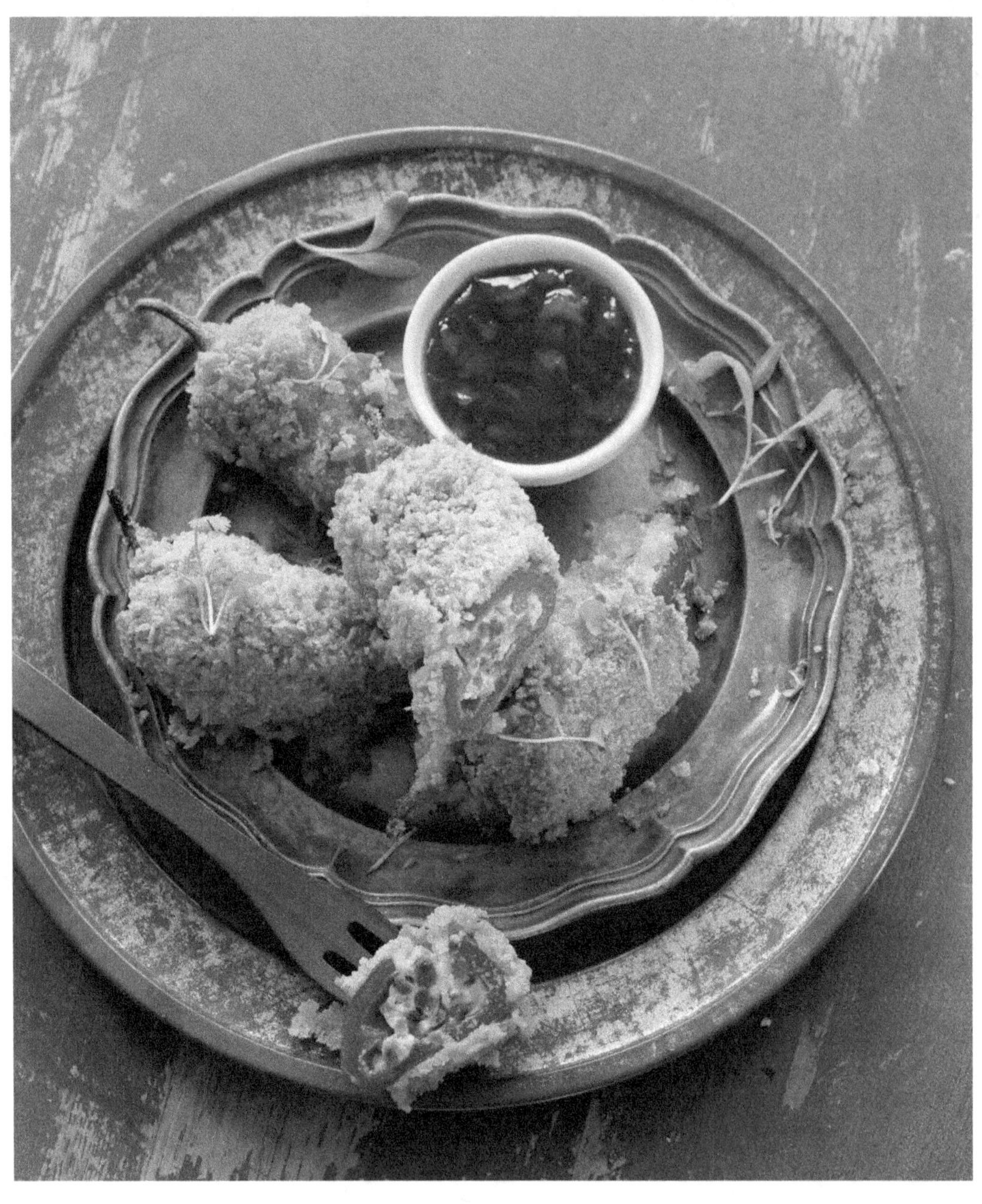

### 300. Air Fried Cauliflower Ranch Chips

**Difficulty:** Easy
**Preparation Time:** 5 minutes
**Cooking Time:** 12 minutes
**Servings:** 2
**Ingredients:**

- Raw cauliflower, grated - ½ cup (1/4 green)
- Parsley - ¼ tsp (1/8 green)
- Basil - ¼ tsp (1/8 green)
- Dill - ¼ tsp (1/8 green)
- Chives - ¼ tsp (1/8 green)
- Garlic powder - ¼ tsp (1/8 condiment)
- Onion powder - ¼ tsp (1/8 condiment)
- Pepper, ground - ¼ tsp (1/8 condiment)
- Parmesan cheese - ¼ cup (1/8 healthy fat)
- Cooking spray – as required (1/2 healthy fat)

**Directions:**

1. Preheat the air fryer to 230°C.
2. Using a medium bowl, mix all the ingredients.
3. Line the air fryer baking tray with parchment paper.
4. Scoop 1 tbsp mixture and place it on the parchment paper without overlapping one another.
5. Bake for 12 minutes by flipping side halfway through.
6. Serve hot.

**Nutrition:**

- 65 Calories
- 3.6g Fat
- 4g Protein

### 301. Cheesy Broccoli Bites

**Difficulty:** Average
**Preparation Time:** 5 minutes
**Cooking Time:** 40 minutes
**Servings:** 2
**Ingredients:**

- Frozen broccoli – 3 cups (2 greens)
- Scallions, thinly sliced - ¼ cup (1/2 green)
- Eggs – 2 (1 healthy fat)
- Cottage cheese – 1 cup (1/2 healthy fat)
- Mozzarella cheese, grated - ¾ cup (1/2 healthy fat)
- Parmesan cheese, shredded - ¼ cup (1/4 healthy fat)
- Olive oil – 1 tsp (1/2 condiment)
- Garlic powder - ½ tsp (1/2 condiment)
- Salt – 1/8 tsp (1/4 condiment)
- Water – 2 cups (1 healthy fat)

**Directions:**

1. Preheat the air fryer to 190°C.
2. Place the broccoli in an air fryer, save bowl, and pour water.
3. Air fryer it for 10 minutes until the broccoli becomes tender.
4. Drain the water and transfer the broccoli into the blender.
5. Blitz it until it chopped well.
6. Now add cottage cheese, scallions, parmesan, mozzarella, eggs, olive oil, salt, and garlic into the blender.
7. Pulse it until it gets mixed well.
8. Transfer it to 12 muffin tins evenly after greasing them.
9. Place it in the air fryer and bake for 30 minutes until the filling becomes firm and its top turns to a golden brown.
10. After baking, remove them from the air fryer.
11. Allow it to settle down the heat and serve.

**Nutrition:**

- 366 Calories

- 15.1g Fat
- 41g Protein

### 302.Brine & Spinach Egg Muffins Air Fried

**Difficulty:** Difficult
**Preparation Time:** 10 minutes
**Cooking Time:** 25 minutes
**Servings:** 2
**Ingredients:**
**For Egg Muffin**

- Eggs – 4 (2 healthy fat)
- Liquid egg whites – 1 cup (1/2 healthy fat)
- Greek yogurt, plain, low fat - ¼ cup (1/2 healthy fat)
- Salt - ¼ tsp (1/4 condiment)

**For Brie, Spinach & Mushroom Mix**

- Brie – 1 oz (1/2 green)
- Spinach, frozen, coarsely chopped – 5 oz (2 greens)
- Mushrooms, chopped – 1 cup. (1/2 green)

**Directions:**

1. Thaw the frozen spinach for 10 minutes.
2. Wash all the vegetables separately and pat dry.
3. Preheat the air fryer to 190°C.
4. In a large bowl, combine Greek yogurt, egg whites, eggs, cheese, and salt.
5. Add all the vegetables in the bowl mix and combine well.
6. Take 12 muffin tins and lightly spray with cooking oil.
7. Transfer the mixture evenly into the muffin tins.
8. Place them in the air fryer and bake for 25 minutes until the center portion becomes hard.
9. Do a toothpick test by inserting it in the center and check if it comes out clean.
10. Take it out from the air fryer and allow it to settle down the heat before serving.
11. Enjoy your muffin.

**Nutrition:**

- 278 Calories
- 13.1g Fat
- 33g Protein

### 303.Cheddar Herb Pizza Bites

**Difficulty:** Average
**Preparation Time:** 5 minutes
**Cooking Time:** 10 minutes
**Servings:** 2
**Ingredients:**

- Buttermilk Cheddar Herb Biscuit – 2 sachets (1 condiment)
- Almond milk, unsweetened - ½ cup (1/2 healthy fat)
- Olive oil – 1 tsp (1/2 condiment)
- Basil leaves, julienned - ½ cup (1/2 green)
- Mozzarella stick, cut into 6 small pieces – 2 oz. (1 healthy fat)
- Tomatoes, sliced – 1 medium (1 green)
- Balsamic vinegar – 1 tbsp (1/2 condiment)

**Directions:**

1. Preheat the air fryer to 230°C.
2. Combine the Buttermilk Cheddar Herb Biscuit, olive oil, and almond milk in a large bowl until they become a smooth paste.
3. Take 6 muffin tin and spray lightly with cooking oil.
4. Distribute the mixture evenly into the muffin tin.
5. Place the muffin tin on the air fryer grill tray, topped with mozzarella and sliced tomato.
6. Sprinkle basil on top and bake for 10 minutes, until the biscuit mixture becomes brown and cheese starts to bubble.

7.Drop balsamic vinegar on top before serving.

**Nutrition:**

- 203 Calories
- 7g Fat
- 13g Protein

### 304.Pumpkin Chocolate Cheesecake

**Difficulty:** Difficult
**Preparation Time:** 10 minutes
**Cooking Time:** 40 minutes
**Servings:** 2
**Ingredients:**

- Essential Decadent Double Chocolate Brownie – 4 sachets (2 healthy fat)
- Butter, unsalted, melted – 1 tbsp (1/2 healthy fat)
- Coldwater – 4 tbsp (1 condiment)
- Greek yogurt, plain, low fat – 2 cups (1/2 healthy fat)
- Cream cheese, light, softened – 5 tbsp (2 healthy fat)
- Pumpkin puree – 6 tbsp (3 lean)
- Egg – 2 (1 healthy fat)
- Stevia – 4 packets (1/4 condiment)
- Vanilla extract – 1 tsp (1/2 condiment)
- Pumpkin pie spice – 1 tsp (1/2 condiment)
- Salt – 1/8 tsp (1/4 condiment)

**Directions:**

1. Mix the Decadent Double Chocolate Brownie, water, and butter in a medium bowl thoroughly.
2. Preheat the air fryer to 175°C.
3. Grease 4 air fry oven-safe springform pan and evenly place the chocolate brownie mixture.
4. Push the mixture firmly to the bottom of the pan to form a thin crust.
5. Bake it for 15 minutes.
6. Now combine the rest of the ingredients in a medium-size bowl until they become a smooth paste.
7. Transfer it evenly to the springform pans.
8. Reduce the baking temperature to 150°C and bake it for 30-35 minutes until the center becomes firm and the edges start to brown.
9.Pull it from the air fryer and allow them to settle down the temperature.
10.Serve fresh.

**Nutrition:**

- 518 Calories
- 28g Fat
- 29g Protein

### 305.Cloud Garlic Bread Breakfast

**Difficulty:** Difficult
**Preparation Time:** 10 minutes
**Cooking Time:** 30 minutes
**Servings:** 2
**Ingredients:**

- Eggs, medium (separate yellow and white) – 2 (1 healthy fat)
- Cream cheese, low fat - 1½ tbsp (1 healthy fat)
- Sweetener, no-calorie - ½ pkt (1/2 condiment)
- Tartar cream - ¼ tsp (1/4 condiment)

**For Garlic Bread**

- Butter, unsalted, melted – 1tsp (1/2 healthy fat)
- Garlic powder – 1/8 tsp (1/4 condiment)
- Italian seasoning - ¼ tsp (1/4 condiment)
- Salt – 1/8 tsp (1/4 condiment)

**Directions:**

1. Combine thoroughly cream cheese, egg yolks, and the sweetener in a medium bowl.

2.    Beat egg whites in a large bowl along with tartar cream until the whites become stiff peaks.

3.    Now carefully fold the yellow yolk mixture into the egg whites without breaking the whites.

4.    Line a parchment paper in the air fryer baking tray and place 4 scoops of the mixture without overlapping one another.

5.Set the temperature to 150°C and bake for 20 minutes.

6.  Take out the bread, and brush butter on top and sprinkle the seasoning, garlic powder, and salt.

7.  Place it again into the air fryer and bake for further 10 minutes until the top becomes golden brown.

8.  After baking, allow it to settle down the heat before serving.

**Nutrition:**

- 115 Calories
- 8.8g Fat
- 6g Protein

### 306.Portbello Mushrooms Stuffed with Cheese

**Difficulty:** Difficult
**Preparation Time:** 15 minutes
**Cooking Time:** 17 minutes
**Servings:** 2
**Ingredients:**

- Portabella mushroom caps, large – 4 (2 leans)
- Soy sauce – 1 tbsp (1/2 condiment)
- Lemon juice – 1 tbsp (1/2 condiment)
- Olive oil, divided – 1 tsp (1/4 condiment)
- Mozzarella cheese, low fat, grated – 2 cups (1 healthy fat)
- Tomato, fresh, diced - ½ cup (1/2 green)
- Clove Garlic, finely grated – 1 clove (1/4 green)
- Cilantro, fresh, chopped – 1 tbsp (1/4 green)

**Directions:**

1.  Make bowls by scooping the flesh from the interior of the mushroom caps.

2.  Set the air fryer temperature to 200°C and preheat.

3.  Mix the soy sauce, lemon juice, and half a portion of olive oil in a small bowl.

4.  Marinate the mixture on the mushroom cap both inside and outside.

5.  Line foil coated baking paper in the air fryer tray.

6.  Place the marinated mushroom cap in the tray and bake for 10 minutes until they become tender.

7.  Now combine tomatoes, mozzarella, garlic, remaining olive oil, and Italian seasoning in a medium bowl.

8.  Fill the mushroom caps with the mixture evenly.

9.  Bake it in the air fryer for 7 minutes, until the cheese starts to melt.

10.Sprinkle cilantro on top and serve.

**Nutrition:**

- 250 Calories
- 4.4g Fat
- 40g Protein

### 307.Crispy Roasted Broccoli

**Difficulty:** Easy
**Preparation Time:** 10 minutes
**Cooking Time:** 8 minutes
**Servings:** 1
**Ingredients:**

- 1/4 Tsp. Masala (1/2 condiment)
- 1/2 Tsp. red chili powder (1 condiment)
- 1/2 Tsp. salt (1 condiment)
- 1/4 Tsp. turmeric powder (1/2 condiment)

• 1 Tbsp. chickpea flour (1 healthy fat)
• 1 Tbsp. yogurt (2 healthy fats)
• 1/2 Pound broccoli (1 green)

**Directions:**

1. Cut broccoli up into florets. Immerse in a bowl of water with two teaspoons of salt for at least half an hour to remove impurities.
2. Take out broccoli florets from water and let drain. Wipe down thoroughly.
3. Mix all other ingredients to create a marinade.
4. Toss broccoli florets in the marinade. Cover and chill for 15-30 minutes.
5. Preheat the Instant Crisp Air Fryer to 390 degrees. Place marinated broccoli florets into the fryer, lock the air fryer lid, set the temperature to 350°F, and set the time to 10 minutes. Florets will be crispy when done.

**Nutrition:**

• 96 Calories
• 1.3g Fat
• 7g Protein

## 308. Air Fryer Mint Cookies

**Difficulty:** Average
**Preparation Time:** 5 minutes
**Cooking Time:** 15 minutes
**Servings:** 2
**Ingredients:**

• Essentials Decadent Double Chocolate Brownie – 2 sachets (1 condiment)
• Essential Chocolate Mint Cookie Bars (2 healthy fats)
• Almond milk, unsweetened – 2 tbsp (1 healthy fat)
• Egg white – 2 (1/2 healthy fat)

**Directions:**

1. Preheat the air fryer to 180°C.
2. In a mixer blender, crush the chocolate mint bars.
3. Combine chocolate brownie, crushed chocolate mint bars, almond milk, and egg whites in a large bowl.
4. Evenly transfer the mix to 8 cookies ramekins.
5. Place it in the air fryer grill tray and bake for 15 minutes until the top becomes firm.
6. Allow it to settle down the heat and serve.

**Nutrition:**

• 187 Calories
• 4.1g Fat
• 5g Protein

## 309. Brownie Pies in Peanut Butter

**Difficulty:** Average
**Preparation Time:** 10 minutes
**Cooking Time:** 20 minutes
**Servings:** 2
**Ingredients:**

• Decadent Double Chocolate Brownie – 2 pkt (1 condiment)
• Baking powder - ¼ tsp (1/4 condiment)
• Liquid egg substitute – 3 tbsp (1 healthy fat)
• Vanilla almond milk, unsweetened, divided – 6 tbsp (2 healthy fats)
• Vegetable oil – 1 tsp (1/4 condiment)
• Peanut butter, powdered - ¼ cup (1/2 healthy fat)

**Directions:**

1. Preheat the air fryer to 180°C.
2. Mix the Decadent Double Chocolate Brownie mixture, egg substitute, baking powder, oil, half of the milk in a large bowl until it becomes a smooth paste.
3. Take 4 muffin tin and spray cooking oil.
4. Evenly fill ¾ portion of the muffin tin and bake in the air fryer for 20 minutes.

5.When the center becomes firm, insert a toothpick and check whether it comes out clean so that you can confirm the doneness of the muffin.

6.Remove it from the air fryer and allow them to cool down.

7.Now mix the remaining milk and powdered peanut butter in a medium bowl.

8.Slice the muffin horizontally and spread the peanut butter paste onto one half.

9.Situate the other half on top and serve.

**Nutrition:**

- 281 Calories
- 9.8g Fat
- 7g Protein

### 310.Red Pepper & Kale Egg Muffins Air Fried

**Difficulty:** Average
**Preparation Time:** 10 minutes
**Cooking Time:** 25 minutes
**Servings:** 2
**Ingredients:**
**For Egg Muffin**

- Eggs – 4 (1 healthy fat)
- Liquid egg whites – 1 cup (1/2 healthy fat)
- Greek yogurt, plain, low fat - ¼ cup (1/4 healthy fat)
- Salt - ¼ tsp (1/4 condiment)

**For Red Bell Pepper, Goat Cheese & Kale Mix**

- Red bell pepper, cored and chopped – 6 oz. (3 greens)
- Kale, frozen, chopped – 5 oz (2 greens)
- Goat cheese – 1 oz (1/2 healthy fat)

**Directions:**

1. Thaw the frozen cauliflower rice for 10 minutes.
2. Preheat the air fryer to 190°C.
3. In a large bowl, combine Greek yogurt, egg whites, eggs, cheese, and salt.

4. Add all the vegetables to the bowl mix to combine well.

5. Take 12 muffin tins and lightly spray with cooking oil.

6. Transfer the mixture evenly into the muffin tins.

7. Place them in the air fryer and bake for 25 minutes until the center portion becomes hard.

8. Do a toothpick test by inserting it in the center and check if it comes out clean.

9. Take it out from the air fryer and allow it to settle down the heat before serving.

10.Enjoy your muffin.

**Nutrition:**

- 323 Calories
- 15.4g Fat
- 34g Protein

### 311.Jalapeno Cheese Balls

**Difficulty:** Average
**Preparation Time:** 10 minutes
**Cooking Time:** 8 minutes
**Servings:** 1
**Ingredients:**

- 1 Ounce cream cheese (2 healthy fats)
- 1/6 Cup shredded mozzarella cheese (1/3 healthy fat)
- 1/6 Cup shredded Cheddar cheese (1/3 healthy fat)
- 1/2 Jalapeños, finely chopped (1 green)
- 1/2 Cup breadcrumbs (1 healthy fat)
- 2 eggs (4 healthy fats)
- 1/2 Cup all-purpose flour (1 healthy fat)
- Salt (1/2 condiment)
- Pepper (1/2 condiment)

**Directions:**

1.Combine the cream cheese, mozzarella, Cheddar, and jalapeños in a medium bowl. Mix well.

2.Form the cheese mixture into balls about an inch thick. You may also use a small ice cream scoop. It works well.

3.Arrange the cheese balls on a sheet pan and place in the freezer for 15 minutes. It will help the cheese balls maintain their shape while frying.

4.Spray the Instant Crisp Air Fryer basket with cooking oil. Place the breadcrumbs in a small bowl. In another small bowl, beat the eggs. In the third small bowl, combine the flour with salt and pepper to taste, and mix well. Remove the cheese balls from the freezer. Plunge the cheese balls in the flour, then the eggs, and then the breadcrumbs.

5.Place the cheese balls in the Instant Crisp Air Fryer. Spray with cooking oil. Lock the air fryer lid—Cook for 8 minutes.

6.Open the Instant Crisp Air Fryer and flip the cheese balls. I recommend flipping them instead of shaking, so the balls maintain their form. Cook an additional 4 minutes. Cool before serving.

**Nutrition:**
- 96 Calories
- 6g Fat
- 4g Protein

### 312.Cloud Focaccia Bread

**Breakfast**

**Difficulty:** Difficult

**Preparation Time:** 10 minutes

**Cooking Time:** 30 minutes

**Servings:** 2

**Ingredients:**
- Eggs, medium (separate yellow and white) – 2 (1 healthy fat)
- Cream cheese, low fat - 1½ tbsp (1 healthy fat)
- Sweetener, no-calorie - ½ pkt (1/2 condiment)
- Tartar cream - ¼ tsp (1/4 condiment)

**For Focaccia Bread**
- Olive oil – ½ tsp
- Rosemary - ½ tsp (1/2 green)
- Salt – 1/8 tsp (1/4 condiment)

**Directions:**
1.Combine thoroughly cream cheese, egg yolks, and the sweetener in a medium bowl.

2.Beat egg whites in a large bowl along with tartar cream until the whites become stiff peaks.

3.Now carefully fold the yellow yolk mixture into the egg whites without breaking the whites.

4.Line a parchment paper in the air fryer baking tray and place 4 scoops of the mixture without overlapping one another.

5.Set the temperature to 150°C and bake for 20 minutes.

6.Take out the bread, and brush olive oil on top and sprinkle Rosemary and salt.

7.Place it again into the air fryer and bake for further 10 minutes until the top becomes golden brown.

8.After baking, allow it to settle down the heat before serving.

**Nutrition:**
- 90 Calories
- 6.5g Fat
- 6g Protein

### 313.Asparagus Risotto with Chicken

**Difficulty:** Difficult

**Preparation Time:** 20 minutes

**Cooking Time:** 38 minutes

**Servings:** 2

**Ingredients:**

- Chicken breast – 1 lb. (2 lean)
- Pepper ground - ½ tsp (1/4 condiment)
- Salt - ¼ tsp (1/4 condiment)
- Butter, melted – 1 tbsp (1/2 healthy fat)
- Cauliflower, finely grated - ¾ lb. (1 green)
- Asparagus, finely chopped - ¼ lb. (1/2 green)
- Chicken stock - ¼ cup (1/2 condiment)
- Nutritional yeast flakes – 2 tbsp (1 condiment)

**Directions:**

1. Soak the chicken in running water and pat dry.
2. Preheat the air fryer to 180°C.
3. Season the chicken with pepper and salt.
4. Place it in an air fryer safe casserole and pour melted butter over it.
5. Air fry it for 30 minutes until the internal temperature of the meat reaches 70°C.
6. Pull it out from the air fryer and let it cool.
7. Now place the asparagus and cauliflower rice in the air fryer tray.
8. Pour the chicken stock over it and air fry for 8 minutes until the veggies become tender.
9. After cooking, remove the risotto and mix the yeast.
10. Cut the chicken and serve along with the risotto.

**Nutrition:**

- 382 Calories
- 8.6g Fat
- 60g Protein

### 314. Bell-Pepper Wrapped in Tortilla

**Difficulty:** Easy
**Preparation Time:** 5 minutes
**Cooking Time:** 15 minutes
**Servings:** 1
**Ingredients:**

- 1/4 Small red bell pepper (1/2 greens)
- 1/4 Tablespoon water (1/2 condiment)
- 1 large tortilla (1 healthy fat)
- 1-piece commercial vegan nuggets, chopped (3 leans)
- Mixed greens for garnish (6 greens)

**Directions:**

1. Preheat the Instant Crisp Air Fryer to 400°F.
2. In a skillet heated over medium heat, water sautés the vegan nuggets and bell peppers. Set aside.
3. Place filling inside the corn tortillas.
4. Fold the tortillas, place them inside the Instant Crisp Air Fryer, and cook for 15 minutes until the tortilla wraps are crispy.
5. Serve with mixed greens on top.

**Nutrition:**

- 548 Calories
- 21g Fat
- 46g Protein

### 315. Crispy Cauliflowers

**Difficulty:** Easy
**Preparation Time:** 10 minutes
**Cooking Time:** 10 minutes
**Servings:** 4
**Ingredients:**

- 2 Cup cauliflower florets, diced (6 greens)
- 1/2 Cup almond flour (1 healthy fat)
- 1/2 Cup coconut flour (1 healthy fat)
- Salt and pepper to taste (1/2 condiment)
- 1 Tsp. mixed herbs (1 green)
- 1 Tsp. chives, chopped (1 green)
- 1 Egg (1 lean)
- 1 Tsp. cumin (1 condiment)
- 1/2 Tsp. garlic powder (1 condiment)
- 1 Cup water (1 condiment)
- Oil for frying (1 condiment)

**Directions:**

1.Combine the egg, salt, garlic, water, cumin, chives, mixed herbs, pepper, and flour in a mixing bowl.

2.Stir in the cauliflower to the mixture and then fry them in oil until they become golden in color.

3.Serve.

**Nutrition:**

•3.3g Protein

•10.4g Fat

•259 Calories

### 316.Chicken Salad

**Difficulty:** Easy

**Preparation Time:** 15 minutes

**Cooking Time:** 40 minutes

**Servings:** 2

**Ingredients:**

**Salad making:**

- Eggplant, chopped - ½ cup. (1/2 green)
- Zucchini, chopped - ½ cup. (1/2 green)
- Cherry tomatoes halved - ½ cup. (1/2 green)
- Romaine lettuce – 3 cups (2 greens)
- Parmesan cheese, shredded - ¼ cup (1/4 healthy fat)
- Chicken breast - ¾ lb. (1 lean)
- Salt - ¼ tsp (1/4 condiment)
- Pepper ground - ¼ tsp (1/4 condiment)

**Dressing:**

- Fresh lemon juice - ½ tsp (1/2 condiment)
- Dijon mustard - ¼ tsp (1/4 condiment)
- Worcestershire sauce - ½ tsp (1/4 condiment)
- Clove garlic – 1 (1/4 condiment)
- Salt - ½ tsp (1/4 condiment)
- Pepper ground - ¼ tsp (1/4 condiment)
- Parmesan cheese, shredded – 1 tbsp (1/2 healthy fat)

- Mayonnaise, light – 1 tbsp (1/2 healthy fat)
- Olive oil, extra virgin - 1½ tsp (1 condiment)

**Directions:**

- Preheat the air fryer to 200°C.
- Clean, wash, and drain the chicken breast.
- Rub salt, pepper on the chicken breast, and keep aside for 15 minutes for marinating.
- Line a baking paper in the air fryer tray and spray some cooking on to it.
- Place zucchini and eggplant on the baking paper.
- Start baking by shaking intermittently for 20 minutes until they become tender.
- For preparing the dressing, combine all the ingredients in the dressing section in a medium bowl.
- Put the tomatoes, lettuce, air fried veggies in the dressing mixture, and toss well.
- Place the marinated chicken on the air fryer grill tray and broil for 20 minutes until the inside meat temperature reaches 75°C.
- After cooking, remove it and allow it to cool down.
- Slice the chicken and serve along with the dressing.

**Nutrition:**

- 370 Calories
- 14.3g Fat
- 45g Protein

### 317.Coconut Battered Cauliflower Bites

**Difficulty:** Average

**Preparation Time:** 5 minutes

**Cooking Time:** 20 minutes

**Servings:** 1

**Ingredients:**

•Salt and pepper to taste (2 condiments)

•1 flax egg or one tablespoon flaxseed meal + 3 tablespoon water (1 healthy fat)
•1 small cauliflower, cut into florets (2 greens)
•1 teaspoon mixed spice (1 condiment)
•1/2 teaspoon mustard powder (1 condiment)
•2 tablespoons maple syrup (2 healthy fats)
•1 clove of garlic, minced (1 green)
•2 tablespoons soy sauce (2 condiments)
•1/3 Cup oats flour (1/2 healthy fat)
•1/3 Cup plain flour (1/2 healthy fat)
•1/3 Cup desiccated coconut (1/2 lean)

**Directions:**

1. In a mixing bowl, mix oats, flour, and desiccated coconut. Season with salt and pepper to taste. Set aside.
2. In another bowl, place the flax egg and add a pinch of salt to taste. Set aside.
3. Season the cauliflower with mixed spice and mustard powder.
4. Dredge the florets in the flax egg first, then in the flour mixture.
5. Place inside the Instant Crisp Air Fryer, lock the air fryer lid and cook at 400°F or 15 minutes.
6. Meanwhile, place the maple syrup, garlic, and soy sauce in a saucepan and heat over medium flame. Wait for it to boil and adjust the heat to low until the sauce thickens.
7. After 15 minutes, take out the Instant Crisp Air Fryer's florets and place them in the saucepan.
8. Toss to coat the florets and place inside the Instant Crisp Air Fryer and cook for another 5 minutes.

**Nutrition:**

•154 Calories
•2.3g Fat
•4.6g Protein



## 318. Lemon Garlic Oregano Boneless Chicken

**Difficulty:** Average
**Preparation Time:** 5 minutes
**Cooking Time:** 44 minutes
**Servings:** 2

**Ingredients:**

•Chicken breast boneless, skinless - ½ lb. (1 lean)
•Lemon juice – 1 tbsp (1/2 condiment)
•Clove Garlic, minced – 1 (1/2 condiment)
•Oregano fresh, minced – 1 tbsp (1/2 green)
•Black pepper, ground - ¼ tsp (1/4 condiment)
•Salt - ¼ tsp (1/4 condiment)
•Asparagus ends trimmed – 1 lb. (2 greens)
•Water – 1 cup (1/2 condiment)

**Directions:**

1. Soak, wash, and pat dry chicken.
2. Situate the chicken in a big bowl and marinate with pepper, lemon juice, salt, garlic, and oregano.
3. Place the marinated chicken in the air fry grill tray.
4. Broil at 175°C for 40 minutes until the meat's internal temperature reaches 70°C.
5. After broiling, remove it from the air fryer and set it aside.
6. Now place the asparagus in the air fry ray and pour 1 cup water.
7. Air fry at 175°C for 4 minutes until the asparagus becomes tender.
8. Remove it from the air fryer and drain the water.
9. Slice the chicken and serve along with asparagus.

**Nutrition:**

•258 Calories
•11g Fat
•29g Protein

# Lunch Recipes

### 319.Lemon Butter Scallops
**Preparation Time:** 15 minutes
**Cooking Time:** 30 minutes
**Servings:** 1
**Ingredients:**
- 1 lemon
- 1 lb. scallops
- ½ cup butter
- ¼ cup parsley, chopped

**Directions:**
1.Juice the lemon into a Ziploc bag.
2.Wash your scallops, dry them, and season to taste. Put them in the bag with the lemon juice. Refrigerate for an hour.
3.Remove the bag from the refrigerator and leave for about twenty minutes until it returns to room temperature. Transfer the scallops into a foil pan that is small enough to be placed inside the fryer.
4.Pre-heat the fryer at 400°F and put the rack inside.
5.Place the foil pan on the rack and cook for five minutes.
6.In the meantime, melt the butter in a saucepan over a medium heat. Zest the lemon over the saucepan, then add in the chopped parsley. Mix well.
7.Take care when removing the pan from the fryer. Transfer the contents to a plate and drizzle with the lemon-butter mixture. Serve hot.

**Nutrition:**
Calories: 420
Fat: 12g
Protein: 23g
Sugar: 13g

### 320.Cheesy Lemon Halibut
**Preparation Time:** 10 minutes
**Cooking Time:** 20 minutes
**Servings:** 2
**Ingredients:**
- 1 lb. halibut fillet
- ½ cup butter
- 2 ½ tbsp. mayonnaise
- 2 ½ tbsp. lemon juice
- ¾ cup parmesan cheese, grated

**Directions:**
1.Pre-heat your fryer at 375°F.
2.Spritz the halibut fillets with cooking spray and season as desired.
3.Put the halibut in the fryer and cook for twelve minutes.
4.In the meantime, combine the butter, mayonnaise, and lemon juice in a bowl with a hand mixer. Ensure a creamy texture is achieved.
5.Stir in the grated parmesan.
6.When the halibut is ready, open the drawer and spread the butter over the fish with a butter knife. Allow to cook for a further two minutes, then serve hot.

**Nutrition:**
Calories: 432
Fat: 18g
Protein: 14g
Sugar: 12g

### 321.Spicy Mackerel
**Preparation Time:** 10 minutes
**Cooking Time:** 20 minutes
**Servings:** 2
**Ingredients:**
- 2 mackerel fillets
- 2 tbsp. red chili flakes
- 2 tsp. garlic, minced
- 1 tsp. lemon juice

**Directions:**

1.Season the mackerel fillets with the red pepper flakes, minced garlic, and a drizzle of lemon juice. Allow to sit for five minutes.

2.Preheat your fryer at 350°F.

3.Cook the mackerel for five minutes, before opening the drawer, flipping the fillets, and allowing to cook on the other side for another five minutes.

4.Plate the fillets, making sure to spoon any remaining juice over them before serving.

**Nutrition:**

Calories: 240

Fat: 4g

Protein: 16g

Sugar: 3g

### 322.Thyme Scallops

**Preparation Time:** 5 minutes

**Cooking Time:** 12 minutes

**Servings:** 1

**Ingredients:**

- 1 lb. scallops
- Salt and pepper
- ½ tbsp. butter
- ½ cup thyme, chopped

**Directions:**

1.Wash the scallops and dry them completely. Season with pepper and salt, then set aside while you prepare the pan.

2.Grease a foil pan in several spots with the butter and cover the bottom with the thyme. Place the scallops on top.

3.Pre-heat the fryer at 400°F and set the rack inside.

4.Place the foil pan on the rack and allow to cook for seven minutes.

5.Take care when removing the pan from the fryer and transfer the scallops to a serving dish. Spoon any remaining butter in the pan over the fish and enjoy.



**Nutrition:**

Calories: 291

Fat: 9g

Protein: 17g

Sugar: 5g

### 323.Chinese Pancetta Mix

**Difficulty:** Average

**Preparation Time:** 10 minutes

**Cooking Time:** 12 minutes

**Servings:** 4

**Ingredients:**

2 eggs (1 healthy fat)

2 pounds Pancetta, cut into medium cubes (1 lean)

1 cup cornstarch (1/2 condiment)

1 tsp. sesame oil (1/2 condiment)

Salt and black pepper to the taste (1/2 condiment)

A pinch of Chinese five-spice (1/2 condiment)

3 tbsp. canola oil (1/2 healthy fat)

Sweet ketchup for serving (1/2 condiment)

**Directions:**

In a bowl, mix five spices with salt, pepper, and cornstarch and mix.

Scourge eggs with the sesame oil and beat well.

Dip the bacon cubes into the cornstarch mixture, then dip the eggs and place them in the air fryer you greased with canola oil.

Bake at 340 ° F for 12 minutes, shaking the fryer once.

Serve the bacon for lunch with the sweet ketchup on the side.

**Nutrition:**

125 Calories

7.9g Fat

8.3g Protein

## 324.Crispy Calamari

**Preparation Time:** 5 minutes
**Cooking Time:** 15 minutes
**Servings:** 4
**Ingredients:**
- 1 lb. fresh squid
- Salt and pepper
- 2 cups flour
- 1 cup water
- 2 cloves garlic, minced
- ½ cup mayonnaise

**Directions:**
1.Remove the skin from the squid and discard any ink. Slice the squid into rings and season with some salt and pepper.
2.Put the flour and water in separate bowls. Dip the squid firstly in the flour, then into the water, then into the flour again, ensuring that it is entirely covered with flour.
3.Pre-heat the fryer at 400°F. Put the squid inside and cook for six minutes.
4.In the meantime, prepare the aioli by combining the garlic with the mayonnaise in a bowl.
5.Once the squid is ready, plate up and serve with the aioli.

**Nutrition:**
Calories: 247
Fat: 3g
Protein: 18g
Sugar: 3g

## 325.Filipino Bistek

**Preparation Time:** 5 minutes
**Cooking Time:** 10 minutes
**Servings:** 4
**Ingredients:**
- 2 milkfish bellies, deboned and sliced into 4 portions
- ¾ tsp. salt
- ¼ tsp. ground black pepper
- ¼ tsp. cumin powder
- 2 tbsp. calamansi juice
- 2 lemongrasses, trimmed and cut crosswise into small pieces
- ½ cup tamari sauce
- 2 tbsp. fish sauce
- 2 tbsp. sugar
- 1 tsp. garlic powder
- ½ cup chicken broth
- 2 tbsp. olive oil

**Directions:**
1.Dry the fish using some paper towels.
2.Put the fish in a large bowl and coat with the rest of the ingredients. Allow to marinate for 3 hours in the refrigerator.
3.Cook the fish steaks on an Air Fryer grill basket at 340°F for 5 minutes.
4.Turn the steaks over and allow to grill for an additional 4 minutes. Cook until medium brown.
5.Serve with steamed white rice.

**Nutrition:**
Calories: 259
Fat: 3g
Protein: 10g
Sugar: 2g

## 326.Saltine Fish Fillets

**Preparation Time:** 10 minutes
**Cooking Time:** 15 minutes
**Servings:** 4
**Ingredients:**
- 1 cup crushed saltines
- ¼ cup extra-virgin olive oil
- 1 tsp. garlic powder
- ½ tsp. shallot powder
- 1 egg, well whisked
- 4 white fish fillets

•Salt and ground black pepper to taste
•Fresh Italian parsley to serve
**Directions:**
1.In a shallow bowl, combine the crushed saltines and olive oil.
2.In a separate bowl, mix together the garlic powder, shallot powder, and the beaten egg.
3.Sprinkle a good amount of salt and pepper over the fish, before dipping each fillet into the egg mixture.
4.Coat the fillets with the crumb mixture.
5.Air fry the fish at 370°F for 10 - 12 minutes.
6.Serve with fresh parsley.
**Nutrition:**
Calories: 502
Fat: 4g
Protein: 11g
Sugar: 9g

# Dinner Recipes

## 327. Air Fryer Sweet & Sour Chicken

**Preparation Time**: 5 minutes
**Cooking Time**: 10 minutes
**Servings**: 2
**Ingredients**
Chicken
•4 cups chicken breasts /thighs: cut into one-inch pieces
•Cornstarch: 2 tablespoons
Sweet & Sour Sauce
•Cornstarch: 2 tablespoons
•Pineapple juice: 1 cup
•Water: 2 tablespoons
•Stevia: 1 tbsp
•Soy sauce: 1 tablespoon
•Rice wine vinegar: 3 tablespoons
•Ground ginger: 1/4 teaspoon
Optional
•1/4 cup pineapple chunks
•3-4 drops of red food coloring (for traditional orange look)
**Directions:**
1.Let the air fryer preheat to 400 degrees.
2.Coat the chicken in cornstarch, until the chicken is coated completely.
3.Put the chicken in the air fryer and let it cook for 7, 9 minutes. Take out from air fryer
4.In the meantime, in a saucepan, add pineapple juice, ginger, stevia, soy sauce, and rice wine vinegar and cook. Let it simmer for five minutes.
5.Make cornstarch slurry and add in the sauce. Let it simmer for one minute.
6.Coat cooked chicken pieces and Servings with steamed vegetables

**Nutrition**: Cal 302|Fat: 8g| Carbs 18g|Protein 22g

## 328. Low Carb Air-Fried Calzones

**Preparation Time**: 15 minutes
**Cooking Time**: 27 minutes
**Servings**: 2
**Ingredients**
•Cooked chicken breast: 1/3 cup(shredded)
•One teaspoon olive oil
•Spinach leaves(baby): 3 cups
•Whole-wheat pizza dough, freshly prepared
•Marinara sauce: 1/3 cup(lower-sodium)
•Diced red onion:1/4 cup
•Skim mozzarella cheese: 6 Tbsp.
•Cooking spray
**Directions:**
1.In a medium skillet, over a medium flame, add oil, onions. Sauté until soft. Then add spinach leaves, cook until wilted. Turn off the heat and add chicken and marinara sauce.
2.Cut the dough into two pieces.
3.Add 1/4 of the spinach mix on each circle dough piece.
4.Add skim shredded cheese on top. Fold the dough over and crimp the edges.
5.Spray the calzones with cooking spray.
6.Put calzones in the air fryer. Cook for 12 minutes, at 325°F until dough is light brown. Turn the calzone over and cook for eight more minutes.
**Nutrition**: Calories 348|Fat 12g | Protein 21g |Carbohydrate 18g

### 329.Air Fryer Popcorn Chicken

**Preparation Time:** 10 minutes
**Cooking Time:** 20 minutes
**Servings:** 2
**Ingredients**
**For Marinade**
•8 cups, chicken tenders, cut into bite-size pieces
•Freshly ground black pepper: 1/2 tsp
•Almond milk: 2 cups
•Salt: 1 tsp
•paprika: 1/2 tsp
**Dry Mix**
•Salt: 3 tsp
•Flour: 3 cups
•Paprika: 2 tsp
•Oil spray
•Freshly ground black pepper: 2 tsp
**Directions:**
1.In a bowl, add all marinade ingredients and chicken. Mix well, and put it in a Zip lock bag and refrigerator for two hours for the minimum, or six hours.
2.In a large bowl, add all the dry ingredients.
3.Coat the marinated chicken to the dry mix. Into the marinade again then for the second time in the dry mixture.
4.Spray the air fryer basket with olive oil and place the breaded chicken pieces in one single layer. Spray oil over the chicken pieces too.
5.Cook at 370 degrees for 10 minutes, tossing halfway through.
6.Serve immediately with salad greens or dipping sauce.
**Nutrition**: Calories 340 |Proteins 20g |Carbs 14g |Fat 10g |

### 330.Air Fried Cheesy Chicken Omelet

**Preparation Time**: 5 minutes
**Cooking Time:** 18 minutes
**Servings:** 2
**Ingredients**
•Cooked Chicken Breast: half cup(diced)divided
•Four eggs
•Onion powder: 1/4 tsp, divided
•Salt: 1/2 tsp., divided
•Pepper: 1/4 tsp., divided
•Shredded cheese: 2 tbsp. divided
•Granulated garlic: 1/4 tsp, divided
**Directions:**
1Take two ramekins, grease with olive oil.
2Add two eggs in each ramekin. Add cheese with seasoning.
3Blend to combine. Add 1/4 cup of cooked chicken on top.
4Cook for 14-18 minutes, in the air fryer at 330 F, or until fully cooked.
**Nutrition**: Calories 185 |Proteins 20g |Carbs 10g |Fat 5g |

### 331.Air-Fried Tortilla Hawaiian Pizza

**Preparation Time:** 10 minutes
**Cooking Time:** 20 minutes
**Servings:** 1
**Ingredients**
•Mozzarella Cheese
•Tortilla wrap
•Tomato sauce: 1 tbsp.
•Toppings
•Cooked chicken shredded or hotdog: 2 tbsp.
•Pineapple pieces: 3 tbsp.
•Ham: half slice, cut into pieces
•Cheese slice cut into pieces

**Directions**:

1.Lay tortilla flat on a plate, add tomato sauce and spread it.

2.Add some shredded mozzarella, add toppings. Top with cheese slices

3.Put in the air fryer and cook for five or ten minutes at 160 C.

4.Take out from the air fryer and slice it. Serve hot with baby spinach.

**Nutrition**: Calories 178 |Proteins 21g |Carbs 15g |Fat 15g |

### 332.Air Fryer Personal Mini Pizza

**Preparation Time**: 2 minutes

**Cooking Time:** 5 minutes

**Servings:** 1

**Ingredients**

•Sliced olives: 1/4 cup

•One pita bread

•One tomato

•Shredded cheese: 1/2 cup

**Directions:**

1.Let the air fryer preheat to 350 F

2.Lay pita flat on a plate. Add cheese, slices of tomatoes, and olives.

3.Cook for five minutes at 350 F

4.Take the pizza out of the air fryer.

5.Slice it and enjoy

**Nutrition**: Calories: 344kcal | Carbohydrates: 37g | Protein: 18g | Fat: 13g |

### 333.Air Fryer Chicken Nuggets

**Preparation Time**: 15 minutes

**Cooking Time**: 15 minutes

**Servings**: 4

**Ingredients**

•Olive oil spray

•Skinless boneless: 2 chicken breasts, cut into bite pieces

•Half tsp. of kosher salt& freshly ground black pepper, to taste

•Grated parmesan cheese: 2 tablespoons

•Italian seasoned breadcrumbs: 6 tablespoons (whole wheat)

•Whole wheat breadcrumbs: 2 tablespoons

•olive oil: 2 teaspoons

**Directions**:

1.Let the air fryer preheat for 8 minutes, to 400 F

2.In a big mixing bowl, add panko, parmesan cheese, and breadcrumbs and mix well.

3.Sprinkle kosher salt and pepper on chicken and olive oil, mix well.

4.Take a few pieces of chicken, dunk them to breadcrumbs mixture.

5.Put these pieces in an air fryer and spray with olive oil.

6.Cook for 8 minutes, turning halfway through

7.Enjoy with kale chips.

**Nutrition**: Calories: 188kcal, Carbohydrates: 8g, Protein: 25g, Fat: 4.5g

### 334.5-Ingredient Air Fryer Lemon Chicken

**Preparation Time**: 5 minutes

**Cooking Time**: 15 minutes

**Servings**: 4

**Ingredients**

•Whole-wheat crumbs: 1 and 1/2 cups

•Six pieces of chicken tenderloins

•Two eggs

•Two half lemons and lemon slices

•Kosher salt to taste

**Directions**:

1.In a dish, whisk the eggs.

2.In a separate dish, add the breadcrumbs

3.With egg, coat the chicken and roll in breadcrumbs.

4.Add the breaded chicken in the air fryer

5.Cook for 14 minutes at 400 F, flip the chicken halfway through.

6.Take out from air fryer and squeeze lemon juice and sprinkle with kosher salt and Serve with lemon slices.

**Nutrition**: Cal 240| Fat: 12g| Net Carbs: 13g|Protein: 27g

### 335.Low Carb Chicken Tenders

**Preparation Time**: 10 minutes
**Cooking Time**: 20 minutes
**Servings**: 3
**Ingredients**

- Chicken tenderloins: 4 cups
- Eggs: one
- Superfine Almond Flour: ½ cup
- Powdered Parmesan cheese: ½ cup
- Kosher Sea salt: ½ teaspoon
- (1-teaspoon) freshly ground black pepper
- (1/2 teaspoon) Cajun seasoning,

**Directions:**

1.On a small plate, pour the beaten egg.

2.Mix all ingredients in a zip lock bag the cheese. Almond flour freshly ground black pepper & kosher salt and other seasonings.

3.Spray the air fryer with oil spray.

4.To avoid clumpy fingers with breading and egg. Use different hands for egg and breading. Dip each tender in egg and then in bread until they are all breaded.

5.Using a fork to place one tender at a time. Bring it in the zip lock bag and shake the bag forcefully. make sure all the tenders are covered in almond mixture

6.Using the fork to take out the tender and place it in your air fryer basket.

7.Spray oil on the tenders.

8.Cook for 12 minutes at 350F, or before 160F registers within. Raise temperature to 400F to shade the surface for 3 minutes.

9.Serve with sauce.

174

**Nutrition**: Calories 280 |Proteins 20g |Carbs 6g|Fat 10g |Fiber 5g

### 336.Cheesy Cauliflower Tots

**Preparation Time**: 15 minutes
**Cooking Time:** 12 minutes
**Servings**: 4
**Ingredients**

- 1 large head cauliflower
- 1 cup shredded mozzarella cheese
- 1/2 cup grated Parmesan cheese
- 1 large egg
- 1/4 teaspoon garlic powder
- 1/4 teaspoon dried parsley
- 1/8 teaspoon onion powder

**Directions:**

1.Fill a big pot with 2 cups of water on the stovetop, and insert a steamer in the oven. Put to boil bath.

2.Break the cauliflower into flower and placed on a steamer box—cover pot and lid.

3.Let steam the cauliflower for 7 minutes until the fork-tender. Put in the cheesecloth or clean kitchen towel from the steamer basket and let it cool.

4.Push on the sink to eliminate as much extra humidity as possible. If not all of the moisture is removed, the mixture will be too soft to form into tots.

5.Mash down to a smooth consistency with a blade.

6.In a large mixing bowl, put the cauliflower and add the mozzarella, parmesan, egg, garlic powder, parsley, and onion powder. Remove until well combined. The blend should be smooth but easy to mold.

7.Take 2 tablespoons of the mixture and roll the mixture into a tot form. Repeat with mixture leftover. Put the basket into the air fryer.

8.Set the temperature to 320 ° F and adjust the timer for 12 minutes.

9.Turn the tots halfway through the period of cooking.

10.Cauliflower tots should be golden when fully cooked. Serve warm.

**Nutrition**: calories: 181| protein 13.5g|fiber 3.0g| carbohydrates: 6.6 g |fat: 9.5 g|

### 337.Tasty Kale & Celery Crackers

**Preparation Time**: 10 minutes

**Cooking Time**: 20 minutes

**Servings**: 2

**Ingredients**

•One cups flax seed, ground

•1 cups flax seed, soaked overnight and drained

•2 bunches kale, chopped

•1 bunch basil, chopped

•½ bunch celery, chopped

•2 garlic cloves, minced

•1/3 cup olive oil

**Directions**:

1.Mix the ground flaxseed with the celery, kale, basil, and garlic in your food processor and mix well.

2.Add the oil and soaked flaxseed, then mix again, scatter in the pan of your air fryer, break into medium crackers and cook for 20 minutes at 380 degrees F.

3.Serve as an appetizer and break into cups.

4.Enjoy

**Nutrition**: calories 143|fat 1g| fiber 2g| carbs 8g| Protein 4g

### 338.Parmesan Sweet Potato Casserole

**Preparation Time**: 15 minutes

**Cooking Time**: 35 minutes

**Servings**: 2

**Ingredients:**

•2 sweet potatoes, peeled

•½ yellow onion, sliced

•½ cup cream

•¼ cup spinach

•2 oz. Parmesan cheese, shredded

•½ teaspoon salt

•1 tomato

•1 teaspoon olive oil

**Directions:**

1.Chop the sweet potatoes.

2.Chop the tomato.

3.Chop the spinach.

4.Spray the air fryer tray with the olive oil.

5.Then place on the layer of the chopped sweet potato.

6.Add the layer of the sliced onion.

7.After this, sprinkle the sliced onion with the chopped spinach and tomatoes.

8.Sprinkle the casserole with the salt and shredded cheese.

9.Pour cream.

10.Preheat the air fryer to 390 F.

11.Cover the air fryer tray with the foil.

12.Cook the casserole for 35 minutes.

13.When the casserole is cooked – serve it.

*14.*Enjoy!

**Nutrition:** Calories: 93 Fat: 1.8g Fiber: 3.4g Carbs: 20.3g Protein: 1.8g

### 339.Spicy Zucchini Slices

**Preparation Time**: 10 minutes

**Cooking Time**: 6 minutes

**Servings**: 2

**Ingredients:**

•1 teaspoon cornstarch

•1 zucchini

•½ teaspoon chili flakes

•1 tablespoon flour

•1 egg

•¼ teaspoon salt

**Directions:**

1.Slice the zucchini and sprinkle with the chili flakes and salt.

2.Crack the egg into the bowl and whisk it.

3.Dip the zucchini slices in the whisked egg.

4.Combine together cornstarch with the flour. Stir it.

5.Coat the zucchini slices with the cornstarch mixture.

6.Preheat the air fryer to 400 F.

7.Place the zucchini slices in the air fryer tray.

8.Cook the zucchini slices for 4 minutes.

9.After this, flip the slices to another side and cook for 2 minutes more.

10. Serve the zucchini slices hot.

*11.* Enjoy!

**Nutrition:** Calories: 67 Fat: 2.4g Fiber: 1.2g Carbs: 7.7g Protein: 4.4g

### 340.Cheddar Potato Gratin

**Preparation Time**: 15 minutes

**Cooking Time:** 20 minutes

**Servings:** 2

**Ingredients:**

•2 potatoes

•1/3 cup half and half

•1 tablespoon oatmeal flour

•¼ teaspoon ground black pepper

•1 egg

•2 oz. Cheddar cheese

**Directions:**

1.Wash the potatoes and slice them into thin pieces.

2.Preheat the air fryer to 365 F.

3.Put the potato slices in the air fryer and cook them for 10 minutes.

4.Meanwhile, combine the half and half, oatmeal flour, and ground black pepper.

176

5.Crack the egg into the liquid and whisk it carefully.

6.Shred Cheddar cheese.

7.When the potato is cooked – take 2 ramekins and place the potatoes on them.

8.Pour the half and half mixture.

9.Sprinkle the gratin with shredded Cheddar cheese.

10.Cook the gratin for 10 minutes at 360 F.

11.Serve the meal immediately.

*12.*Enjoy!

**Nutrition:** Calories: 353 Fat: 16.6g Fiber: 5.4g Carbs: 37.2g Protein: 15g

### 341.Salty Lemon Artichokes

**Preparation Time**: 15 minutes

**Cooking Time:** 45 minutes

**Servings:** 2

**Ingredients:**

•1 lemon

•2 artichokes

•1 teaspoon kosher salt

•1 garlic head

•2 teaspoons olive oil

**Directions:**

1.Cut off the edges of the artichokes.

2.Cut the lemon into the halves.

3.Peel the garlic head and chop the garlic cloves roughly.

4.Then place the chopped garlic in the artichokes.

5.Sprinkle the artichokes with the olive oil and kosher salt.

6.Then squeeze the lemon juice into the artichokes.

7.Wrap the artichokes in the foil.

8.Preheat the air fryer to 330 F.

9.Place the wrapped artichokes in the air fryer and cook for 45 minutes.

10. When the artichokes are cooked – discard the foil and serve.

*11.* Enjoy!
**Nutrition:** Calories: 133 Fat: 5g Fiber: 9.7g Carbs: 21.7g Protein: 6g

## 342.Asparagus & Parmesan

**Preparation Time**: 10 minutes
**Cooking Time:** 6 minutes
**Servings:** 2
**Ingredients:**
- 1 teaspoon sesame oil
- 11 oz. asparagus
- 1 teaspoon chicken stock
- ½ teaspoon ground white pepper
- 3 oz. Parmesan

**Directions:**
1.Wash the asparagus and chop it roughly.
2.Sprinkle the chopped asparagus with the chicken stock and ground white pepper.
3.Then sprinkle the vegetables with the sesame oil and shake them.
4.Place the asparagus in the air fryer basket.
5.Cook the vegetables for 4 minutes at 400 F.
6.Meanwhile, shred Parmesan cheese.
7.When the time is over – shake the asparagus gently and sprinkle with the shredded cheese.
8.Cook the asparagus for 2 minutes more at 400 F.
9.After this, transfer the cooked asparagus in the serving plates.
*10.* Serve and taste it!
**Nutrition:** Calories: 189 Fat: 11.6g Fiber: 3.4g Carbs: 7.9g Protein: 17.2g

## 343.Carrot Lentil Burgers

**Preparation Time**: 10 minutes
**Cooking Time:** 12 minutes
**Servings:** 2
**Ingredients:**
- 6 oz. lentils, cooked
- 1 egg
- 2 oz. carrot, grated
- 1 teaspoon semolina
- ½ teaspoon salt
- 1 teaspoon turmeric
- 1 tablespoon butter

**Directions:**
1.Crack the egg into the bowl and whisk it.
2.Add the cooked lentils and mash the mixture with the help of the fork.
3.Then sprinkle the mixture with the grated carrot, semolina, salt, and turmeric.
4.Mix it up and make the medium burgers.
5.Put the butter into the lentil burgers. It will make them juicy.
6.Preheat the air fryer to 360 F.
7.Put the lentil burgers in the air fryer and cook for 12 minutes.
8.Flip the burgers into another side after 6 minutes of cooking.
9.Then chill the cooked lentil burgers and serve them.
*10.* Enjoy!
**Nutrition:** Calories: 404 Fat: 9g Fiber: 26.9g Carbs: 56g Protein: 25.3g

## 344.Corn on Cobs

**Preparation Time**: 10 minutes
**Cooking Time:** 10 minutes
**Servings:** 2
**Ingredients:**
- 2 fresh corn on cobs
- 2 teaspoon butter
- 1 teaspoon salt
- 1 teaspoon paprika
- ¼ teaspoon olive oil

**Directions:**
1.Preheat the air fryer to 400 F.

2.Rub the corn on cobs with the salt and paprika.

3.Then sprinkle the corn on cobs with the olive oil.

4.Place the corn on cobs in the air fryer basket.

5.Cook the corn on cobs for 10 minutes.

6.When the time is over – transfer the corn on cobs in the serving plates and rub with the butter gently.

7.Serve the meal immediately.

8.Enjoy!

**Nutrition:** Calories: 122 Fat: 5.5g Fiber: 2.4g Carbs: 17.6g Protein: 3.2g

### 345.Sugary Carrot Strips

**Preparation Time**: 10 minutes

**Cooking Time:** 10 minutes

**Servings:** 2

**Ingredients:**

•2 carrots

•1 teaspoon stevia

•1 teaspoon olive oil

•1 tablespoon soy sauce

•1 teaspoon honey

•½ teaspoon ground black pepper

**Directions:**

1.Peel the carrot and cut it into the strips.

2.Then put the carrot strips in the bowl.

3.Sprinkle the carrot strips with the olive oil, soy sauce, honey, and ground black pepper.

4.Shake the mixture gently.

5.Preheat the air fryer to 360 F.

6.Cook the carrot for 10 minutes.

7.After this, shake the carrot strips well.

8.Enjoy!

**Nutrition:** Calories: 67 Fat: 2.4g Fiber: 1.7g Carbs: 11.3g Protein: 1.1g

### 346.Onion Green Beans

**Preparation Time**: 10 minutes

**Cooking Time:** 12 minutes

**Servings:** 2

**Ingredients:**

•11 oz. green beans

•1 tablespoon onion powder

•1 tablespoon olive oil

•½ teaspoon salt

•¼ teaspoon chili flakes

**Directions:**

1.Wash the green beans carefully and place them in the bowl.

2.Sprinkle the green beans with the onion powder, salt, chili flakes, and olive oil.

3.Shake the green beans carefully.

4.Preheat the air fryer to 400 F.

5.Put the green beans in the air fryer and cook for 8 minutes.

6.After this, shake the green beans and cook them for 4 minutes more at 400 F.

7.When the time is over – shake the green beans.

8.Serve the side dish and enjoy!

**Nutrition:** Calories: 1205 Fat: 7.2g Fiber: 5.5g Carbs: 13.9g Protein: 3.2g

### 347.Mozzarella Radish Salad

**Preparation Time**: 10 minutes

**Cooking Time:** 20 minutes

**Servings:** 2

**Ingredients:**

•8 oz. radish

•4 oz. Mozzarella

•1 teaspoon balsamic vinegar

•½ teaspoon salt

•1 tablespoon olive oil

•1 teaspoon dried oregano

**Directions:**

1.Wash the radish carefully and cut it into the halves.

2.Preheat the air fryer to 360 F.

3.Put the radish halves in the air fryer basket.
4.Sprinkle the radish with the salt and olive oil.
5.Cook the radish for 20 minutes.
6.Shake the radish after 10 minutes of cooking.
7.When the time is over – transfer the radish to the serving plate.
8.Chop Mozzarella roughly.
9.Sprinkle the radish with Mozzarella, balsamic vinegar, and dried oregano.
10.                Stir it gently with the help of 2 forks.
11.                 Serve it immediately.
**Nutrition:** Calories: 241 Fat: 17.2g Fiber: 2.1g Carbs: 6.4g Protein: 16.9g

### 348.Cremini Mushroom

**Preparation Time**: 10 minutes
**Cooking Time:** 6 minutes
**Servings:** 2
**Ingredients:**
•7 oz. cremini mushrooms
•2 tablespoon coconut milk
•1 tablespoon butter
•1 teaspoon chili flakes
•½ teaspoon balsamic vinegar
•½ teaspoon curry powder
•½ teaspoon white pepper
**Directions:**
1.Wash the mushrooms carefully.
2.Then sprinkle the mushrooms with the chili flakes, curry powder, and white pepper.
3.Preheat the air fryer to 400 F.
4.Toss the butter in the air fryer basket and melt it.
5.Put the mushrooms in the air fryer and cook for 2 minutes.
6.Shake the mushrooms well and sprinkle with the coconut milk and balsamic vinegar.
7.Cook the mushrooms for 4 minutes more at 400 F.
8.Then skewer the mushrooms on the wooden sticks and serve.
9.Enjoy!
**Nutrition:** Calories 116 Fat: 9.5g Fiber: 1.3g Carbs: 5.6g Protein: 3g

### 349.Eggplant Ratatouille

**Preparation Time**: 15 minutes
**Cooking Time:** 15 minutes
**Servings:** 2
**Ingredients:**
•1 eggplant
•1 sweet yellow pepper
•3 cherry tomatoes
•1/3 white onion, chopped
•½ teaspoon garlic clove, sliced
•1 teaspoon olive oil
•½ teaspoon ground black pepper
•½ teaspoon Italian seasoning
**Directions:**
1.Preheat the air fryer to 360 F.
2.Peel the eggplants and chop them.
3.Put the chopped eggplants in the air fryer basket.
4.Chop the cherry tomatoes and add them to the air fryer basket.
5.Then add chopped onion, sliced garlic clove, olive oil, ground black pepper, and Italian seasoning.
6.Chop the sweet yellow pepper roughly and add it to the air fryer basket.
7.Shake the vegetables gently and cook for 15 minutes.
8.Stir the meal after 8 minutes of cooking.
9.Transfer the cooked ratatouille in the serving plates.
10. Enjoy!

**Nutrition:** Calories: 149 Fat: 3.7g Fiber: 11.7g Carbs: 28.9g Protein: 5.1g

### 350.Cheddar Portobello Mushrooms

**Preparation Time**: 15 minutes
**Cooking Time:** 6 minutes
**Servings:** 2
**Ingredients:**
•2 Portobello mushroom hats
•2 slices Cheddar cheese
•¼ cup panko breadcrumbs
•½ teaspoon salt
•½ teaspoon ground black pepper
•1 egg
•1 teaspoon oatmeal
•2 oz. bacon, chopped cooked
**Directions:**
1.Crack the egg into the bowl and whisk it.
2.Combine the ground black pepper, oatmeal, salt, and breadcrumbs in the separate bowl.
3.Dip the mushroom hats in the whisked egg.
4.After this, coat the mushroom hats in the breadcrumb mixture.
5.Preheat the air fryer to 400 F.
6.Place the mushrooms in the air fryer basket tray and cook for 3 minutes.
7.After this, put the chopped bacon and sliced cheese over the mushroom hats and cook the meal for 3 minutes.
8.When the meal is cooked – let it chill gently.
9.Enjoy!
**Nutrition:** Calories: 376 Fat: 24.1g Fiber: 1.8g Carbs: 14.6g Protein: 25.2g

### 351.Salty Edamame

**Preparation Time**: 15 minutes
**Cooking Time:** 6 minutes
**Servings:** 2
**Ingredients:**

•1 cup of edamame, inside a shell
•The salt, for taste
**Directions:**
1.Over a medium-low heat, place a large saucepan. Add 2 quarts of edamame and water. Cover and simmer for about 5-8 minutes, until tender.
2.Drain and add salt to sprinkle.
**Nutrition:** Calories: 376 Fat: 24.1g Fiber: 1.8g Carbs: 14.6g Protein: 25.2g

# Snack and Appetizer Recipes

### 352.Greek Tuna Salad Bites

**Preparation Time:** 5 Minutes
**Cooking Time:** 10 Minutes
**Servings:** 6
**Ingredients:**

- Cucumbers (2 medium)
- White tuna (2 - 6 oz. cans.)
- Lemon juice (half of 1 lemon)
- Red bell pepper (.5 cup)
- Sweet/red onion (.25 cup)
- Black olives (.25 cup)
- Garlic (2 tablespoon.)
- Olive oil (2 tablespoon.)
- Fresh parsley (2 tablespoon.)
- Dried oregano - salt & pepper (as desired)

**Directions:**

1.Drain and flake the tuna. Juice the lemon. Dice/chop the onions, olives, pepper, parsley, and garlic. Slice each of the cucumbers into thick rounds (skin off or on).
2.In a mixing container, combine the rest of the fixings.
3.Place a heaping spoonful of salad onto the rounds and enjoy for your next party or just a snack.

**Nutrition:**

Calories: 400
Fats: 22 g
Carbs: 26 g
Fiber Content: 8 g
Protein: 30 g

### 353.Bulgur Lamb Meatballs

**Preparation Time:** 10 minutes
**Cooking Time:** 15 minute
**Servings:** 6
**Ingredients:**

- 1 and ½ cups Greek yogurt
- ½ teaspoon cumin, ground
- 1 cup cucumber, shredded
- ½ teaspoon garlic, minced
- A pinch of salt and black pepper
- 1 cup bulgur
- 2 cups water
- 1 pound lamb, ground
- ¼ cup parsley, chopped
- ¼ cup shallots, chopped
- ½ teaspoon allspice, ground
- ½ teaspoon cinnamon powder
- 1 tablespoon olive oil

**Directions:**

1.In a bowl, combine the bulgur with the water, cover the bowl, leave aside for 10 minutes, drain and transfer to a bowl.
2.Add the meat, the yogurt and the rest of the ingredients except the oil, stir well and shape medium meatballs out of this mix.
3.Heat up a pan with the oil over medium-high heat, add the meatballs, cook them for 7 minutes on each side, arrange them all on a platter and serve as an appetizer.

**Nutrition:**

Calories 300;
Fat 9.6 g;
Fiber 4.6 g;
Carbs 22.6 g;
Protein 6.6 g

### 354.Cucumber Bites

**Preparation Time:** 10 minutes
**Cooking Time:** 0 minutes
**Servings:** 12
**Ingredients:**

- 1 English cucumber, sliced into 32 rounds
- 10 ounces hummus
- 16 cherry tomatoes, halved

•1 tablespoon parsley, chopped

•1 ounce feta cheese, crumbled

**Directions:**

1.Spread the hummus on each cucumber round, divide the tomato halves on each, sprinkle the cheese and parsley on to and serve as an appetizer.

**Nutrition:**

Calories 162;

Fat 3.4 g;

Fiber 2 g;

Carbs 6.4 g;

Protein 2.4 g

## 355.Tomato Salsa

**Preparation Time: 5 minutes**

**Cooking Time: 0 minutes**

**Servings: 6**

**Ingredients:**

•1 garlic clove, minced

•4 tablespoons olive oil

•5 tomatoes, cubed

•1 tablespoon balsamic vinegar

•¼ cup basil, chopped

•1 tablespoon parsley, chopped

•1 tablespoon chives, chopped

•Salt and black pepper to the taste

•Pita chips for serving

**Directions:**

1.In a bowl, mix the tomatoes with the garlic and the rest of the ingredients except the pita chips, stir, divide into small cups and serve with the pita chips on the side.

**Nutrition:**

Calories 160;

Fat 13.7 g;

Fiber 5.5 g;

Carbs 10.1 g;

Protein 2.2

## 356.Olives and Cheese Stuffed Tomatoes

**Preparation Time: 10 minutes**

**Cooking Time: 0 minutes**

**Servings: 24**

**Ingredients:**

•24 cherry tomatoes, top cut off and insides scooped out

•2 tablespoons olive oil

•¼ teaspoon red pepper flakes

•½ cup feta cheese, crumbled

•2 tablespoons black olive paste

•¼ cup mint, torn

**Directions:**

1.In a bowl, mix the olives paste with the rest of the ingredients except the cherry tomatoes and whisk well.

2.Stuff the cherry tomatoes with this mix, arrange them all on a platter and serve as an appetizer.

**Nutrition:**

Calories 136;

Fat 8.6 g;

Fiber 4.8 g;

Carbs 5.6 g;

Protein 5.1 g

## 357.Feta Artichoke Dip

**Preparation Time: 10 minutes**

**Cooking Time: 30 minutes**

**Servings: 8**

**Ingredients:**

•8 ounces artichoke hearts, drained and quartered

•¾ cup basil, chopped

•¾ cup green olives, pitted and chopped

•1 cup parmesan cheese, grated

•5 ounces feta cheese, crumbled

**Directions:**

1.In your food processor, mix the artichokes with the basil and the rest of the ingredients, pulse well, and transfer to a baking dish.
2.Introduce in the oven, bake at 375° F for 30 minutes and serve as a party dip.
**Nutrition:**
Calories 186;
Fat 12.4 g;
Fiber 0.9 g;
Carbs 2.6 g;
Protein 1.5 g

### 358.Cucumber Rolls
**Preparation Time: 5 minutes**
**Cooking Time: 0 minutes**
**Servings: 6**
**Ingredients:**
•1 big cucumber, sliced lengthwise
•1 tablespoon parsley, chopped
•8 ounces canned tuna, drained and mashed
•Salt and black pepper to the taste
•1 teaspoon lime juice
**Directions:**
1.Arrange cucumber slices on a working surface, divide the rest of the ingredients, and roll.
2.Arrange all the rolls on a platter and serve as an appetizer.
**Nutrition:**
Calories 200
Fat 6 g
Fiber 3.4 g
Carbs 7.6 g
Protein 3.5 g

### 359.Chili Mango and Watermelon Salsa
**Preparation Time: 5 minutes**
**Cooking Time: 0 minutes**
**Servings: 12**
**Ingredients:**
•1 red tomato, chopped
•Salt and black pepper to the taste
•1 cup watermelon, seedless, peeled and cubed
•1 red onion, chopped
•2 mangos, peeled and chopped
•2 chili peppers, chopped
•¼ cup cilantro, chopped
•3 tablespoons lime juice
•Pita chips for serving
**Directions:**
1.In a bowl, mix the tomato with the watermelon, the onion and the rest of the ingredients except the pita chips and toss well.
2.Divide the mix into small cups and serve with pita chips on the side.
**Nutrition:**
Calories 62;
Fat 4g;
Fiber 1.3 g;
Carbs 3.9 g;
Protein 2.3 g

### 360.Creamy Spinach and Shallots Dip
**Preparation Time: 10 minutes**
**Cooking Time: 0 minutes**
 **Servings: 4**
**Ingredients:**
•1 pound spinach, roughly chopped
•2 shallots, chopped
•2 tablespoons mint, chopped
•¾ cup cream cheese, soft
•Salt and black pepper to the taste
**Directions:**

1.In a blender, combine the spinach with the shallots and the rest of the ingredients, and pulse well.

2.Divide into small bowls and serve as a party dip.

**Nutrition:**

Calories 204;

Fat 11.5 g;

Fiber 3.1 g;

Carbs 4.2 g;

Protein 5.9 g

### 361.Hummus with Ground Lamb

**Preparation Time:** 10 minutes

**Cooking Time:** 15 minute

**Servings:** 8

**Ingredients:**

•10 ounces hummus

•12 ounces lamb meat, ground

•½ cup pomegranate seeds

•¼ cup parsley, chopped

•1 tablespoon olive oil

•Pita chips for serving

**Directions:**

1.Heat up a pan with the oil over medium-high heat, add the meat, and brown for 15 minutes stirring often.

2.Spread the hummus on a platter, spread the ground lamb all over, also spread the pomegranate seeds and the parsley and serve with pita chips as a snack.

**Nutrition:**

Calories 133;

Fat 9.7 g;

Fiber 1.7 g;

Carbs 6.4 g;

Protein 5

### 362.Cucumber Sandwich Bites

**Preparation Time:** 5 minutes

**Cooking Time:** 0 minutes

**Servings:** 12

**Ingredients:**

•1 cucumber, sliced

•8 slices whole wheat bread

•2 tablespoons cream cheese, soft

•1 tablespoon chives, chopped

•¼ cup avocado, peeled, pitted and mashed

•1 teaspoon mustard

•Salt and black pepper to the taste

**Directions:**

1.Spread the mashed avocado on each bread slice, also spread the rest of the ingredients except the cucumber slices.

2.Divide the cucumber slices on the bread slices, cut each slice in thirds, arrange on a platter and serve as an appetizer.

**Nutrition:**

Calories 187;

Fat 12.4 g;

Fiber 2.1 g;

Carbs 4.5 g;

Protein 8.2 g

### 363.Wrapped Plums

**Preparation Time: 5 minutes**

**Cooking Time: 0 minutes**

**Servings: 8**

**Ingredients:**

•2 ounces prosciutto, cut into 16 pieces

•4 plums, quartered

•1 tablespoon chives, chopped

•A pinch of red pepper flakes, crushed

**Directions:**

3.Wrap each plum quarter in a prosciutto slice, arrange them all on a platter, sprinkle the chives, pepper flakes all over, and serve.

**Nutrition:**

Calories 30;

Fat 1 g;

Fiber 0 g;

Carbs 4 g;
Protein 2 g

### 364.Mediterranean Chicken Salad

**Preparation Time**: 15 minutes
**Cooking Time:** 30 minutes
**Servings:** 4
**Ingredients:**
For Chicken:
•1 3/4 lb. boneless, skinless chicken breast
•1/4 teaspoon each of pepper and salt (or as desired)
•1 1/2 tablespoon of butter, melted
For Mediterranean Salad:
•1 cup of sliced cucumber
•6 cups of romaine lettuce, that is torn or roughly chopped
•10 pitted Kalamata olives
•1 pint of cherry tomatoes
•1/3 cup of reduced-fat feta cheese
•1/4 teaspoon each of pepper and salt (or lesser)
•1 small lemon juice (it should be about 2 tablespoons)
**Directions:**
1.Preheat your oven or grill to about 3500F.
2.Season the chicken with salt, butter, and black pepper
3.Roast or grill chicken until it reaches an internal temperature of 1650F in about 25 minutes.
4.Once your chicken breasts are cooked, remove and keep aside to rest for about 5 minutes before you slice it.
5.Combine all the salad ingredients you have and toss everything together very well.
6.Serve the chicken with a Mediterranean salad.
**Nutrition:**
Calories: 340 Cal

Prot: 45 g
Carb : 9 g
Fat: 14 g

### 365.Jalapeno Lentil Burgers

**Preparation Time**: 15 minutes
**Cooking Time:** 10 minutes
**Servings:** 5
**Ingredients:**
•Dried red lentils; half cup; rinsed
•Chickpeas; 1 to 12 ounces can; rinsed
•Ground cumin; one teaspoon
•Chili powder; one teaspoon
•Sea salt; one teaspoon
•Packed cilantro; half cup
•Garlic cloves minced
•Jalapeno finely chopped
•Red onion; half, small; minced
•Red bell pepper
•Carrot; shredded
•Oat bran/oat flour; 1/4 cup (gluten-free)
•Lettuce/hamburger buns
For Pico:
•Ripe mango (1) diced
•Ripe avocado (1) diced
•Red onion; half, small; finely diced
•Chopped cilantro; half cup
•Fresh lime juice; half teaspoon
•Sea salt
**Directions:**
1.Put all ingredients in a large bowl and mix.
2.Stir in the salt to compare.
3.Put a medium saucepan on medium heat, add lentils plus 1 1/2 cups of water, then bring water to a boil, cover it afterward, lower the heat to low, and then simmer lentils until the water is absorbed.
4.Drain, and set aside some extra water.

5.In a food processor, put the cooked lentils, chickpeas, garlic, sea salt, cilantro, chili powder and cumin, and blend until the beans and lentils are smooth.

6.Add tomato, red pepper, jalapeno, and carrot to compare.

7.Divide into 6 equal parts and use your hands to create dense patties.

8.Heat skillet over a medium-high flame; apply 1/2 tablespoon of olive oil

9.Place a few burgers in at a time and cook on either side for a couple of minutes, just until crisp and golden brown.

10.Repeat with remaining patties and add olive oil whenever desired.

11.Place the patties in a bun or lettuce and finish with mango avocado pico.

**Nutrition:**
Carbohydrates: 34.9 g
Calories: 225 Cal
Sugar: 7.7 g
Fats: 6.1 g

### 366.Avocado Dip

**Preparation Time: 5 minutes**
**Cooking Time: 0 minutes**
**Servings: 8**
**Ingredients:**
•½ cup heavy cream
•1 green chili pepper, chopped
•Salt and pepper to the taste
•4 avocados, pitted, peeled and chopped
•1 cup cilantro, chopped
•¼ cup lime juice
**Directions:**
1.In a blender, combine the cream with the avocados and the rest of the ingredients and pulse well.
2.Divide the mix into bowls and serve cold as a party dip.



**Nutrition:**
Calories 200;
Fat 14.5 g;
Fiber 3.8 g;
Carbs 8.1 g;
Protein 7.6 g

### 367. Goat Cheese and Chives Spread

**Preparation Time: 10 minutes**
**Cooking Time: 0 minute**
**Servings: 4**
**Ingredients:**
•2 ounces goat cheese, crumbled
•¾ cup sour cream
•2 tablespoons chives, chopped
•1 tablespoon lemon juice
•Salt and black pepper to the taste
•2 tablespoons extra virgin olive oil
**Directions:**
1.In a bowl, mix the goat cheese with the cream and the rest of the ingredients and whisk really well.
2.Keep in the fridge for 10 minutes and serve as a party spread.
**Nutrition:**
Calories 220;
Fat 11.5 g;
Fiber 4.8 g;
Carbs 8.9 g;
Protein 5.6 g

### 368.Grandma's Rice

**Preparation Time**: 15 minutes
**Cooking Time:** 2 hours
**Servings:** 4
**Ingredients:**
•40 g butter
•1 tbsp brown sugar
•1/2 cup arborio rice
•3 cups milk

•1/2 tbsp. ground cinnamon
•1/8 tbsp. ground nutmeg
•1 tbsp. vanilla paste
•1/2 cup raisins
•300 ml. cream

**Directions:**
1.Preheat oven to 300F.
2.Grease a 1-liter ability oven-safe plate.
3.Heat butter in a saucepan and add sugar and rice.
4.Stir for 1 minute to thoroughly coat the rice.
5.Remove from heat and wish in milk, spices, and vanilla.
6.Stir through raisins then pour into prepared dish.
7.Bake for 30 minutes, then remove from the oven and stir well.
8.Drizzle over the cream and return to the oven for an additional hour.
9.Check that the rice is cooked through.
10.Return to the oven for 15-30 minutes if required.
11.Serve with extra cream and nutmeg.

**Nutrition:**
Fat: 20 g
Protein: 23 g
Cholesterol: 25 mg
Carbohydrates: 30 g
Sodium: 1000 mg

### 369.Baked Beef Zucchini

**Preparation Time**: 10 minutes
**Cooking Time:** 40 minutes
**Servings:** 4
**Ingredients:**
•2 large zucchinis
•1 cup minced beef
•1 cup mushroom, chopped
•1 tomato, chopped
•1/2 cup spinach, chopped

•1 tbsp. chives, minced
•2 tbsp. olive oil
•Salt and pepper to taste
•1 tbsp. almond butter
•1 tsp. garlic powder
•1 cup cheddar cheese, grated
•1/3 tsp. ginger powder

**Directions:**
1.Preheat the oven to 400 degrees F.
2.Add aluminum foil on a baking sheet.
3.Cut the zucchini in half. Scoop out the seeds and make pockets to stuff it later.
4.In a pan, add the olive oil.
5.Toss the beef until brown.
6.Add the mushroom, tomato, chives, salt, pepper, garlic, ginger, and spinach.
7.Cook for 2 minutes. Take off the heat.
8.Stuff the zucchinis using the mix.
9.Add them onto the baking sheet. Sprinkle the cheese on top.
10.Add the butter on top. Bake for 30 minutes. Serve warm.

**Nutrition:**
Fat: 12.8 g
Cholesterol: 79.7 mg
Sodium: 615.4 mg
Potassium: 925.8 mg
Carbohydrate: 26.8 g

### 370.Baked Tuna with Asparagus

**Preparation Time**: 10 minutes
**Cooking Time:** 10 minutes
**Servings:** 2
**Ingredients:**
•2 tuna steak
•1 cup asparagus, trimmed
•1 tsp. almond butter
•1 tsp. rosemary
•1/2 tsp. oregano

•1/2 tsp. garlic powder

•1tsp. lemon juice

•1/2 tsp. ginger powder

•1 tbsp. olive oil

•1 tsp. red chili powder

•Salt and pepper to taste

**Directions:**

1.Marinate the tuna using oregano, lemon juice, salt, pepper, red chili powder, garlic, ginger, and let it sit for 10 minutes.

2.In a pan, add the olive oil.

3.Fry the tuna steaks 2 minutes per side.

4.In another pan, melt the almond butter.

5.Toss the asparagus with salt, pepper, and rosemary for 3 minutes.

6.Serve.

**Nutrition:**

Fat: 4.7 g

Cholesterol: 0.0 mg

Sodium: 98.5 mg

Potassium: 171.6 mg

Carbohydrate: 3.2 g

### 371.Cocoa Brownies

**Preparation Time**: 10 minutes

**Cooking Time**: 30 minutes

**Servings:** 12

**Ingredients:**

•1 egg

•2 tablespoons butter, grass-fed

•2 teaspoons vanilla extract, pure

•¼ teaspoon baking powder

•¼ cup cocoa powder

•1/3 cup heavy cream

•¾ cup almond butter

•Pinch sea salt

**Directions:**

1.Break your egg into a bowl, whisking until smooth.

2.Add in all of your wet ingredients, mixing well.

3.Mix all dry ingredients into a bowl.

4.Sift your dry ingredients into your wet ingredients, mixing to form a batter.

5.Get out a baking pan, greasing it before pouring in your mixture.

6.Heat your oven to 350 and bake for twenty-five minutes.

7.Allow it to cool before slicing and serve at room temperature or warm.

**Nutrition:**

Calories: 184

Protein: 1 g

Fat: 20 g

Carbohydrates: 1 g

### 372.Sweet Almond Bites

**Preparation Time**: 30 minutes

**Cooking Time:** 90 minutes

**Servings:** 12

**Ingredients:**

•18 ounces butter, grass fed

•2 ounces heavy cream

•½ cup Stevia

•2/3 cup cocoa powder

•1 teaspoon vanilla extract, pure

•4 tablespoons almond butter

Direction:

1.Use a double boiler to melt your butter before adding in all of your remaining ingredients.

2.Place the mixture into molds, freezing for two hours before serving.

**Nutrition:**

Calories: 350

Protein: 2 g

Fat: 38 g

## 373.Lamb Stuffed Avocado

**Preparation Time**: 10 minutes
**Cooking Time:** 40 minutes
**Servings:** 4
**Ingredients:**
•2 avocados
•1 1/2 cup minced lamb
•1/2 cup cheddar cheese, grated
•1/2 cup parmesan cheese, grated
•2 tbsp. almond, chopped
•1 tbsp. coriander, chopped
•2 tbsp. olive oil
•1 tomato, chopped
•1 jalapeno, chopped
•Salt and pepper to taste
•1 tsp. garlic, chopped
•1-inch ginger, chopped
**Directions:**
1.Cut the avocados in half. Remove the pit and scoop out some flesh to stuff it later.
2.In a skillet, add half of the oil.
3.Toss the ginger, garlic for 1 minute.
4.Add the lamb and toss for 3 minutes.
5.Add the tomato, coriander, parmesan, jalapeno, salt, pepper, and cook for 2 minutes.
6.Take off the heat. Stuff the avocados.
7.Sprinkle the almonds, cheddar cheese, and add olive oil on top.
8.Add to a baking sheet and bake for 30 minutes. Serve.
**Nutrition:**
Fat: 19.5 g
Cholesterol: 167.5 mg
Sodium: 410.7 mg
Potassium: 617.1 mg
Carbohydrate: 13.1 g

## 374.Strawberry Cheesecake Minis

**Preparation Time**: 30 minutes
**Cooking Time:** 120 minutes
**Servings:** 12
**Ingredients:**
•1 cup coconut oil
•1 cup coconut butter
•½ cup strawberries, sliced
•½ teaspoon lime juice
•2 tablespoons cream cheese, full fat
•Stevia to taste
**Directions:**
1.Blend your strawberries together.
2.Soften your cream cheese, and then add in your coconut butter.
3.Combine all ingredients together, and then pour your mixture into silicone molds.
4.Freeze for at least two hours before serving.
**Nutrition:**
Calories: 372
Protein: 1 g
Fat: 41 g
Carbohydrates: 2 g

## 375.Chocolate Orange Bites

**Preparation Time**: 20 minutes
**Cooking Time:** 120 minutes
**Servings:** 6
**Ingredients:**
•10 ounces coconut oil
•4 tablespoons cocoa powder
•¼ teaspoon orange extract
•Stevia to taste
**Directions:**
1.Melt half of your coconut oil using a double boiler, and then add in your stevia and orange extract.
2.Get out candy molds, pouring the mixture into it. Fill each mold halfway, and then place in the fridge until they set.

3.Melt the other half of your coconut oil, stirring in your cocoa powder and stevia, making sure that the mixture is smooth with no lumps.

4.Pour into your molds, filling them up all the way, and then allow it to set in the fridge before serving.

**Nutrition:**

Calories: 188 g

Protein: 1 g

Fat: 21g

Carbohydrates: 5 g

## 376.Nutmeg Nougat

**Preparation Time**: 30 minutes

**Cooking Time:** 60 minutes

**Servings:** 12

**Ingredients:**

•1 cup heavy cream

•1 cup cashew butter

•1 cup coconut, shredded

•½ teaspoon nutmeg

•1 teaspoon vanilla extract, pure

•Stevia to taste

**Directions:**

1.Melt your cashew butter using a double boiler, and then stir in your vanilla extract, dairy cream, nutmeg, and stevia. Make sure it's mixed well.

2.Remove from heat, allowing it to cool down before refrigerating it for half an hour.

3.Shape into balls, and coat with shredded coconut. Chill for at least two hours before serving.

**Nutrition:**

Calories: 341

Fat: 34 g

Carbohydrates: 5 g

## 377.Fluffy Bites

**Preparation Time**: 20 minutes

**Cooking Time:** 60 minutes

**Servings:** 12

**Ingredients:**

•2 teaspoons cinnamon

•2/3 cup sour cream

•2 cups heavy cream

•1 teaspoon scraped vanilla bean

•¼ teaspoon cardamom

•4 egg yolks

•Stevia to taste

**Directions:**

1.Start by whisking your egg yolks until creamy and smooth.

2.Get out a double boiler, and add your eggs with the rest of your ingredients. Mix well.

3.Remove from heat, allowing it to cool until it reaches room temperature.

4.Refrigerate for an hour before whisking well.

5.Pour into molds, and freeze for at least an hour before serving.

**Nutrition:**

Calories: 363

Protein: 2 g

Fat: 40 g

Carbohydrates: 1 g

## 378.Caramel Cones

**Preparation Time**: 25 minutes

**Cooking Time:** 120 minutes

**Servings:** 6

**Ingredients:**

•2 tablespoons heavy whipping cream

•2 tablespoons sour cream

•1 tablespoon caramel sugar or stevia

•1 teaspoon sea salt, fine

•1/3 cup butter, grass-fed

•1/3 cup coconut oil

•Stevia to taste

**Directions:**

1.Soften your coconut oil and butter, mixing together.

2.Mix all ingredients to form a batter, and then place them in molds.

3.Top with a little salt, and keep refrigerated until serving.

**Nutrition:**

Calories: 100

Fat: 12 g

Carbohydrates: 1 g

### 379.Easy Vanilla Bombs

**Preparation Time**: 20 minutes

**Cooking Time:** 45 minutes

**Servings:** 14

**Ingredients:**

•1 cup macadamia nuts, unsalted

•¼ cup coconut oil / ¼ cup butter

•2 teaspoons vanilla extract, sugar-free

•20 drops liquid Stevia

•2 tablespoons erythritol, powdered

**Directions:**

1.Pulse your macadamia nuts in a blender, and then combine all of your ingredients together. Mix well.

2.Get out mini muffin tins with a tablespoon and a half of the mixture.

3.Refrigerate it for a half hour before serving.

**Nutrition:**

Calories: 125

Fat: 5 g

Carbohydrates: 5 g

### 380.Mozzarella Sticks

**Preparation Time**: 8 minutes

**Cooking Time:** 2 minutes

**Servings:** 2

**Ingredients:**

•1 large whole egg

•3 sticks mozzarella cheese in half (frozen overnight)

•2 tablespoon grated parmesan cheese

•1/2 cup almond flour

•1/4 cup coconut oil

•2 1/2 teaspoons Italian seasoning blend

•1 tablespoon chopped parsley

•1/2 teaspoon salt

**Directions:**

1.Heat the coconut oil in a cast-iron skillet of medium size over low-medium heat.

2.Crack the egg in a small bowl in the meantime and beat it well.

3.Take another bowl of medium size and add parmesan cheese, almond flour, and seasonings to it. Whisk together the ingredients until a smooth mixture is prepared.

4.Take the overnight frozen mozzarella stick and dip in the beaten egg, then coat it well with the dry mixture. Do the same with all the remaining cheese sticks.

5.Place all the coated sticks in the preheated skillet and cook them for 2 minutes or until they start giving a golden-brown look from all sides.

6.Remove from the skillet once cooked properly and place over a paper towel so that any extra oil gets absorbed.

7.Sprinkle parsley over the sticks if you desire and serve with keto marinara sauce.

**Nutrition:**

Calories: 430

Fat: 39 g

Carbohydrates: 10 g

Protein: 20 g

### 381.Sweet Chai Bites

**Preparation Time**: 20 minutes
**Cooking Time:** 45 minutes
**Servings:** 6
**Ingredients:**
- 1 cup cream cheese
- 1 cup coconut oil
- 2 ounces butter, grass-fed
- 2 teaspoons ginger
- 2 teaspoons cardamom
- 1 teaspoon nutmeg
- 1 teaspoon cloves
- 1 teaspoon vanilla extract, pure
- 1 teaspoon Darjeeling black tea
- Stevia to taste

**Directions:**
1. Melt your coconut oil and butter before adding in your black tea. Allow it to set for one to two minutes.
2. Add in your cream cheese, removing your mixture from heat.
3. Add in all of your spices, and stir to combine.
4. Pour into molds, and freeze before serving.

**Nutrition:**
Calories: 178
Protein: 1 g
Fat: 19 g

### 382.Coconut Fudge

**Preparation Time**: 20 minutes
**Cooking Time:** 60 minutes
**Servings:** 12
**Ingredients:**
- 2 cups coconut oil
- ½ cup dark cocoa powder
- ½ cup coconut cream
- ¼ cup almonds, chopped
- ¼ cup coconut, shredded

- 1 teaspoon almond extract
- Pinch of salt
- Stevia to taste

**Directions:**
1. Pour your coconut oil and coconut cream in a bowl, whisking with an electric beater until smooth. Once the mixture becomes smooth and glossy, do not continue.
2. Begin to add in your cocoa powder while mixing slowly, making sure that there aren't any lumps.
3. Add in the rest of your ingredients, and mix well.
4. Line a pan with parchment paper, and freeze until it sets.
5. Slice into squares before serving.

**Nutrition:**
Calories: 172
Fat: 20 g
Carbohydrates: 3 g

### 383.Cinnamon Bites

**Preparation Time**: 20 minutes
**Cooking Time:** 95 minutes
**Servings:** 6
**Ingredients:**
- 1/8 teaspoon nutmeg
- 1 teaspoon vanilla extract
- ¼ teaspoon cinnamon
- 4 tablespoons coconut oil
- ½ cup butter, grass-fed
- 8 ounces cream cheese
- Stevia to taste

**Directions:**
1. Soften your coconut oil and butter, mixing in your cream cheese.
2. Add all of your remaining ingredients, and mix well.
3. Pour into molds, and freeze until set.

**Nutrition:**
Calories: 178
Protein: 1g
Fat: 19 g

### 384. Yogurt Mint

**Preparation Time:** 5 minutes
**Cooking Time:** 10 minutes
**Servings:** 2
**Ingredients:**

- 1 cup of water
- 5 cups of milk
- ¾ cup plain yogurt
- ¼ cup fresh mint
- 1 tbsp. maple syrup

**Directions:**

1. Add 1-cup water to the Instant Pot Pressure Cooker.
2. Press the STEAM function button and adjust to 1 minute.
3. Once done, add the milk, then press the YOGURT function button and allow boiling.
4. Add yogurt and fresh mint, and then stir well.
5. Pour into a glass and add maple syrup.
6. Enjoy.

**Nutrition:**
Calories: 25
Fat: 0.5 g
Carbs: 5 g
Protein: 2 g

### 385. Chocolate Bars

**Preparation Time:** 10 minutes
**Cooking Time:** 20 minutes
**Servings:** 16
**Ingredients:**

- 15 oz cream cheese, softened
- 15 oz unsweetened dark chocolate
- 1 tsp vanilla
- 10 drops liquid stevia

**Directions:**

1. Grease 8-inch square dish and set aside.
2. In a saucepan, dissolve chocolate over low heat.
3. Add stevia and vanilla and stir well.
4. Remove pan from heat and set aside.
5. Add cream cheese into the blender and blend until smooth.
6. Add melted chocolate mixture into the cream cheese and blend until just combined.
7. Transfer mixture into the prepared dish, spread evenly, and place in the refrigerator until firm.
8. Slice and serve.

**Nutrition:**
Calories: 230
Fat: 24 g
Carbs: 7.5 g
Sugar: 0.1 g
Protein: 6 g
Cholesterol: 29 mg

### 386. Blueberry Muffins

**Preparation Time:** 15 minutes
**Cooking Time:** 35 minutes
**Servings:** 12
**Ingredients:**

- 2 eggs
- 1/2 cup fresh blueberries
- 1 cup heavy cream
- 2 cups almond flour
- 1/4 tsp lemon zest
- 1/2 tsp lemon extract
- 1 tsp baking powder
- 5 drops stevia
- 1/4 cup butter, melted

**Directions:**

1. Heat the cooker to 350 F. Line muffin tin with cupcake liners and set aside.
2. Add eggs into the bowl and whisk until mix.
3. Add remaining ingredients and mix to combine.

4.Pour mixture into the prepared muffin tin and bake for 25 minutes.

5.Serve and enjoy.

**Nutrition:** Calories: 190 Fat: 17 g Carbs: 5 g Sugar: 1 g Protein: 5 g Cholesterol: 55 mg

### 387.Chocolate Fondue

**Preparation Time:** 5 minutes

**Cooking Time:** 10 minutes

**Servings:** 2

**Ingredients:**

•1 cup water

•½ tsp. sugar or stevia

•½ cup coconut cream

•¾ cup dark chocolate, chopped

**Directions:**

1.Pour the water into your Instant Pot.

2.To a heatproof bowl, add the chocolate, sugar, and coconut cream.

3.Place in the Instant Pot.

4.Seal the lid, select MANUAL, and cook for 2 minutes. When ready, do a quick release and carefully open the lid. Stir well and serve immediately.

**Nutrition:**

Calories: 216

Fat: 17 g

Carbs: 11 g

Protein: 2 g

### 388.Apple Crisp

**Preparation Time:** 10 minutes

**Cooking Time:** 13 minutes

**Servings:** 2

**Ingredients:**

•2 apples, sliced into chunks

•1 tsp. cinnamon

•¼ cup rolled oats

•1/4 cup brown sugar   or stevia

•½ cup of water

**Directions:**

1.Put all the listed **Ingredients:** in the pot and mix well.

2.Seal the pot, choose MANUAL mode, and cook at HIGH pressure for 8 minutes.

3.Release the pressure naturally and let sit for 5 minutes or until the sauce has thickened.

4.Serve and enjoy.

**Nutrition:**

Calories: 218

Fat: 5 mg

Carbs: 54 g

### 389.Raspberry Compote

**Preparation Time:** 11 minutes

**Cooking Time:** 30 minutes

**Servings:** 2

**Ingredients:**

•1 cup raspberries

•½ cup Swerve

•1 tsp freshly grated lemon zest

•1 tsp vanilla extract

•2 cups water

**Directions:**

1.Press the SAUTÉ button on your Instant Pot, then add all the listed Ingredients.

2.Stir well and pour in 1 cup of water.

3.Cook for 5 minutes, continually stirring, then pour in 1 more cup of water and press the CANCEL button.

4.Secure the lid properly, press the MANUAL button, and set the timer to 15 minutes on LOW pressure.

5.When the timer buzzes, press the CANCEL button and release the pressure naturally for 10minutes.

6.Move the pressure handle to the "venting" position to release any remaining pressure and open the lid.

7.Let it cool before serving.

**Nutrition:**
Calories: 48
Fat: 0.5 g
Carbs: 5 g
Protein: 1 g

### 390.Braised Apples

**Preparation Time:** 5 minutes
**Cooking Time:** 12 minutes
**Servings:** 2
**Ingredients:**
•2 cored apples
•½ cup of water
•½ cup red wine
•3 tbsp. sugar  or stevia
•½ tsp. ground cinnamon
**Directions:**
1.In the bottom of Instant Pot, add the water and place apples.
2.Pour wine on top and sprinkle with sugar and cinnamon. Close the lid carefully and cook for 10 minutes at HIGH PRESSURE.
3.When done, do a quick pressure release.
4.Transfer the apples onto serving plates and top with cooking liquid.
5.Serve immediately.
**Nutrition:**
Calories: 245
Fat: 0.5 g
Carbs: 53 g
Protein: 1 g

### 391.Rice Pudding

**Preparation Time:** 5 minutes
**Cooking Time:** 12 minutes
**Servings:** 2
**Ingredients:**
•½ cup short grain rice
•¼ cup of sugar  or stevia
•1 cinnamon stick
•1½ cup milk

•1 slice lemon peel
•Salt to taste
**Directions:**
1.Rinse the rice under cold water.
2.Put the milk, cinnamon stick, sugar, salt, and lemon peel inside the Instant Pot Pressure Cooker.
3.Close the lid, lock in place, and make sure to seal the valve. Press the PRESSURE button and cook for 10 minutes on HIGH.
4.When the timer beeps, choose the QUICK PRESSURE release. This will take about 2 minutes.
5.Remove the lid. Open the pressure cooker and discard the lemon peel and cinnamon stick. Spoon in a serving bowl and serve.
**Nutrition:**
Calories: 111
Fat: 6 g
Carbs: 21 g
Protein: 3 g

### 392.Rhubarb Dessert

**Preparation Time:** 4 minutes
**Cooking Time:** 5 minutes
**Servings:** 2
**Ingredients:**
•3 cups rhubarb, chopped
•1 tbsp. ghee, melted
•1/3 cup water
•1 tbsp. stevia
•1 tsp. vanilla extract
**Directions:**
1.Put all the listed **Ingredients:** in your Instant Pot, cover, and cook on HIGH for 5 minutes.
2.Divide into small bowls and serve cold.
3.Enjoy!
**Nutrition:**
Calories: 83
Fat: 2 g
Carbs: 2 g

Protein: 2 g

### 393.Wine Figs

**Preparation Time:** 5 minutes
**Cooking Time:** 3 minutes
**Servings:** 2
**Ingredients:**
•½ cup pine nuts
•1 cup red wine
•1 lb. figs
•Sugar, as needed
**Directions:**
1.Slowly pour the wine and sugar into the Instant Pot.
2.Arrange the trivet inside it; place the figs over it. Close the lid and lock. Ensure that you have sealed the valve to avoid leakage.
3.Press MANUAL mode and set timer to 3 minutes.
4.After the timer reads zero, press CANCEL and quick-release pressure.
5.Carefully remove the lid.
6.Divide figs into bowls, and drizzle wine from the pot over them.
7.Top with pine nuts and enjoy.
**Nutrition:**
Calories: 95
Fat: 3 g
Carbs: 5 g
Protein: 2 g

### 394.Chia Pudding

**Preparation Time**: 20 minutes
**Cooking Time:** 0 minutes
**Servings:** 2
**Ingredients:**
•4 tbsp chia seeds
•1 cup unsweetened coconut milk
•1/2 cup raspberries
**Directions:**
1.Add raspberry and coconut milk into a blender and blend until smooth.
2.Pour mixture into the glass jar.
3.Add chia seeds in a jar and stir well.
4.Seal the jar with a lid, shake well, and place in the refrigerator for 3 hours.
5.Serve chilled and enjoy.
**Nutrition:** Calories: 360 Fat: 33 g Carbs: 13 g Sugar: 5 g Protein: 6 g Cholesterol: 0 mg

### 395.Lemon Curd

**Preparation Time:** 10 minutes
**Cooking Time:** 10 minutes
**Servings:** 2
**Ingredients:**
•4 tbsp. butter
•1 cup sugar  or stevia
•2/3 cup lemon juice
•3 eggs
•2 tsp. lemon zest
•1 ½ cups of water
**Directions:**
1.Whisk the butter and sugar thoroughly until smooth.
2.Add 2 whole eggs and incorporate just the yolk of the other egg.
3.Add the lemon juice.
4.Transfer the mixture into the two jars and tightly seal the tops
5.Pour 1 ½ cups of water into the bottom of the Instant Pot and place in steaming rack. Put the jars on the rack and cook on HIGH PRESSURE for 10 minutes.
6.Natural-release the pressure for 10 minutes before quick releasing the rest.
7.Stir in the zest and put the lids back on the jars.
**Nutrition:**
Calories: 45
Fat: 1 g

Carbs: 8 g

Protein: 1 g

### 396.Poached Pears

**Preparation Time:** 8 minutes

**Cooking Time:** 10 minutes

**Servings:** 2

**Ingredients:**

•1 tbsp. lime juice

•2 tsp. lime zest

•1 cinnamon stick

•2 whole pears, peeled

•1 cup of water

•Fresh mint leaves for garnish

**Directions:**

1.Add all **Ingredients:** except for the mint leaves to the Instant Pot.

2.Seal the Instant Pot and choose the MANUAL button.

3.Cook on HIGH for 10 minutes.

4.Perform a natural pressure release.

5.Remove the pears from the pot.

6.Serve in bowls and garnish with mint on top.

**Nutrition:**

Calories: 59

Fat: 0.1 g

Carbs: 14 g

Protein: 0.3 g

### 397.Avocado Pudding

**Preparation Time**: 20 minutes

**Cooking Time:** 0 minutes

**Servings:** 8

**Ingredients:**

•2 ripe avocados, pitted and cut into pieces

•1 tbsp. fresh lime juice

•14 oz. can coconut milk

•2 tsp. liquid stevia

•2 tsp. vanilla

**Directions:**

1.Inside the blender. Add all ingredients and blend until smooth.

2.Serve immediately and enjoy.

**Nutrition:** Calories: 317 Fat: 30 g Carbs: 9 g Sugar: 0.5 g Protein: 3 g Cholesterol: 0 mg

### 398.Delicious Brownie Bites

**Preparation Time**: 20 minutes

**Cooking Time:** 0 minutes

**Servings:** 13

**Ingredients:**

•1/4 cup unsweetened chocolate chips

•1/4 cup unsweetened cocoa powder

•1 cup pecans, chopped

•1/2 cup almond butter

•1/2 tsp. vanilla

•1/4 cup monk fruit sweetener

•1/8 tsp. pink salt

**Directions:**

1.Add pecans, sweetener, vanilla, almond butter, cocoa powder, and salt into the food processor and process until well combined.

2.Transfer brownie mixture into the large bowl. Add chocolate chips and fold well.

3.Make small round shape balls from brownie mixture and place onto a baking tray.

4.Place in the freezer for 20 minutes.

5.Serve and enjoy.

**Nutrition:** Calories: 108 Fat: 9 g Carbs: 4 g Sugar: 1 g Protein: 2 g Cholesterol: 0 mg

### 399.Pumpkin Balls

**Preparation Time**: 15 minutes

**Cooking Time:** 0 minutes

**Servings:** 18

**Ingredients:**

•1 cup almond butter

•5 drops liquid stevia

•2 tbsp. coconut flour

•2 tbsp. pumpkin puree

•1 tbsp. pumpkin pie spice

**Directions:**
1.Mix together pumpkin puree in a large bowl, and almond butter until well combined.
2.Add liquid stevia, pumpkin pie spice, and coconut flour and mix well.
3.Make small balls from mixture and place onto a baking tray.
4.Place in the freezer for 1 hour.
5.Serve and enjoy.
**Nutrition:** Calories: 96 Fat: 8 g Carbs: 4 g Sugar: 1 g Protein: 2 g Cholesterol: 0 mg

## 400.Smooth Peanut Butter Cream

**Preparation Time**: 10 minutes
**Cooking Time:** 0 minutes
**Servings:** 8
**Ingredients:**
•1/4 cup peanut butter
•4 overripe bananas, chopped
•1/3 cup cocoa powder
•1/4 tsp. vanilla extract
•1/8 tsp. salt
**Directions:**
1.In the blender add all the listed ingredients and blend until smooth.
2.Serve immediately and enjoy.
**Nutrition:** Calories: 101 Fat: 5 g Carbs: 14 g Sugar: 7 g Protein: 3 g Cholesterol: 0 mg

## 401.Vanilla Avocado Popsicles

**Preparation Time**: 20 minutes
**Cooking Time:** 0 minutes
**Servings:** 6
**Ingredients:**
•2 avocadoes
•1 tsp vanilla
•1 cup almond milk
•1 tsp liquid stevia
•1/2 cup unsweetened cocoa powder

**Directions:**
1.In the blender add all the listed ingredients and blend smoothly.
2.Pour blended mixture into the Popsicle molds and place in the freezer until set.
3.Serve and enjoy.
**Nutrition:** Calories: 130 Fat: 12 g Carbs: 7 g Sugar: 1 g Protein: 3 g Cholesterol: 0 mg

## 402.Chocolate Popsicle

**Preparation Time**: 20 minutes
**Cooking Time:** 10 minutes
**Servings:** 6
**Ingredients:**
•4 oz. unsweetened chocolate, chopped
•6 drops liquid stevia
•1 1/2 cups heavy cream
**Directions:**
1.Add heavy cream into the microwave-safe bowl and microwave until just begins the boiling.
2.Add chocolate into the heavy cream and set aside for 5 minutes.
3.Add liquid stevia into the heavy cream mixture and stir until chocolate is melted.
4.Pour mixture into the Popsicle molds and place in freezer for 4 hours or until set.
5.Serve and enjoy.
**Nutrition:** Calories: 198 Fat: 21 g Carbs: 6 g Sugar: 0.2 g Protein: 3 g Cholesterol: 41 mg

## 403.Raspberry Ice Cream

**Preparation Time**: 10 minutes
**Cooking Time:** 0 minutes
**Servings:** 2
**Ingredients:**
•1 cup frozen raspberries
•1/2 cup heavy cream
•1/8 tsp stevia powder
**Directions:**

1.Blend all the listed ingredients in a blender until smooth.

2.Serve immediately and enjoy.

**Nutrition:** Calories: 144 Fat: 11 g Carbs: 10 g Sugar: 4 g Protein: 2 g Cholesterol: 41 mg

## 404.Bread Dough and Amaretto Dessert

**Preparation Time:** 15 minutes

**Cooking Time:** 8 Minutes

**Servings:** 12

**Ingredients:**

- 1 lb. bread dough
- 1 cup sugar  or stevia
- ½ cup butter
- 1 cup heavy cream
- 12 oz. chocolate chips
- 2 tbsp. amaretto liqueur

**Directions:**

1.Turn dough, cut into 20 slices and cut each piece in halves.

2.Sweep dough pieces with spray sugar, butter, put into air fryer's basket and cook them at 350°F for 5 minutes. Turn them, cook for 3 minutes still. Move to a platter.

3.Melt the heavy cream in pan over medium heat, put chocolate chips and turn until they melt.

4.Put in liqueur, turn and move to a bowl.

5.Serve bread dippers with the sauce.

**Nutrition:**

Calories: 179

Total Fat: 18g

Total carbs: 17g

## 405.Wrapped Pears

**Preparation Time:** 10 minutes

**Cooking Time:** 10 Minutes

**Servings:** 4

**Ingredients:**

- 4 puff pastry sheets
- 14 oz. vanilla custard
- 2 pears
- 1 egg
- ½ tbsp. cinnamon powder
- 2 tbsp. sugar or stevia

**Directions:**

1.Put wisp pastry slices on flat surface, add spoonful of vanilla custard at the center of each, add pear halves and wrap.

2.Sweep pears with egg, cinnamon and spray sugar, put into air fryer's basket and cook at 320°F for 15 minutes.

3.Split parcels on plates.

4.Serve.

**Nutrition:**

Calories: 285

Total Fat: 14g

Total carbs: 30g

## 406.Air Fried Bananas

**Preparation Time:** 5 minutes

**Cooking Time:** 10 Minutes

**Servings:** 4

**Ingredients:**

- 3 tbsp. butter
- 2 eggs
- 8 bananas
- ½ cup corn flour
- 3 tbsp. cinnamon sugar
- 1 cup panko

**Directions:**

1.Warm up pan with the butter over medium heat, put panko, turn and cook for 4 minutes then move to a bowl.

2.Spin each in flour, panko, egg blend, assemble them in air fryer's basket, grime with cinnamon sugar and cook at 280° F for 10 minutes.

3.Serve immediately.

**Nutrition:**
Calories: 337
Total Fat: 3g
Total carbs: 23g

### 407.Cocoa Cake

**Preparation Time:** 5 minutes
**Cooking Time:** 17 Minutes
**Servings:** 6
**Ingredients:**
•oz. butter
•3 eggs
•3 oz. stevia
•1 tbsp. cocoa powder
•3 oz. flour
•½ tbsp. lemon juice
**Directions:**
1.Mix in 1 tablespoon butter with cocoa powder in a bowl and beat.
2.Mix in the rest of the butter with eggs, flour, sugar and lemon juice in another bowl, blend properly and move half into a cake pan
3.Put half of the cocoa blend, spread, add the rest of the butter layer and crest with remaining cocoa.
4.Put into air fryer and cook at 360° F for 17 minutes.
5.Allow to cool before slicing.
6.Serve.
**Nutrition:**
Calories: 221
Total Fat: 5g
Total carbs: 12g

### 408.Apple Bread

**Preparation Time:** 5 minutes
**Cooking Time:** 40 Minutes
**Servings:** 6
**Ingredients:**
•3 cups apples
•1 cup stevia
•1 tbsp. vanilla
•2 eggs
•1 tbsp. apple pie spice
•2 cups white flour
•1 tbsp. baking powder
•1 stick butter
•1 cup water
**Directions:**
1.Mix in egg with 1 butter stick, stevia, apple pie spice and turn using mixer.
2.Put apples and turn properly.
3.Mix baking powder with flour in another bowl and turn.
4.Blend the 2 mixtures, turn and move it to spring form pan.
5.Get spring form pan into air fryer and cook at 320°F for 40 minutes
6.Slice.
7.Serve.
**Nutrition:**
Calories: 401
Total Fat: 9g
Total carbs: 29g

### 409.Banana Bread

**Preparation Time:** 5 minutes
**Cooking Time:** 40 Minutes
**Servings:** 6
**Ingredients:**
•¾ cup sugar or stevia
•1/3 cup butter
•1 tbsp. vanilla extract
•1 egg
•2 bananas
•1 tbsp. baking powder
•1 and ½ cups flour
•½ tbsp. baking soda
•1/3 cup milk

•1 and ½ tbsp. cream of tartar
•Cooking spray
**Directions:**
1.Mix in milk with cream of tartar, vanilla, egg, sugar, bananas and butter in a bowl and turn whole.
2.Mix in flour with baking soda and baking powder.
3.Blend the 2 mixtures, turn properly, move into oiled pan with cooking spray, put into air fryer and cook at 320°F for 40 minutes.
4.Remove bread, allow to cool, slice.
5.Serve.
**Nutrition:**
Calories: 540
Total Fat: 16g
Total carbs: 28g

### 410.Mini Lava Cakes

**Preparation Time:** 5 minutes
**Cooking Time:** 20 Minutes
**Servings:** 3
**Ingredients:**
•1 egg
•4 tbsp. sugar or stevia
•2 tbsp. olive oil
•4 tbsp. milk
•4 tbsp. flour
•1 tbsp. cocoa powder
•½ tbsp. baking powder
•½ tbsp. orange zest
**Directions:**
1.Mix in egg with sugar, flour, salt, oil, milk, orange zest, baking powder and cocoa powder, turn properly. Move it to oiled ramekins.
2.Put ramekins in air fryer and cook at 320°F for 20 minutes.
3.Serve warm.

**Nutrition:**
Calories: 329
Total Fat: 8.5g
Total carbs: 12.4g

### 411.Papaya Cream

**Preparation Time: 10 minutes**
**Cooking Time: 0 minutes**
**Servings: 2**
**Ingredients:**
•1 cup papaya, peeled and chopped
•1 cup heavy cream
•1 tablespoon stevia
•½ teaspoon vanilla extract
**Directions:**
1.In a blender, combine the cream with the papaya and the other ingredients, pulse well, divide into cups and serve cold.
**Nutrition:**
Calories 182
Fat 3.1
Fiber 2.3
Carbs 3.5
Protein 2

### 412.Ricotta Ramekins

**Preparation Time: 10 minutes**
**Cooking Time: 1 hour**
**Servings: 4**
**Ingredients:**
•6 eggs, whisked
•1 and ½ pounds ricotta cheese, soft
•½ pound stevia
•1 teaspoon vanilla extract
•½ teaspoon baking powder
•Cooking spray
**Directions:**
1.In a bowl, mix the eggs with the ricotta and the other ingredients except the cooking spray and whisk well.

2.Grease 4 ramekins with the cooking spray, pour the ricotta cream in each and bake at 360 degrees F for 1 hour.

3.Serve cold.

**Nutrition:**

Calories 180

Fat 5.3

Fiber 5.4

Carbs 11.5

Protein 4

### 413.Strawberry Sorbet

**Preparation Time: 15 minutes**

**Cooking Time: 10 minutes**

**Servings: 6**

**Ingredients:**

- 1 cup strawberries, chopped
- 1 tablespoon of liquid honey
- 2 tablespoons water
- 1 tablespoon lemon juice

**Directions:**

1.Preheat the water and liquid honey until you get homogenous liquid.

2.Blend the strawberries until smooth and combine them with honey liquid and lemon juice.

3.Transfer the strawberry mixture in the ice cream maker and churn it for 20 minutes or until the sorbet is thick.

4.Scoop the cooked sorbet in the ice cream cups.

**Nutrition:**

Calories 30,

Fat 0.4 g,

Fiber 1.4 g,

Carbs 14.9 g,

Protein 0.9 g

### 414.Crispy Apples

**Preparation Time:** 10 minutes

**Cooking Time:** 10 Minutes

**Servings:** 4

**Ingredients:**

- 2 tbsp. cinnamon powder
- 5 apples
- ½ tbsp. nutmeg powder
- 1 tbsp. maple syrup
- ½ cup water
- 4 tbsp. butter
- ¼ cup flour
- ¾ cup oats
- ¼ cup brown sugar or stevia

**Directions:**

1.Get the apples in a pan, put in nutmeg, maple syrup, cinnamon and water.

2.Mix in butter with flour, sugar, salt and oat, turn, put spoonful of blend over apples, get into air fryer and cook at 350°F for 10 minutes.

3.Serve while warm.

**Nutrition:**

Calories: 387

Total Fat: 5.6g

Total carbs: 12.4g

### 415.Ginger Cheesecake

**Preparation Time:** 20 minutes

**Cooking Time:** 20 Minutes

**Servings:** 6

**Ingredients:**

- 2 tbsp. butter
- ½ cup ginger cookies
- 16 oz. cream cheese
- 2 eggs
- ½ cup sugar or stevia
- 1 tbsp. rum
- ½ tbsp. vanilla extract
- ½ tbsp. nutmeg

**Directions:**

1.Spread pan with the butter and sprinkle cookie crumbs on the bottom.
2.Whisk cream cheese with rum, vanilla, nutmeg and eggs, beat properly and sprinkle the cookie crumbs.
3.Put in air fryer and cook at 340° F for 20 minutes.
4.Allow cheese cake to cool in fridge for 2 hours before slicing.
5.Serve.

**Nutrition:**
Calories: 312
Total Fat: 9.8g
Total carbs: 18g

### 416.Cocoa Cookies

**Preparation Time:** 10 minutes
**Cooking Time:** 14 Minutes
**Servings:** 12
**Ingredients:**
•6 oz. coconut oil
•6 eggs
•3 oz. cocoa powder
•2 tbsp. vanilla
•½ tbsp. baking powder
•4 oz. cream cheese
•5 tbsp. sugar or stevia
**Directions:**
1.Mix in eggs with coconut oil, baking powder, cocoa powder, cream cheese, vanilla in a blender and sway and turn using a mixer.
2.Get it into a lined baking dish and into the fryer at 320°F and bake for 14 minutes.
3.Split cookie sheet into rectangles.
4.Serve.
**Nutrition:**
Calories: 149
Total Fat: 2.4g
Total carbs: 27.2g

### 417.Vanilla Apple Pie

**Preparation Time: 15 minutes**
**Cooking Time: 50 minutes**
**Servings: 8**
**Ingredients:**
•3 apples, sliced
•½ teaspoon ground cinnamon
•1 teaspoon vanilla extract
•1 tablespoon Erythritol
•7 oz yeast roll dough
•1 egg, beaten
**Directions:**
1.Roll up the dough and cut it on 2 parts.
2.Line the springform pan with baking paper.
3.Place the first dough part in the springform pan.
4.Then arrange the apples over the dough and sprinkle it with Erythritol, vanilla extract, and ground cinnamon.
5.Then cover the apples with remaining dough and secure the edges of the pie with the help of the fork.
6.Make the small cuts in the surface of the pie.
7.Brush the pie with beaten egg and bake it for 50 minutes at 375F.
8.Cool the cooked pie well and then remove from the springform pan.
9.Cut it on the servings.
 **Nutrition:**
Calories 140,
Fat 3.4 g,
Fiber 3.4 g,
Carbs 23.9 g,
Protein 2.9 g

### 418.Apple Couscous Pudding

**Preparation Time: 10 minutes**
**Cooking Time: 25 minutes**
**Servings: 4**

**Ingredients:**
- ½ cup couscous
- 1 and ½ cups milk
- ¼ cup apple, cored and chopped
- 3 tablespoons stevia
- ½ teaspoon rose water
- 1 tablespoon orange zest, grated

**Directions:**
1. Heat up a pan with the milk over medium heat,
2. add the couscous and the rest of the ingredients, whisk, simmer for 25 minutes, divide into bowls and serve.

**Nutrition:**
Calories 150
Fat 4.5
Fiber 5.5
Carbs 7.5
Protein 4

### 419. Cinnamon Pears

**Preparation Time: 2 hours**
**Cooking Time: 0 minutes**
**Servings: 6**
**Ingredients:**
- 2 pears
- 1 teaspoon ground cinnamon
- 1 tablespoon Erythritol
- 1 teaspoon liquid stevia
- 4 teaspoons butter

**Directions:**
1. Cut the pears on the halves.
2. Then scoop the seeds from the pears with the help of the scooper.
3. In the shallow bowl mix up together Erythritol and ground cinnamon.
4. Sprinkle every pear half with cinnamon mixture and drizzle with liquid stevia.
5. Then add butter and wrap in the foil.
6. Bake the pears for 25 minutes at 365F.

7. Then remove the pears from the foil and transfer in the serving plates.

**Nutrition:**
Calories 96,
Fat 4.4 g,
Fiber 1.4 g,
Carbs 3.9 g,
Protein 0.9 g

### 420. Creamy Strawberries

**Preparation Time: 15 minutes**
**Cooking Time: 10 minutes**
**Servings: 6**
**Ingredients:**
- 6 tablespoons almond butter
- 1 tablespoon Erythritol
- 1 cup milk
- 1 teaspoon vanilla extract
- 1 cup strawberries, sliced

**Directions:**
1. Pour milk in the saucepan.
2. Add Erythritol, vanilla extract, and almond butter.
3. With the help of the hand mixer mix up the liquid until smooth and bring it to boil.
4. Then remove the mixture from the heat and let it cool.
5. The cooled mixture will be thick.
6. Put the strawberries in the serving glasses and top with the thick almond butter dip.

**Nutrition:**
Calories 192,
Fat 14.4 g,
Fiber 3.4 g,
Carbs 10.9 g,
Protein 1.9 g

### 421. Almonds and Oats Pudding

**Preparation Time: 10 minutes**
**Cooking Time: 15 minutes**

**Servings:** 4

**Ingredients:**

- 1 tablespoon lemon juice
- Zest of 1 lime
- 1 and ½ cups almond milk
- 1 teaspoon almond extract
- ½ cup oats
- 2 tablespoons stevia
- ½ cup silver almonds, chopped

**Directions:**

1.In a pan, combine the almond milk with the lime zest and the other ingredients, whisk, bring to a simmer and cook over medium heat for 15 minutes.

2.Divide the mix into bowls and serve cold.

**Nutrition:**

Calories 174

Fat 12.1

Fiber 3.2

Carbs 3.9

Protein 4.8

## 422.Cherry Compote

**Preparation Time:** 2 hours

**Cooking Time:** 0 minutes

**Servings:** 6

**Ingredients:**

- 2 peaches, pitted, halved
- 1 cup cherries, pitted
- ½ cup grape juice
- ½ cup strawberries
- 1 tablespoon liquid honey
- 1 teaspoon vanilla extract
- 1 teaspoon ground cinnamon

**Directions:**

1.Pour grape juice in the saucepan.

2.Add vanilla extract and ground cinnamon. Bring the liquid to boil.

3.After this, put peaches, cherries, and strawberries in the hot grape juice and bring to boil.

4.Remove the mixture from heat, add liquid honey, and close the lid.

5.Let the compote rest for 20 minutes.

6.Carefully mix up the compote and transfer in the serving plate.

**Nutrition:**

Calories 80,

Fat 0.4 g,

Fiber 2.4 g,

Carbs 19.9 g,

Protein 0.9 g

## 423.Brownies

**Preparation Time:** 10 minutes

**Cooking Time:** 22 Minutes

**Servings:** 4

**Ingredients:**

- 1 egg
- 1/3 cup cocoa powder
- 1/3 cup sugar  or stevia
- 7 tbsp. butter
- ½ tbsp. vanilla extract
- ¼ cup white flour
- ¼ cup walnuts
- ½ tbsp. baking powder
- 1 tbsp. peanut butter

**Directions:**

1.Warm pan with 6 tablespoons butter and the sugar over medium heat, turn, cook for 5 minutes, move to a bowl, put salt, egg, cocoa powder, vanilla extract, walnuts, baking powder and flour, turn mix properly and into a pan.

2.Mix peanut butter with one tablespoon butter in a bowl, heat in microwave for some seconds, turn properly and sprinkle brownies blend over.

3.Put in air fryer and bake at 320° F and bake
for 17 minutes.
4.Allow brownies to cool, cut.
5.Serve.
**Nutrition:**
Calories: 438
Total Fat: 18g
Total carbs: 16.5g

### 424.Blueberry Scones

**Preparation Time:** 10 minutes
**Cooking Time:** 10 Minutes
**Servings:** 10
**Ingredients:**
•1 cup white flour
•1 cup blueberries
•2 eggs
•½ cup heavy cream
•½ cup butter
•5 tbsp. sugar or stevia
•2 tbsp. vanilla extract
•2 tbsp. baking powder
**Directions:**
1.Mix in flour, baking powder, salt and
blueberries in a bowl and turn.
2.Mix heavy cream with vanilla extract, sugar,
butter and eggs and turn properly.
3.Blend the 2 mixtures, squeeze till dough is
ready, obtain 10 triangles from mix, put on
baking sheet into air fryer and cook them at
320°F for 10 minutes.
4.Serve cold.
**Nutrition:**
Calories: 525
Total Fat: 21g
Total carbs: 37g

### 425. Brussels Sprouts and Rhubarb Mix

**Preparation Time**: 5 minutes
**Cooking Time:** 20 minutes
**Servings:** 4
Ingredients
•1 pound Brussels sprouts, trimmed and halved
•½ pound rhubarb, sliced
•2 tablespoons avocado oil
•Juice of 1 lemon
•A pinch of salt and black pepper
•1 tablespoon chives, chopped
•1 teaspoon chili paste
Directions
1.In a pan that fits the air fryer, mix the sprouts with the rhubarb and the other ingredients, toss, put the pan in the fryer and cook at 390 degrees F for 20 minutes.
2.Divide between plates and serve as a side dish.
**Nutrition:**  Calories 200, Fat 9, Fiber 2, Carbs 6, Protein 9

### 426. Creamy Cauliflower

**Preparation Time**: 5 minutes
**Cooking Time:** 20 minutes
**Servings:** 4
Ingredients
•1 pound cauliflower florets
•1 cup cream cheese, soft
•½ cup mozzarella, shredded
•½ cup coconut cream
•4 bacon strips, cooked and chopped
•Salt and black pepper to the taste
Directions
1.In the air fryer's pan, mix the cauliflower with the cream cheese and the other ingredients, toss, introduce the pan in the machine and cook at 400 degrees F for 20 minutes.
2.Divide between plates and serve as a side dish.
**Nutrition:**  Calories 203, Fat 13, Fiber 2, Carbs 5, Protein 9

### 427. Cumin Cauliflower

**Preparation Time**: 5 minutes
**Cooking Time:** 20 minutes
**Servings:** 4
Ingredients
•1 pound cauliflower florets
•1 teaspoon cumin, ground
•Juice of 1 lime
•1 tablespoon butter, melted
•A pinch of salt and black pepper
•1 tablespoon chives, chopped
•¼ teaspoon cloves, ground
Directions
1.In the air fryer, mix the cauliflower with the cumin, lime juice and the other ingredients, toss and cook at 390 degrees F for 20 minutes.
2.Divide between plates and serve as a side dish.
**Nutrition:**  Calories 182, Fat 8, Fiber 2, Carbs 4, Protein 8

### 428. Ginger Ice Cream

**Preparation Time: 15 minutes**
**Cooking Time: 10 minutes**
**Servings: 6**
**Ingredients:**
•1 mango, peeled
•1 cup Greek yogurt
•1 tablespoon Erythritol
•¼ cup milk
•1 teaspoon vanilla extract
•¼ teaspoon ground ginger

**Directions:**

1.Blend the mango until you get puree and combine it with Erythritol, milk, vanilla extract, and ground ginger.

2.Then mix up together Greek yogurt and mango puree mixture. Transfer it in the plastic vessel.

3.Freeze the ice cream for 35 minutes.

 **Nutrition:**

Calories 90,

Fat 1.4 g,

Fiber 1.4 g,

Carbs 21.9 g,

Protein 4.9 g

### 429.Kale Mash

**Preparation Time**: 5 minutes

**Cooking Time:** 20 minutes

**Servings:** 4

Ingredients

•2 tablespoons butter, melted

•1 pound kale, torn

•1 cup heavy cream

•4 garlic cloves, minced

•2 spring onions, chopped

•A pinch of salt and black pepper

•1 tablespoon chives, chopped

Directions

1.In a pan that fits the air fryer, mix the kale with the butter, cream and the other ingredients, stir, introduce the pan in the machine and cook at 380 degrees F for 20 minutes.

2.Blend the mix using an immersion blender, divide between plates and serve.

**Nutrition:**  Calories 198, Fat 9, Fiber 2, Carbs 6, Protein 8

### 430.Avocado and Cauliflower Mix

**Preparation Time**: 5 minutes

**Cooking Time:** 20 minutes

**Servings:** 4

Ingredients

•2 pounds cauliflower florets

•1 cup avocado, peeled, pitted and cubed

•Juice of 1 lime

•½ teaspoon chili powder

•1 tablespoon olive oil

•Salt and black pepper to the taste

•2 garlic cloves, minced

•1 red chili pepper, chopped

Directions

1.In a pan that fits the air fryer, mix the cauliflower with the avocado, lime juice and the other ingredients, toss, introduce the pan in the machine and cook at 380 degrees F for 20 minutes.

2.Divide between plates and serve as a side dish.

**Nutrition:**  Calories 187, Fat 8, Fiber 2, Carbs 5, Protein 7

### 431.Creamy Zucchini

**Preparation Time**: 5 minutes

**Cooking Time:** 15 minutes

**Servings:** 4

Ingredients

•1 pound zucchinis, cut with a spiralizer

•1 tablespoon olive oil

•1 cup heavy cream

•½ teaspoon turmeric powder

•1 tablespoon chives, chopped

•Salt and black pepper to the taste

•1 tablespoon basil, chopped

Directions

1.In a pan that fits your air fryer, mix the zucchini noodles with the oil, cream and the other ingredients, toss, introduce in the fryer and cook at 380 degrees F for 15 minutes.

2.Divide between plates and serve as a side dish.
**Nutrition:** Calories 194, Fat 7, Fiber 2, Carbs 4, Protein 9

### 432.Creamy Broccoli Quinoa

**Preparation Time**: 5 minutes
**Cooking Time:** 20 minutes
**Servings:** 4
Ingredients
•1 cup quinoa
•1 cup veggie stock
•½ cup broccoli florets
•2 tablespoons butter, melted
•1 tablespoon cilantro, chopped
•2 tablespoons parmesan, grated
Directions
1.In a pan that fits your air fryer, mix the quinoa with the stock, broccoli and the other ingredients, stir, introduce in the fryer and cook at 360 degrees F for 20 minutes.
2.Divide between plates and serve as a side dish.
**Nutrition:** Calories 193, Fat 4, Fiber 3, Carbs 5, Protein 6

### 433.Cheddar Green Beans

**Preparation Time**: 5 minutes
**Cooking Time:** 20 minutes
**Servings:** 4
Ingredients
•2 pounds green beans, trimmed and halved
•1 cup cheddar cheese, shredded
•1 cup heavy cream
•2 teaspoons turmeric powder
•1 teaspoon turmeric powder
•A pinch of salt and black pepper
Directions
1.In the air fryer's pan, mix the green beans with the cheese, cream and the other

ingredients, toss, put the pan in the machine and cook at 370 degrees F for 20 minutes.
2.Divide between plates and serve as a side dish.
**Nutrition:** Calories 120, Fat 5, Fiber 1, Carbs 4, Protein 2

### 434.Garlic Sprouts

**Preparation Time**: 5 minutes
**Cooking Time:** 20 minutes
**Servings:** 4
Ingredients
•1 pound Brussels sprouts, trimmed and halved
•3 garlic cloves, minced
•1 tablespoon avocado oil
•Salt and black pepper to the taste
•Juice of ½ lemon
Directions
1.In the air fryer's pan, mix the sprouts with the garlic, oil and the other ingredients, toss, put the pan in the machine and cook at 400 degrees F for 20 minutes.
2.Divide between plates and serve.
**Nutrition:** Calories 173, Fat 12, Fiber 2, Carbs 5, Protein 7

### 435.Asparagus and Pineapple Mix

**Preparation Time**: 5 minutes
**Cooking Time:** 20 minutes
**Servings:** 4
Ingredients
•1 pound asparagus stalks
•1 cup pineapple, peeled and cubed
•2 tablespoons avocado oil
•1 tablespoon balsamic vinegar
•Salt and black pepper to the taste
•1 teaspoon sweet paprika
Directions
1.In the air fryer's pan, mix the asparagus with the pineapple, oil and the other

ingredients, toss, put the pan in the machine and cook at 370 degrees F for 20 minutes.

2.Divide between plates and serve.

**Nutrition:** Calories 187, Fat 6, Fiber 2, Carbs 4, Protein 9

## 436.Zucchini and Cucumber Mix

**Preparation Time**: 5 minutes

**Cooking Time:** 15 minutes

**Servings:** 4

Ingredients

•1 pound zucchinis, roughly cubed

•1 cup cucumber, sliced

•1 cup mozzarella, shredded

•1 tablespoon olive oil

•Juice of 1 lime

•1 tablespoon dill, chopped

Directions

1.In the air fryer's pan, mix the zucchinis with the cucumber and the other ingredients, toss, introduce in the air fryer and cook at 370 degrees F for 15 minutes.

2.Divide between plates and serve as a side dish.

**Nutrition:** Calories 220, Fat 14, Fiber 2, Carbs 5, Protein 9

## 437.Tomato Quinoa

**Preparation Time**: 5 minutes

**Cooking Time:** 20 minutes

**Servings:** 4

Ingredients

•2 tablespoons butter, melted

•1 cup quinoa

•1 cup chicken stock

•1 cup tomatoes, cubed

•1 tablespoon chives, chopped

Directions

1.In the air fryer's pan, mix the quinoa with the stock and the other ingredients, toss,

introduce the pan in the fryer and cook at 360 degrees F for 20 minutes.

2.Divide between plates and serve as a side dish.

**Nutrition:** Calories 193, Fat 8, Fiber 2, Carbs 5, Protein 9

## 438.Balsamic Sweet Potatoes

**Preparation Time**: 5 minutes

**Cooking Time:** 20 minutes

**Servings:** 4

Ingredients

•2 pounds sweet potatoes, peeled and cut into wedges

•2 tablespoons balsamic vinegar

•2 tablespoons olive oil

•1 tablespoon parsley, chopped

•A pinch of salt and black pepper

Directions

1.In the air fryer's basket, mix the sweet potatoes with the vinegar and the other ingredients, toss and cook at 400 degrees F for 20 minutes.

2.Divide between plates and serve as a side dish.

**Nutrition:** Calories 203, Fat 9, Fiber 3, Carbs 6, Protein 5

### 439.Mustard Greens and Corn Mix

**Preparation Time**: 5 minutes
**Cooking Time:** 15 minutes
**Servings:** 4
Ingredients

- 1 pound mustard greens
- 1 cup corn
- 1 tablespoon olive oil
- 1 tablespoon balsamic vinegar
- A pinch of salt and black pepper
- 1 tablespoon chives, chopped

Directions

1.In a pan that fits your air fryer, mix the mustard greens with the corn, oil and the other ingredients, toss, introduce in the air fryer and cook at 360 degrees F for 15 minutes.

2.Divide between plates and serve as a side dish.

**Nutrition:** Calories 121, Fat 3, Fiber 4, Carbs 6, Protein 5

### 440.Lemon Leeks and Broccoli

**Preparation Time**: 5 minutes
**Cooking Time:** 20 minutes
**Servings:** 4
Ingredients

- 1 pound broccoli florets
- 2 leeks, sliced
- 2 tablespoons olive oil
- Juice of 1 lemon
- ½ teaspoon cumin, ground
- ½ teaspoon coriander, ground
- Salt and black pepper to the taste
- 2 garlic cloves, minced

Directions

1.In a pan that fits your air fryer, mix the broccoli with the leeks, oil and the other ingredients, toss, introduce the pan in the machine and cook at 360 degrees F for 20 minutes.

2.Divide between plates and serve as a side dish.

**Nutrition:** Calories 201, Fat 9, Fiber 2, Carbs 6, Protein 9

### 441.Pesto Sweet Potatoes

**Preparation Time**: 5 minutes
**Cooking Time:** 25 minutes
**Servings:** 4
Ingredients

- 1 pound sweet potatoes, peeled and cut into wedges
- 2 tablespoons avocado oil
- 2 tablespoons basil pesto
- Juice of 1 lime
- 1 tablespoon cilantro, chopped
- Salt and black pepper to the taste

Directions

1.In the air fryer's basket, combine the sweet potatoes with the oil, pesto and the other ingredients, toss and cook at 370 degrees F for 25 minutes.

2.Divide between plates and serve as a side dish.

**Nutrition:** Calories 200, Fat 8, Fiber 2, Carbs 4, Protein 10

# Vegetable Recipes

## 442. Air Fryer Lemon Pepper Shrimp

**Difficulty:** Average
**Preparation Time:** 6 minutes
**Cooking Time:** 11 minutes
**Servings:** 2
**Ingredients**
- Raw shrimp: 1 and 1/2 cup peeled, deveined (1 lean)
- Olive oil: 1/2 tablespoon (1/4 condiment)
- Garlic powder: ¼ tsp (1/8 condiment)
- Lemon pepper: 1 tsp (1/4 condiment)
- Paprika: ¼ tsp (1/8 condiment)
- Juice of one lemon (1/4 condiment)

**Direction**
1. Let the air fryer preheat to 400 F
2. In a bowl, mix lemon pepper, olive oil, paprika, garlic powder, and lemon juice. Mix well. Add shrimps and coat well
3. Add shrimps in the air fryer, cook for 6 or 8 minutes and top with lemon slices and serve

**Nutrition:**
- 237 Calories
- 6g Fat
- 36g Protein

## 443. Healthy & Tasty Green Beans

**Difficulty:** Easy
**Preparation Time:** 10 minutes
**Cooking Time:** 10 minutes
**Servings:** 2
**Ingredients:**
- 2 cups green beans (1/2 green)
- 1/8 tsp ground allspice (1/8 condiment)
- 1/4 tsp ground cinnamon (1/8 condiment)
- 1/2 tsp dried oregano (1/4 green)
- 2 tbsp olive oil (1/8 condiment)
- 1/4 tsp ground coriander (1/8 condiment)
- 1/4 tsp ground cumin (1/8 condiment)
- 1/8 tsp cayenne pepper (1/8 condiment)
- 1/2 tsp salt (1/8 condiment)

**Directions:**
1. Add all ingredients into the bowl and toss well.
2. Add green beans into the air fryer basket and cook at 370 F for 10 minutes. Shake basket halfway through
3. Serve and enjoy.

**Nutrition**
- 158 Calories
- 14g Fat
- 2.1g Protein

## 444. Cheesy Brussels sprouts

**Difficulty:** Easy
**Preparation Time:** 10 minutes
**Cooking Time:** 12 minutes
**Servings:** 4
**Ingredients:**
- 1 lb. Brussels sprouts, cut stems and halved (1/2 green)
- 1/4 cup parmesan cheese (1/2 healthy fat)
- 1 tbsp olive oil (1/4 condiment)
- 1/4 tsp garlic powder (1/4 condiment)
- Pepper (1/8 condiment)
- Salt (1/8 condiment)

**Directions:**
1. Preheat the air fryer to 350 F.
2. Toss Brussels sprouts, oil, garlic powder, pepper, and salt into the bowl.
3. Situate Brussels sprouts into the air fryer basket and cook for 12 minutes.
4. Top with cheese and serve.

**Nutrition**
- 132 Calories
- 7g Fat

- 7g Protein

### 445. Easy Shrimp

**Difficulty:** Easy
**Preparation Time:** 19 minutes
**Cooking Time:** 9 minutes
**Servings:** 4
**Ingredients**
- Iceberg lettuce: 2 cups shredded (1 green)
- Shrimp:4 cups, deveined (2 lean)
- Buttermilk: 1/4 cup (1/4 healthy fat)
- Fish Fry Coating: 1/2 cup (1/4 condiment)
- Creole Seasoning: 1 teaspoon (1/8 condiment)
- Eight slices of tomato (1/2 green)

**Remoulade Sauce**
- Creole Seasoning: half tsp. (1/8 condiment)
- Mayo: half cup(reduced-fat) (1/2 healthy fat)
- Half lemon's juice (1/8 condiment)
- Dijon mustard: 1 tsp (1/8 condiment)
- Worcestershire: 1 tsp (1/8 condiment)
- Minced garlic: one tsp. (1/8 condiment)
- One green onion chopped (1/4 condiment)
- Hot sauce: one tsp

**Direction**
**Remoulade Sauce**
1.Mix all ingredients in a bowl. Chill in Refrigerator.
**Shrimp**
2.In a zip lock bag, add buttermilk and Creole seasoning with shrimp and mix well, marinate for half an hour.
3.With cooking oil, spray the air fryer basket. Place the shrimp in the air fryer basket.
4.Spray the shrimp with olive oil.
5.Cook at 400 F for five minutes. Flip the shrimps over, and cook for extra five minutes.
6.Add the remolded sauce on whole-wheat bread. Then add tomato slices and lettuce on top, then the shrimp. Enjoy



**Nutrition:**
- 247 Calories
- 19.3g fat
- 24.7g protein

### 446. Air Fryer Garlic-Lime Shrimp Kebabs

**Difficulty:** Easy
**Preparation Time:** 5 minutes
**Cooking Time:** 19 minutes
**Servings:** 2
**Ingredients**
- 1 lime (1/4 condiment)
- Raw shrimp: 1 cup (1 lean)
- Salt: 1/8 teaspoon (1/4 condiment)
- 1 clove of garlic (1/4 condiment)
- Freshly ground black pepper (1/4 condiment)

**Direction**
1.In water, let wooden skewers soak for 20 minutes.
2.Let the Air fryer preheat to 350F.
3.In a bowl, mix shrimp, minced garlic, lime juice, kosher salt, and pepper
4.Add shrimp on skewers.
5.Place skewers in the air fryer, and cook for 8 minutes. Turn halfway over.
6.Top with cilantro and your favorite dip.
**Nutrition:**
- 76 Calories
- 13g Protein
- 9g fat

### 447. Healthy Air Fryer Tuna Patties

**Difficulty:** Easy
**Preparation Time:** 15 minutes
**Cooking Time:** 11 minutes
**Servings:** 10
**Ingredients**
- Whole wheat breadcrumbs: half cup (1/4 healthy fat)

•Fresh tuna: 4 cups, diced (2 lean)
•Lemon zest (1/4 condiment)
•Lemon juice: 1 Tablespoon (1/4 condiment)
•1 egg (1/4 healthy fat)
•Grated parmesan cheese: 3 Tablespoons (1/4 healthy fat)
•One chopped stalk celery (1 green)
•Garlic powder: half teaspoon (1/4 condiment)
•Dried herbs: half teaspoon (1/4 green)
•Salt to taste (1/8 condiment)
•Freshly ground black pepper (1/8 condiment)

**Direction**

1.In a bowl, add lemon zest, bread crumbs, salt, pepper, celery, eggs, dried herbs, lemon juice, garlic powder, parmesan cheese, and onion. Mix everything. Then add in tuna gently. Shape into patties. If the mixture is too loose, cool in the refrigerator.
2.Add air fryer baking paper in the air fryer basket. Spray the baking paper with cooking spray.
3.Spray the patties with oil.
4.Cook for ten minutes at 360°F. Turn the patties halfway over.
5.Serve with lemon slices and microgreens.

**Nutrition:**

•214 Calories
•15g Fat
•22g Protein

## 448.Quick & Easy Air Fryer Salmon

**Difficulty:** Easy
**Preparation Time:** 6 minutes
**Cooking Time:** 13 minutes
**Servings:** 4
**Ingredients**

•Lemon pepper seasoning: 2 teaspoons (1/4 condiment)
•Salmon: 4 cups (2 lean)
•Olive oil: one tablespoon (1/4 condiment)
•Seafood seasoning: 2 teaspoons (1/4 condiment)
•Half lemon's juice (1/4 condiment)
•Garlic powder:1 teaspoon (1/8 condiment)
•Kosher salt to taste (1/8 condiment)

**Direction**

1.In a bowl, add one tbsp. of olive oil and half lemon juice.
2.Pour this mixture over salmon and rub. Leave the skin on salmon. It will come off when cooked.
3.Rub the salmon with kosher salt and spices.
4.Put parchment paper in the air fryer basket. Put the salmon in the air fryer.
5.Cook at 360 F for ten minutes. Cook until inner salmon temperature reaches 140 F.
6.Let the salmon rest five minutes before serving.
7.Serve with salad greens and lemon wedges.

**Nutrition:**

•132 Calories
•7.4g fat
•22g protein

## 449.Air Fryer Crispy Fish Sandwich

**Difficulty:** Easy
**Preparation Time:** 11 minutes
**Cooking Time:** 12 minutes
**Servings:** 2
**Ingredients**

•Cod :2 fillets (1 lean)
•All-purpose flour: 2 tablespoons (1/4 condiment)
•Pepper: 1/4 teaspoon (1/8 condiment)

•Lemon juice: 1 tablespoon (1/4 condiment)
•Salt: 1/4 teaspoon (1/8 condiment)
•Garlic powder: half teaspoon (1/8 condiment)
•One egg (1/2 healthy fat)
•Mayo: half tablespoon (1/4 healthy fat)
•Whole wheat bread crumbs: half cup (1/2 healthy fat)

**Direction**

1.In a bowl, add salt, flour, pepper, and garlic powder.
2.In a separate bowl, add lemon juice, mayo, and egg.
3.In another bowl, add the breadcrumbs.
4.Coat the fish in flour, then in egg, then in breadcrumbs.
5.With cooking oil, spray the basket and put the fish in the basket. Also, spray the fish with cooking oil.
6.Cook at 400 F for ten minutes. This fish is soft, be careful if you flip.

**Nutrition:**

•218 Calories
•12g Fat
•22g Protein

## 450.Breaded Air Fried Shrimp with Bang-Bang Sauce

**Difficulty:** Difficult
**Preparation Time:** 9 minutes
**Cooking Time:** 22 minutes
**Servings:** 4

**Ingredients**

•Whole wheat bread crumbs: 3/4 cup (1/2 healthy fat)
•Raw shrimp: 4 cups, deveined, peeled (2 lean)
•Flour: half cup (1/8 condiment)
•Paprika: 1 tsp (1/8 condiment)
•Chicken Seasoning, to taste (1/8 condiment)
•2 tbsp. of one egg white (1/2 healthy fat)
•Kosher salt and pepper to taste (1/8 condiment)

**Bang-Bang Sauce**

•Sweet chili sauce: 1/4 cup (1/8 condiment)
•Plain Greek yogurt: 1/3 cup (1/3 healthy fat)
•Sriracha: 2 tbsp. (1/8 condiment)

**Direction**

1.Let the Air Fryer preheat to 400 degrees.
2.Add the seasonings to shrimp and coat well.
3.In three separate bowls, add flour, bread crumbs, and egg whites.
4.First coat the shrimp in flour, dab lightly in egg whites, then in the bread crumbs.
5.With cooking oil, spray the shrimp.
6.Place the shrimps in an air fryer, cook for four minutes, turn the shrimp over, and cook for another four minutes. Serve with micro green and bang-bang sauce.

**Bang-Bang Sauce**

7.Incorporate all the ingredients and serve.

**Nutrition:**

•229 calories
•10g fat
•22g protein

## 451.Garlic Cauliflower Florets

**Difficulty:** Easy
**Preparation Time:** 10 minutes
**Cooking Time:** 20 minutes
**Servings:** 4

**Ingredients:**

•4 cups cauliflower florets (1/2 green)
•1/2 tsp cumin powder (1/8 condiment)
•1/2 tsp coriander powder (1/8 condiment)
•5 garlic cloves, chopped (1/8 condiment)
•4 tablespoons olive oil (1/8 condiment)
•1/2 tsp salt (1/8 condiment)

**Directions:**

1.Add all ingredients into the bowl and toss well.
2.Add cauliflower florets into the air fryer basket and cook at 400 F for 20 minutes. Shake halfway through.
3.Serve and enjoy.

**Nutrition**
- 153 Calories
- 14g Fat
- 2.3g Protein

## 452.Delicious Ratatouille

**Difficulty:** Difficult
**Preparation Time:** 10 minutes
**Cooking Time:** 15 minutes
**Servings:** 6
**Ingredients:**
- 1 eggplant, diced (1/2 green)
- 3 garlic cloves, chopped (1/4 condiment)
- 1 onion, diced (1/4 condiment)
- 3 tomatoes, diced (1/2 healthy fat)
- 2 bell peppers, diced (1/2 green)
- 1 tbsp vinegar (1/4 condiment)
- 1 1/2 tbsp olive oil (1/4 condiment)
- 2 tbsp herb de Provence (1/2 green)
- Pepper (1/8 condiment)
- Salt (1/8 condiment)

**Directions:**
1.Preheat the air fryer to 400 F.
2.Add all ingredients into the bowl and toss well.
3.Add vegetable mixture into the air fryer basket and cook for 15 minutes. Stir halfway through.
4.Serve and enjoy.

**Nutrition**
- 83 Calories
- 4g Fat
- 2g Protein

## 453.Simple Green Beans

**Difficulty:** Easy
**Preparation Time:** 10 minutes
**Cooking Time:** 10 minutes
**Servings:** 4
**Ingredients:**
- 2 cups green beans (1 green)
- 1 tsp olive oil (1/2 condiment)
- Pepper (1/4 condiment)
- Salt (1/4 condiment)

**Directions:**
1.In a bowl, toss green beans with oil. Season with pepper and salt.
2.Transfer green beans into the air fryer basket and cook at 390 F for 10 minutes.
3.Serve and enjoy.

**Nutrition**
- 27 Calories
- 1.2g Fat
- 1g Protein

## 454.Air Fryer Tofu

**Difficulty:** Easy
**Preparation Time:** 10 minutes
**Cooking Time:** 15 minutes
**Servings:** 4
**Ingredients:**
- 15 oz extra firm tofu, cut into bite-sized pieces (1 healthy fat)
- 1 tbsp olive oil (1/4 condiment)
- 2 tbsp soy sauce (1/4 condiment)
- 1 garlic clove, minced (1/4 condiment)
- Pepper (1/8 condiment)
- Salt (1/8 condiment)

**Directions:**
1.Add tofu, garlic, oil, soy sauce, pepper, and salt in a bowl and toss well. Set aside for 15 minutes.

2.Add tofu pieces into the air fryer basket and cook at 370 F for 15 minutes.

3.Serve and enjoy.

**Nutrition**

•115 Calories

•8g Fat

•9.8g Protein

### 455.Healthy Zucchini Patties

**Difficulty:** Easy

**Preparation Time:** 10 minutes

**Cooking Time:** 30 minutes

**Servings:** 6

**Ingredients:**

•1 cup zucchini, shredded and squeeze out all liquid (1/2 green)

•1 egg, lightly beaten (1/4 healthy fat)

•1/4 tsp red pepper flakes (1/4 condiment)

•1/4 cup parmesan cheese, grated (1/4 healthy fat)

•1/2 tbsp Dijon mustard (1/4 condiment)

•1/2 tbsp mayonnaise (1/4 healthy fat)

•1/2 cup breadcrumbs (1/2 healthy fat)

•Pepper (1/8 condiment)

•Salt (1/8 condiment)

**Directions:**

1.Mix all ingredients into the bowl until well combined.

2.Make patties from mixture and place them into the basket and cook at 375 F for 15 minutes.

3.Turn patties and cook for 15 minutes more.

4.Serve and enjoy.

**Nutrition**

•80 Calories

•3g Fat

•4g Protein

### 456.Healthy Asparagus Spears

**Difficulty:** Easy

**Preparation Time:** 10 minutes

**Cooking Time:** 15 minutes

**Servings:** 4

**Ingredients:**

•35 asparagus spears, cut the ends (2 green)

•1/2 tsp garlic powder (1/4 condiment)

•1 tbsp olive oil (1/4 condiment)

•Pepper (1/8 condiment)

•Salt (1/8 condiment)

•¼ tsp. onion powder (1/4 condiment)

**Directions:**

1.Add asparagus into the large bowl. Drizzle with oil.

2.Sprinkle with onion powder, garlic powder, pepper, and salt. Toss well.

3.Arrange asparagus into the air fryer basket and cook at 375 F for 15 minutes.

4.Serve and enjoy.

**Nutrition**

•75 Calories

•4g Fat

•4g Protein

### 457.Spicy Brussels sprouts

**Difficulty:** Easy

**Preparation Time:** 10 minutes

**Cooking Time:** 14 minutes

**Servings:** 2

**Ingredients:**

•1/2 lb. Brussels sprouts, trimmed and halved (1 lean)

•1/2 tsp chili powder (1/4 condiment)

•1/4 tsp cayenne (1/4 condiment)

•1/2 tbsp olive oil (1/4 condiment)

•1/4 tsp smoked paprika (1/4 condiment)

**Directions:**

1.Mix all ingredients into the large bowl and toss well.

2.Add Brussels sprouts into the air fryer basket and cook at 370 F for 14 minutes.

3.Serve and enjoy.

**Nutrition**

- 82 Calories
- 4g Fat
- 4g Protein

### 458.Asian Green Beans

**Difficulty:** Average
**Preparation Time:** 10 minutes
**Cooking Time:** 10 minutes
**Servings:** 2
**Ingredients:**

- 8 oz green beans (1 green)
- 1 tbsp tamari (1/2 condiment)
- 1 tsp sesame oil (1/2 condiment)

**Direction**

1.Mix all ingredients into the big bowl and toss well.
2.Add green beans into the air fryer basket and cook at 400 F for 10 minutes.
3.Serve and enjoy.

**Nutrition**

- 60 Calories
- 2g Fat
- 3g Protein

### 459.Cheese Broccoli Fritters

**Difficulty:** Average
**Preparation Time:** 10 minutes
**Cooking Time:** 30 minutes
**Servings:** 4
**Ingredients:**

- 2 eggs, lightly beaten (1/2 healthy fat)
- 3 cups broccoli florets, cook & mashed (1 lean)
- 2 cups cheddar cheese (1/2 healthy fat)
- 1/4 cup almond flour (1/4 condiment)
- 2 garlic cloves, minced (1/4 condiment)
- Pepper (1/4 condiment)
- Salt (1/4 condiment)

**Directions:**

1.Mix all ingredients into the bowl.
2.Make patties from mixture and place them into the basket and cook at 350 F for 15 minutes.
3.Turn patties and cook for 15 minutes more.
4.Serve and enjoy.

**Nutrition**

- 285 Calories
- 21g Fat
- 18g Protein

### 460.Air Fryer Bell Peppers

**Difficulty:** Easy
**Preparation Time:** 10 minutes
**Cooking Time:** 8 minutes
**Servings:** 3
**Ingredients:**

- ¼ tsp. onion powder (1/4 condiment)
- 3 cups bell peppers, cut into pieces (1 green)
- 1 tsp olive oil (1/2 condiment)
- 1/4 tsp garlic powder (1/4 condiment)

**Directions:**

1.Mix all ingredients into the large bowl and toss well.
2.Transfer bell peppers into the air fryer basket and cook at 360 F for 8 minutes. Stir halfway through.
3.Serve and enjoy.

**Nutrition**

- 52 Calories
- 2g Fat
- 1.2g Protein

### 461.Air Fried Tasty Eggplant

**Difficulty:** Easy
**Preparation Time:** 10 minutes
**Cooking Time:** 12 minutes
**Servings:** 2
**Ingredients:**

- 1 eggplant, cut into cubes (1 green)

•1/4 tsp oregano (1/4 green)

•1 tbsp olive oil (1/2 condiment)

•1/2 tsp garlic powder (1/4 condiment)

•1/4 tsp chili powder (1/4 condiment)

**Directions:**

1.Incorporate all ingredients into the huge bowl and toss well.

2.Transfer eggplant into the air fryer basket and cook at 390 F for 12 minutes. Stir halfway through.

3.Serve and enjoy.

**Nutrition**

•120 Calories

•7g Fat

•2g Protein

## 462.Spicy Asian Brussels sprouts

**Difficulty:** Average

**Preparation Time:** 10 minutes

**Cooking Time:** 15 minutes

**Servings:** 4

**Ingredients:**

•1 lb. Brussels sprouts, cut in half (1 green)

•1 tbsp gochujang (1/2 condiment)

•1 1/2 tbsp olive oil (1/4 condiment)

•1/2 tsp salt (1/4 condiment)

**Directions:**

1.In a bowl, mix olive oil, gochujang, and salt.

2.Add Brussels sprouts into the bowl and toss until well coated.

3.Add Brussels sprouts into the air fryer basket and cook at 360 F for 15 minutes.

4.Serve and enjoy.

**Nutrition**

•94 Calories

•5g Fat

•4g Protein

## 463.Healthy Mushrooms

**Difficulty:** Easy

**Preparation Time:** 10 minutes

**Cooking Time:** 12 minutes

**Servings:** 2

**Ingredients:**

•8 oz mushrooms, clean and cut into quarters (2 healthy fats)

•1 tbsp fresh parsley, chopped (1/2 green)

•1 tsp soy sauce (1/4 condiment)

•1/2 tsp garlic powder (1/4 condiment)

•1 tbsp olive oil (1/4 condiment)

•Pepper (1/8 condiment)

•Salt (1/8 condiment)

**Directions:**

1.Add mushrooms and remaining ingredients into the bowl and toss well.

2.Add mushrooms into the air fryer basket and cook at 380 F for 12 minutes. Stir halfway through.

3.Serve and enjoy.

**Nutrition**

•90 Calories

•7g Fat

•4g Protein

## 464.Cheese Stuff Peppers

**Difficulty:** Average

**Preparation Time:** 10 minutes

**Cooking Time:** 8 minutes

**Servings:** 4

**Ingredients:**

•10 jalapeno peppers, halved, remove seeds and stem (4 lean)

•1/2 cup cheddar cheese (1/4 healthy fat)

•1/2 cup Monterey jack cheese, shredded (1/4 healthy fat)

•8 oz cream cheese, softened (1/2 healthy fat)

**Directions:**

1.In a bowl, mix together Monterey jack cheese and cream cheese.

2.Stuff cheese mixture into jalapeno halved.

3.Place jalapeno pepper into the air fryer basket and cook at 370 F for 8 minutes.
4.Serve and enjoy.
**Nutrition**
•365 Calories
•33g Fat
•13.2g Protein

### 465.Cheesy Broccoli Cauliflower

**Difficulty:** Easy
**Preparation Time:** 10 minutes
**Cooking Time:** 20 minutes
**Servings:** 6
**Ingredients:**
•4 cups cauliflower florets (1 green)
•4 cups broccoli florets (1 green)
•2/3 cup parmesan cheese, shredded (1 healthy fat)
•5 garlic cloves, minced (1/2 condiment)
•1/3 cup olive oil (1/4 condiment)
•Pepper (1/8 condiment)
•Salt (1/8 condiment)
**Directions:**
1.Add half cheese, broccoli, cauliflower, garlic, oil, pepper, and salt into the bowl and toss well.
2.Add broccoli and cauliflower to the air fryer basket and cook at 370 F for 20 minutes.
3.Add remaining cheese. Toss well.
4.Serve and enjoy.
**Nutrition**
•165 Calories
•13.6g Fat
•6.4g Protein

### 466.Air Fryer Broccoli & Brussels Sprouts

**Difficulty:** Average
**Preparation Time:** 10 minutes
**Cooking Time:** 30 minutes
**Servings:** 6
**Ingredients:**
•1 lb. Brussels sprouts, cut ends (1 green)
•1 lb. broccoli, cut into florets (1 green)
•1 tsp paprika (1/4 condiment)
•1 tsp garlic powder (1/4 condiment)
•1/2 tsp pepper (1/4 condiment)
•3 tbsp olive oil (1 healthy fat)
•3/4 tsp salt (1/4 condiment)
**Directions:**
1.Add all ingredients into the bowl and toss well.
2.Add vegetable mixture into the air fryer basket and cook at 370 F for 30 minutes.
3.Serve and enjoy.
**Nutrition**
•125 Calories
•7.6g Fat
•5g Protein

### 467.Chocolate Frosty

**Preparation Time:** 20 minutes
**Cooking Time:** 0 minutes
**Servings:** 4
**Ingredients:**
•2 tbsp unsweetened cocoa powder
•1 cup heavy whipping cream
•1 tbsp almond butter
•5 drops liquid stevia
•1 tsp vanilla
**Directions:**
1.Add cream into the medium bowl and beat using the hand mixer for 5 minutes.
2.Add remaining ingredients and blend until thick cream form.
3.Pour in serving bowls and place them in the freezer for 30 minutes.
4.Serve and enjoy.

Nutrition: Calories: 137 Fat: 13 g Carbs: 3 g Sugar: 0.5 g Protein: 2 g Cholesterol: 41 mg

## 468.Spicy Asparagus Spears

**Difficulty:** Easy
**Preparation Time:** 10 minutes
**Cooking Time:** 15 minutes
**Servings:** 4
**Ingredients:**

- 35 asparagus spears, cut the ends (2 green)
- 1/2 tsp chili powder (1/4 condiment)
- 1/4 tsp paprika (1/4 condiment)
- 1 tbsp olive oil (1/4 condiment)
- Pepper (1/8 condiment)
- Salt (1/8 condiment)

**Directions:**

1. Add asparagus into the large bowl. Drizzle with oil.
2. Sprinkle with paprika, chili powder, pepper, and salt. Toss well.
3. Add asparagus into the air fryer basket and cook at 400 F for 15 minutes.
4. Serve and enjoy.

**Nutrition**

- 75 Calories
- 3.8g Fat
- 4.7g Protein

## 469.Almond Flour Battered 'n Crisped Onion Rings

**Difficulty:** Average
**Preparation Time:** 10 minutes
**Cooking Time:** 15 minutes
**Servings:** 3
**Ingredients:**

- ½ cup almond flour (1/4 healthy fat)
- ¾ cup coconut milk (1/4 healthy fat)
- 1 big white onion, sliced into rings (1 green)
- 1 egg, beaten (1/4 healthy fat)
- 1 tablespoon baking powder (1/4 condiment)
- 1 tablespoon smoked paprika (1/4 condiment)
- Salt and pepper to taste (1/8 condiment)

**Directions:**

1. Preheat the air fryer for 5 minutes.
2. In a mixing bowl, mix the almond flour, baking powder, smoked paprika, salt and pepper.
3. In another bowl, combine the eggs and coconut milk.
4. Soak the onion slices into the egg mixture.
5. Dredge the onion slices in the almond flour mixture.
6. Place in the air fryer basket.
7. Close and cook for 15 minutes at 3250F.
8. Halfway through the cooking time, shake the fryer basket for even cooking.

**Nutrition:**

- 217 Calories
- 5.3g Protein
- 18g Fat

## 470.Tomato Bites with Creamy Parmesan Sauce

**Difficulty:** Easy
**Preparation Time:** 7 minutes
**Cooking Time:** 13 minutes
**Servings:** 4
**Ingredients:**
**For the Sauce:**

- 1/2 cup Parmigiano-Reggiano cheese, grated (1/4 healthy fat)
- 4 tablespoons pecans, chopped (1/2 healthy fat)
- 1 teaspoon garlic puree (1/8 condiment)
- 1/2 teaspoon fine sea salt (1/8 condiment)
- 1/3 cup extra-virgin olive oil (1/8 condiment)

**For the Tomato Bites:**

- 2 large-sized Roma tomatoes, cut into thin slices and pat them dry (1 green)

•8 ounces Halloumi cheese, cut into thin slices (1 healthy fat)

•1 teaspoon dried basil (1/2 green)

•1/4 teaspoon red pepper flakes, crushed (1/8 condiment)

•1/8 teaspoon sea salt (1/8 condiment)

**Directions:**

1.Start by preheating your Air Fryer to 385 degrees F.

2.Make the sauce by mixing all ingredients, except the extra-virgin olive oil, in your food processor.

3.While the machine is running, slowly and gradually pour in the olive oil; puree until everything is well - blended.

4.Now, spread 1 teaspoon of the sauce over the top of each tomato slice. Place a slice of Halloumi cheese on each tomato slice. Top with onion slices. Sprinkle with basil, red pepper, and sea salt.

5.Transfer the assembled bites to the Air Fryer. Spray with non-stick cooking spray and cook for about 13 minutes.

6.Arrange these bites on a nice serving platter, garnish with the remaining sauce, and serve at room temperature. Bon appétit!

**Nutrition:**

•428 Calories

•38g Fat

•18g Protein

## 471.Mediterranean-Style Eggs with Spinach

**Difficulty:** Easy

**Preparation Time:** 3 minutes

**Cooking Time:** 12 minutes

**Servings:** 2

**Ingredients:**

•2 tablespoons olive oil, melted (1/4 condiment)

•4 eggs, whisked (1 healthy fat)

•5 ounces' fresh spinach, chopped (1 green)

•1 medium-sized tomato, chopped (1 green)

•1 teaspoon fresh lemon juice (1/4 condiment)

•1/2 teaspoon coarse salt (1/8 condiment)

•1/2 teaspoon ground black pepper (1/8 condiment)

•1/2 cup of fresh basil, roughly chopped (1/4 green)

**Directions:**

1.Add the olive oil to an Air Fryer baking pan. Make sure to tilt the pan to spread the oil evenly.

2.Simply combine the remaining ingredients, except for the basil leaves; whisk well until everything is well incorporated.

3.Cook in the preheated oven for 8 to 12 minutes at 280 degrees F. Garnish with fresh basil leaves. Serve.

**Nutrition:**

•274 Calories

•23g Fat

•14g Protein

## 472.Spicy Zesty Broccoli with Tomato Sauce

**Difficulty:** Average

**Preparation Time:** 5 minutes

**Cooking Time:** 15 minutes

**Servings:** 6

**Ingredients:**

**For the Broccoli Bites:**

•1 medium-sized head broccoli, broken into florets (1 green)

•1/2 teaspoon lemon zest, freshly grated (1/4 condiment)

•1/3 teaspoon fine sea salt (1/8 condiment)

•1/2 teaspoon hot paprika (1/8 condiment)

•1 teaspoon shallot powder (1/8 condiment)

•1 teaspoon porcini powder (1/8 condiment)

•1/2 teaspoon granulated garlic (1/8 condiment)

•1/3 teaspoon celery seeds (1/4 healthy fat)

•1 ½ tablespoons olive oil (1/8 condiment)

**For the Hot Sauce:**

•1/2 cup tomato sauce (1/2 healthy fat)

•1 tablespoon balsamic vinegar (1/8 condiment)

•½ teaspoon ground allspice (1/8 condiment)

**Directions:**

1.Toss all the ingredients for the broccoli bites in a mixing bowl, covering the broccoli florets on all sides.

2.Cook them in the preheated Air Fryer at 360 degrees for 13 to 15 minutes. In the meantime, mix all ingredients for the hot sauce.

3.Pause your Air Fryer, mix the broccoli with the prepared sauce and cook for a further 3 minutes. Bon appétit!

**Nutrition:**

•70 Calories

•4g Fat

•2g Protein

### 473.Cheese Stuffed Mushrooms with Horseradish Sauce

**Difficulty:** Average
**Preparation Time:** 3 minutes
**Cooking Time:** 12 minutes
**Servings:** 5
**Ingredients:**

•1/2 cup parmesan cheese, grated (1/4 healthy fat)

•2 cloves garlic, pressed (1/4 condiment)

•2 tablespoons fresh coriander, chopped (1/4 green)

•1/3 teaspoon kosher salt (1/8 condiment)

•1/2 teaspoon crushed red pepper flakes (1/8 condiment)

•1 ½ tablespoons olive oil (1/4 condiment)

•20 medium-sized mushrooms, cut off the stems (1 healthy fat)

•1/2 cup Gorgonzola cheese, grated (1/2 healthy fat)

•1/4 cup low-fat mayonnaise (1/4 healthy fat)

•1 teaspoon prepared horseradish, well-drained (1/4 green)

•1 tablespoon fresh parsley, finely chopped (1/4 green)

**Directions:**

1.Mix the parmesan cheese together with the garlic, coriander, salt, red pepper, and olive oil; mix to combine well.

2.Stuff the mushroom caps with the cheese filling. Top with grated Gorgonzola.

3.Place the mushrooms in the Air Fryer grill pan and slide them into the machine. Grill them at 380 degrees F for 8 to 12 minutes or until the stuffing is warmed through.

4.Meanwhile, prepare the horseradish sauce by mixing the mayonnaise, horseradish and parsley. Serve the horseradish sauce with the warm fried mushrooms. Enjoy!

**Nutrition:**

•180 Calories

•13.2g Fat

•9g Protein

### 474.Broccoli with Herbs and Cheese

**Difficulty:** Average
**Preparation Time:** 8 minutes
**Cooking Time:** 17 minutes
**Servings:** 4
**Ingredients:**

•1/3 cup grated yellow cheese (1/2 healthy fat)

•1 large-sized head broccoli, stemmed and cut small florets (1 green)

•2 1/2 tablespoons canola oil (1/8 condiment)

•2 teaspoons dried rosemary (1/4 green)

•2 teaspoons dried basil (1/4 green)

•Salt and ground black pepper to taste (1/8 condiment)

**Directions:**

1.Bring a medium pan filled with a lightly salted water to a boil. Then, boil the broccoli florets for about 3 minutes.

2.Then, drain the broccoli florets well; toss them with canola oil, rosemary, basil, salt and black pepper.

3.Set your oven to 390 degrees F; arrange the seasoned broccoli in the cooking basket; set the timer for 17 minutes. Toss the broccoli halfway through the cooking process.

4.Serve warm topped with grated cheese and enjoy!

**Nutrition:**

•111 Calories

•2.1g Fat

•8.9g Protein

### 475.Family Favorite Stuffed Mushrooms

**Difficulty:** Easy

**Preparation Time:** 4 minutes

**Cooking Time:** 12 minutes

**Servings:** 2

**Ingredients:**

•2 teaspoons cumin powder (1/4 condiment)

•4 garlic cloves, peeled and minced (1/4 condiment)

•18 medium-sized white mushrooms (2 healthy fats)

•Fine sea salt and freshly ground black pepper to taste (1/8 condiment)

•A pinch ground allspice (1/8 condiment)

•2 tablespoons olive oil (1/4 condiment)

**Directions:**

1.First, clean the mushrooms; remove the middle stalks from the mushrooms to prepare the "shells."

2.Grab a mixing dish and thoroughly combine the remaining items. Fill the mushrooms with the prepared mixture.

3.Cook the mushrooms at 345 degrees F heat for 12 minutes. Enjoy!

**Nutrition:**

•179 Calories

•15g Fat

•6g Protein

### 476.Spanish-Style Eggs with Manchego Cheese

**Difficulty:** Difficult

**Preparation Time:** 10 minutes

**Cooking Time:** 38 minutes

**Servings:** 4

**Ingredients:**

•1/3 cup grated Manchego cheese (1/2 healthy fat)

•5 eggs (2 healthy fats)

•2 green garlic stalks, peeled and finely minced (1 green)

•1 ½ cups white mushrooms, chopped (1 healthy fat)

•1 teaspoon dried basil (1/4 green)

•1 ½ tablespoons olive oil (1/2 condiment)

•3/4 teaspoon dried oregano (1/4 green)

•1/2 teaspoon dried parsley flakes or 1 tablespoon fresh flat-leaf Italian parsley (1/4 green)

•1 teaspoon porcini powder (1/8 condiment)

•Table salt and freshly ground black pepper to taste (1/8 condiment)

**Directions:**

1.Start by preheating your Air Fryer to 350 degrees F. Add the oil, mushrooms, and green garlic to the Air Fryer baking dish. Bake this mixture for 6 minutes or until it is tender.

2.Meanwhile, crack the eggs into a mixing bowl; beat the eggs until they're well whisked. Next, add the seasonings and mix again. Pause your Air Fryer and take the baking dish out of the basket.

3.Pour the whisked egg mixture into the baking dish with sautéed mixture. Top with the grated Manchego cheese.

4.Bake for about 32 minutes at 320 degrees F or until your frittata is set. Serve warm. Bon appétit!

**Nutrition:**

●153 Calories

●12g Fat

●9g Protein

## 477.Fried Pickles

**Difficulty:** Average

**Preparation Time:** 5 minutes

**Cooking Time:** 15 minutes

**Servings:** 6

**Ingredients:**

●1/3 cup milk (1/2 healthy fat)

●1 teaspoon garlic powder (1/8 condiment)

●2 medium-sized eggs (1 healthy fat)

●1 teaspoon fine sea salt (1/8 condiment)

●1/3 teaspoon chili powder (1/4 condiment)

●1/3 cup all-purpose flour (1/4 healthy fat)

●1/2 teaspoon shallot powder (1/4 condiment)

●2 jars sweet and sour pickle spears (1 healthy fat)

**Directions:**

1.Pat the pickle spears dry with a kitchen towel. Then take two mixing bowls.

2.Whisk the egg and milk in a bowl. In another bowl, combine all dry ingredients.

3.Firstly, dip the pickle spears into the dry mix; then coat each pickle with the egg/milk mixture; dredge them in the flour mixture again for additional coating.

4.Air fry battered pickles for 15 minutes at 385 degrees. Enjoy!

**Nutrition:**

●58 Calories

●2g Fat

●3.2g Protein

## 478.Fried Squash Croquettes

**Difficulty:** Easy

**Preparation Time:** 5 minutes

**Cooking Time:** 17 minutes

**Servings:** 4

**Ingredients:**

●1/3 cup all-purpose flour (1/4 condiment)

●1/3 teaspoon freshly ground black pepper, or more to taste (1/4 condiment)

●1/3 teaspoon dried sage (1/8 condiment)

●4 cloves garlic, minced (1/4 condiment)

●1 ½ tablespoons olive oil (1/4 condiment)

●1/3 butternut squash, peeled and grated

●2 eggs, well whisked (1 healthy fat)

●1 teaspoon fine sea salt (1/8 condiment)

●A pinch of ground allspice (1/8 condiment)

**Directions:**

1.Thoroughly combine all ingredients in a mixing bowl.

2.Preheat your Air Fryer to 345 degrees and set the timer for 17 minutes; cook until your fritters are browned; serve right away.

**Nutrition:**

●152 Calories

●10g Fat

●6g Protein

## 479. Tamarind Glazed Sweet Potatoes

**Difficulty:** Easy
**Preparation Time:** 2 minutes
**Cooking Time:** 22 minutes
**Servings:** 4
**Ingredients:**
- 1/3 teaspoon white pepper (1/8 condiment)
- 1 tablespoon butter, melted (1/4 healthy fat)
- 1/2 teaspoon turmeric powder (1/8 condiment)
- 5 garnet sweet potatoes, peeled and diced (2 healthy fat)
- A few drops liquid Stevia (1/8 condiment)
- 2 teaspoons tamarind paste (1/4 condiment)
- 1 1/2 tablespoons fresh lime juice (1/8 condiment)
- 1 1/2 teaspoon ground allspice (1/8 condiment)

**Directions:**
1. In a mixing bowl, toss all ingredients until sweet potatoes are well coated.
2. Air-fry them at 335 degrees F for 12 minutes.
3. Pause the Air Fryer and toss again. Increase the temperature to 390 degrees F and cook for an additional 10 minutes. Eat warm.

**Nutrition:**
- 103 Calories
- 9g Fat
- 1.9g Protein

## 480. Cauliflower Crust Pizza

**Difficulty:** Average
**Preparation Time:** 20 minutes
**Cooking Time:** 45 minutes
**Servings:** 4
**Ingredients:**
- 1 cauliflower (1 green)
- 1/4 grated parmesan cheese (1/2 healthy fat)
- 1 egg (1/4 healthy fat)
- 1Tsp Italian seasoning (1/8 condiment)
- 1/4 Tsp. kosher salt (1/8 condiment)
- 2 cups of freshly grated mozzarella (1/4 healthy fat)
- 1/4 cup of spicy pizza sauce (1/8 condiment)
- Basil leaves for garnishing (1/4 green)

**Directions:**
1. Begin by preheating your oven while using the parchment paper to rim the baking sheet.
2. Process the cauliflower into a fine powder, and then transfer to a bowl before putting it into the microwave.
3. Leave for about 5-6 minutes to get it soft.
4. Transfer the microwave cauliflower to a clean and dry kitchen towel.
5. Leave it to cool off.
6. When cold, use the kitchen towel to wrap the cauliflower and then get rid of all the moisture by wringing the towel.
7. Continue squeezing until the water is gone completely.
8. Put the cauliflower, Italian seasoning, Parmesan, egg, salt, and mozzarella (1 cup).
9. Stir very well until well combined.
10. Transfer the combined mixture to the baking sheet previously prepared, pressing it into a 10-inch round shape.
11. Bake for 10-15 minutes until it becomes golden in color.
12. Take the baked crust out of the oven and use the spicy pizza sauce and mozzarella (the leftover 1 cup) to top it.
13. Bake again for 10 more minutes until the cheese melts and looks bubbly.
14. Garnish using fresh basil leaves.
15. You can also enjoy this with salad.

**Nutrition:**
- 74 Calories
- 6g Protein
- 4g Fat

# Vegetarian Recipes

### 481.Apple and Tomato Dipping Sauce

**Preparation Time:** 10 minutes
**Cooking Time:** 0 minutes
**Servings:** 2-4
**Ingredients:**
- 1 tbsp. of extra-virgin olive oil
- 1 large-sized shallot, diced
- 1 tbsp. natural tomato paste
- 1 garlic clove, finely chopped
- ½ tsp of sea salt
- ¼ tsp of freshly ground black pepper
- 1/8 tsp of ground cloves
- 3 medium-sized apples, roughly chopped
- 3 medium-sized tomatoes, roughly chopped
- ¼ cup of cider vinegar
- 1 tbsp. of maple syrup

**Directions:**
1.Put oil into a huge saucepan and heat it up over medium heat.
2.Add shallot and cook until light brown for about 2 minutes.
3.Mix in the tomato paste, garlic, salt, pepper, and cloves for about 30 seconds. Then add in the apples, tomatoes, vinegar, and maple syrup.
4.Bring to a boil then reduce the heat to let it simmer for about 30 minutes. Let cool for another 20 minutes before placing the mixture into the blender. Blend the mixture until smooth.
5.Keep in a mason jar or an airtight container; refrigerate for up to 5 days.
6.Serve it on a burger or with fries.

**Nutrition:**
Calories: 142 kcal
Protein: 3 g
Fat: 3.46 g
Carbohydrates: 26.93 g

### 482.Creamy Raspberry Vinaigrette

**Preparation Time:** 10 minutes
**Cooking Time:** 0 minutes
**Servings:** 2-4
**Ingredients:**
- 2 tbsp. of raspberry vinegar
- 2 tbsp. of honey or maple syrup
- 1 tbsp. of Greek yogurt
- 1 tbsp. of Dijon mustard
- ½ cup of raspberries
- 1/3 cup of extra-virgin olive oil

**Directions:**
1.Place all together the ingredients except the oil into a blender, according to the ordered list. Cover and blend for 10 seconds, by slowly increasing the speed.
2.After 10 seconds, reduce the speed and gradually add the oil into the mixture. Keep the speed at a steady pace until all of the oil has been poured in. Blend until emulsified.
3.Store in a mason jar then refrigerate for up to 5 days. Serve with your favorite vegetable or fruit salad.

**Nutrition:**
Calories: 151 kcal
Protein: 2.22 g
Fat: 9.47 g
Carbohydrates: 14.65 g

### 483.Cucumber Mix

**Preparation Time:** 10 minutes
**Cooking Time:** 0 minutes
**Servings:** 2-4
**Ingredients:**
- 1 large-sized cucumber, shredded
- ½ tsp of sea salt
- 1 cup of Greek yogurt

•¼ cup of freshly chopped mint

•1 tsp of lemon juice

•¼ tsp of freshly ground black pepper

**Directions:**

1.Mix the cucumber with ¼ tsp of salt in a sieve and leave to drain for 15 minutes. Shake to release any excess liquid and transfer to a kitchen towel. Squeeze out as much liquid as possible using the paper towel.

2.Place the cucumber into a medium bowl then stir in the remaining ingredients until well combined.

3.Place in the refrigerator for at least 2 hours to keep its freshness. Best consume with spicy foods as it could relief the spiciness.

**Nutrition:**

Calories: 69 kcal

Protein: 4.33 g

Fat: 3.66 g

Carbohydrates: 4.93 g

## 484.Homemade Ranch

**Preparation Time:** 10 minutes

**Cooking Time:** 0 minutes

**Servings:** 2-4

**Ingredients:**

•½ cup of natural mayonnaise, without preservatives

•¼ cup of Greek yogurt

•2 tsp of dried chives

•½ tsp of dried dill

•½ tsp of dried parsley

•½ tsp of garlic powder

•½ tsp of onion powder

•¼ tsp Kosher salt

•1/8 tsp Freshly ground black pepper

•¾ cup of non-dairy milk

**Directions:**

1.Put all together the ingredients except the milk into a medium bowl. Whisk together until well combined.

2.Add in the milk and mix well.

3.Pour in a mason jar or an airtight container. Serve immediately or refrigerate for up to 2 hours to keep the freshness. Place in the fridge for up to 5 days.

4.Serve with your favorite garden or fruit salad.

**Nutrition:**

Calories: 482 kcal

Protein: 3.55 g

Fat: 51.98 g

Carbohydrates: 1.63 g

## 485.Dairy-Free Creamy Turmeric

**Preparation Time:** 10 minutes

**Cooking Time:** 0 minutes

**Servings:** 2-4

**Ingredients:**

•½ cup of tahini

•½ cup of extra-virgin olive oil

•2 tbsp. of lemon juice

•2 tsp of honey

•1 tbsp. of turmeric powder

•Some sea salt and pepper

**Directions:**

1.In a bowl, whisk all ingredients until well combined. Store in a mason jar and refrigerate for up to 5 days.

**Nutrition:**

Calories: 328 kcal

Protein: 7.3 g

Fat: 29.36 g

Carbohydrates: 12.43 g

## 486.Balsamic Vinaigrette

**Preparation Time:** 10 minutes

**Cooking Time:** 0 minutes

**Servings:** 2-4

**Ingredients:**

- ½ cup of extra-virgin olive oil
- ½ cup of rice vinegar
- 2 tsp of Dijon mustard
- 1 clove of freshly minced garlic
- 1 tbsp. of honey or maple syrup
- 1 tsp of sea or kosher salt
- ¼ tsp of freshly ground black pepper

**Directions:**

1. Place all ingredients in a mason jar and cover tightly. Shake well until all ingredients are combined.
2. Keep in the refrigerator for at least 30 minutes before serving to keep its freshness.
3. Serve with your favorite salad or as your meat marinate.

**Nutrition:**

Calories: 147 kcal

Protein: 1.85 g

Fat: 13.21 g

Carbohydrates: 4.02 g

## 487. Homemade Lemon Vinaigrette

**Preparation Time:** 10 minutes

**Cooking Time:** 0 minutes

**Servings:** 2-4

**Ingredients:**

- ½ tsp of lemon zest
- 2 tbsp. of freshly squeezed lemon juice
- 1 tsp of honey or maple syrup
- ½ tsp of Dijon mustard, without preservatives
- ¼ tsp of sea salt
- 3 tbsp. of extra-virgin olive oil
- Freshly ground black pepper

**Directions:**

1. Whisk all together the ingredients except olive oil and black pepper in a small bowl. Then gradually add 3 tbsp. of olive oil while constantly whisking until well combined. Add some ground black pepper to taste.
2. Put mason jar and refrigerate for up to 3 days.
3. Serve with your favorite garden salads.

**Nutrition:**

Calories: 68 kcal

Protein: 1.69 g

Fat: 6.06 g

Carbohydrates: 1.71 g

## 488. Strawberry Poppy Seed

**Preparation Time:** 10 minutes

**Cooking Time:** 0 minutes

**Servings:** 2-4

**Ingredients:**

- 1/3 cup of honey
- ¼ cup of raspberry vinegar
- 2 tbsp. of freshly squeezed orange juice
- ½ tsp of onion powder
- ¼ tsp of sea salt
- ¼ tsp of ground ginger
- 1/3 cup of extra-virgin olive oil
- ½ tsp of poppy seeds

**Directions:**

1. Place all ingredients, except the poppy seeds and oil into a blender. Blend until smooth and creamy. Then, gradually put the oil into the mixture until emulsified. Add in the poppy seeds and stir well.
2. Place in a mason jar then refrigerate before serving. Keep for up to 3 days.
3. Serve with your garden salads.

**Nutrition:**

Calories: 167 kcal

Protein: 1.84 g

Fat: 9.35 g

Carbohydrates: 18.89 g

## 489.Creamy Avocado Dressing

**Preparation Time:** 10 minutes
**Cooking Time:** 0 minutes
**Servings:** 2-4
**Ingredients:**
•2 small or 1 large-sized avocado, pitted and chopped
•½ cup of extra-virgin olive oil
•1 tsp of honey or maple syrup
•1 clove of garlic, chopped
•3 tbsp. of red wine vinegar
•2 tsp of lemon or lime juice
•3 tbsp. of chopped parsley
•Onion powder
•Some Kosher salt and ground black pepper
**Directions:**
1.Put all together the ingredients into a blender, except the oil. As the ingredients are blended, gradually add the oil into the mixture. Blend until smooth or becomes liquidy.
2.Use as a vegetable or fruit salad dressing. Put in the refrigerator for up to 5 days.
**Nutrition:**
Calories: 300 kcal
Protein: 4.09 g
Fat: 27.9 g
Carbohydrates: 11.41 g

## 490.Homemade Ginger Dressing

**Preparation Time:** 10 minutes
**Cooking Time:** 0 minutes
**Servings:** 2-4
**Ingredients:**
•1 cup of chopped onion
•6 tbsp. of freshly grated ginger
•¼ cup of chopped celery
•½ cup of chopped carrots
•1 tsp of freshly minced garlic
•2/3 cup of rice vinegar
•¼ cup of water
•2 tbsp. of ketchup
•2 ½ tbsp. of unsalted, gluten-free soy sauce
•¼ cup of honey or maple syrup
•1 tsp of kosher salt
•½ tsp of white pepper
•1 cup of extra-virgin olive oil
**Directions:**
1.Place the onion, ginger, celery, carrots, and garlic into a blender. Blend until the mixture are fine but still lumpy from the small vegetable chunks.
2.Add in the vinegar, water, ketchup, soy sauce, honey or maple syrup, lemon juice, salt, and pepper. Pulse until the ingredients are well combined.
3.Gradually add the oil while blending, until everything is well mixed. The mixture should be runny but still grainy.
4.Serve with your favorite winter salad.
**Nutrition:**
Calories: 389 kcal
Protein: 2.71 g
Fat: 32.08 g
Carbohydrates: 22.14 g

## 491.Soy with Honey and Ginger Glaze

**Preparation Time:** 10 minutes
**Cooking Time:** 0 minutes
**Servings:** 2-4
**Ingredients:**
1.¼ cup of honey
2.2 tbsp. gluten-free soy sauce
3.1 tbsp. of rice vinegar
4.1 tsp of freshly grated ginger
**Directions:**
1.Place all together the ingredients into a small bowl and whisk well.

2. Serve with your favorite vegetables, chickens, or seafood.

2.Keep the glaze in a mason jar, tightly covered, and refrigerate for up to 4 days.
**Nutrition:**
Calories: 90 kcal
Protein: 2.32 g
Fat: 1.54 g
Carbohydrates: 17.99 g

## 492.Creamy Homemade Greek Dressing

**Preparation Time:** 10 minutes
**Cooking Time:** 0 minutes
**Servings:** 2-4
**Ingredients:**
•1/4 cup of white wine vinegar
•2 tbsp. of lemon or lime juice
•1/3 cup of extra-virgin olive oil
•½ cup of high-quality mayonnaise, without preservatives
•2 cloves of garlic, minced
•½ tsp dried basil
•½ tsp dried oregano
•½ tsp parsley
•½ tsp thyme
•2 tsp of honey
•¼ cup non-dairy milk (e.g., almond, rice milk)
•A few tablespoons of water
•Some Kosher salt and pepper
**Directions:**
1.Place all together ingredients in a mason jar and shake, cover tightly, and shake well. Refrigerate for a few hours before serving or serve immediately on your favorite vegetable or fruit salad.

2. Shake well before use. Put in the refrigerator for up to 5 days.

2.You may add a few tablespoons of water to adjust the consistency as per your preference.
**Nutrition:**
Calories: 474 kcal
Protein: 2.08 g
Fat: 50.1 g
Carbohydrates: 5.31 g

## 493.Cucumber and Dill Sauce

**Preparation Time:** 10 minutes
**Cooking Time:** 0 minutes
**Servings:** 2-4
**Ingredients:**
•450g of Greek yogurt
•1 cucumber, peeled and squeezed to remove excess liquid
•1 cup of freshly chopped dill
•¼ cup of lemon juice
•1 tsp of sea salt
**Directions:**
1.In a medium bowl, put together the yogurt, cucumber, and dill then mix until well combined. Add in the lemon juice and salt to taste.
2.Cover and refrigerate for about 1-2 hours before serving to keep its freshness. Best serve with Mediterranean food, chips, fish, or even bread.
**Nutrition:**
Calories: 97 kcal
Protein: 13.49 g
Fat: 2.1 g
Carbohydrates: 6.34 g

## 494.Tomato and Mushroom Sauce

**Preparation Time:** 10 minutes
**Cooking Time:** 0 minutes

**Servings:** 2-4
**Ingredients:**
•1 medium-sized leek, chopped
•2 stalks of celery, chopped
•2 medium-sized carrots, chopped
•450g of button mushrooms, diced
•680g of unsalted tomato puree
•½ cup of water
•2 tsp of dried oregano
•4 cloves of garlic, crushed
•5 tbsp. of coconut milk
•Some sea salt, seasoning
•Black pepper, seasoning
**Directions:**
1.In a large skillet, place a few tablespoons of water and heat over medium heat. Once it sizzles, add in the mushrooms and Sautee for about 5 minutes, stir occasionally.
2.Next, add in the leek, carrots, and celery. Stir well and cook for about 5 minutes or until the vegetables are tender. Add more water if needed.
3.Stir in the tomato puree with ½ cup of water and dried oregano. Bring to a boil and then reduce the heat to let it simmer for about 15 minutes.
4.Take off from heat and mix in the garlic, coconut milk, and salt and pepper to taste.
5.Put in an airtight container, then store for up to 4 days in the refrigerator or freeze for up to 1 month. Serve with your favorite pasta.
**Nutrition:**
Calories: 467 kcal
Protein: 16.91 g
Fat: 3.81 g
Carbohydrates: 109.68 g

## 495.Creamy Siamese Dressing

**Preparation Time:** 10 minutes
**Cooking Time:** 0 minutes
**Servings:** 2-4
**Ingredients:**
•1 cup of mayonnaise
•¼ cup of non-dairy milk (e.g., almond, rice, soymilk)
•¼ cup of unsweetened peanut sauce
•2 tbsp. rice vinegar
•1 tbsp. of honey or maple syrup
•1 tbsps. freshly chopped cilantro
•2 tbsp. of unsalted peanuts
**Directions:**
1.Place all ingredients except the cilantro and peanuts into a blender and blend until smooth and creamy. Then, add in the cilantro and peanuts and pulse the blender a few times until completely crushed and well combined. Put in a mason jar and bring it in the refrigerator.
2.Serve with your favorite garden salad, pasta or as a dipping sauce.
**Nutrition:**
Calories: 525 kcal
Protein: 18.14 g
Fat: 45.55 g
Carbohydrates: 11.01 g

## 496.Tahini Dip

**Preparation Time:** 10 minutes
**Cooking Time:** 0 minutes
**Servings:** 2-4
**Ingredients:**
•1 small grated or finely minced clove of garlic (this is optional)
•¼ cup of tahini
•1 tbsp. of apple cider vinegar
•1 tbsp. of freshly squeezed lemon juice
•1 tbsp. of tamari
•1 tsp of finely grated ginger, or ½ tsp of ground ginger
•½ tsp of maple syrup

•1 tsp of turmeric

•1/3 cup of water

**Directions:**

1.Blend or whisk all ingredients together. Put the dressing in an airtight container then refrigerate for about 5 days.

2.Enjoy!

**Nutrition:**

Calories: 120 kcal

Protein: 4.77 g

Fat: 9.63 g

Carbohydrates: 5.12 g

### 497.Honey Bean Dip

**Preparation Time:** 5 minutes

**Cooking Time:** 0 minutes

**Servings:** 3-4

**Ingredients:**

•2 cherry tomatoes

•2 tablespoons filtered water

•1 tablespoon apple cider vinegar

•1 (14-ounce) can each of kidney beans and black beans

•2 garlic cloves

•¼ teaspoon ground cumin

•¼ teaspoon salt

•2 teaspoons raw honey

•1 teaspoon lime juice

•Pinch cayenne pepper to taste

•Freshly ground black pepper to taste

**Directions:**

1.In a blender or food processor, put together the beans, garlic, tomatoes, water, vinegar, honey, lime juice, cumin, salt, cayenne pepper, and black pepper.

2.Blend until it turns smooth. Add the mix in a bowl.

3.Cover and refrigerate to chill. You can refrigerate for up to 5 days.

**Nutrition:**

Calories 158

Fat 1g

Carbohydrates 33g

Fiber 8g

Protein 9g

### 498.Kale Slaw and Strawberry Salad - Poppyseed Dressing

**Preparation Time:** 10 minutes

**Cooking Time:** 20 minutes

**Servings:** 2

**Ingredients:**

•Chicken breast; 8 ounces; sliced and baked

•Kale; 1 cup; chopped

•Slaw mix; 1 cup (cabbage, broccoli slaw, carrots mixed)

•Slivered almonds; 1/4 cup

•Strawberries; 1 cup; sliced

For the dressing:

•Light mayonnaise; 1 tablespoon

•Dijon mustard

•Olive oil; 1 tablespoon

•Apple cider vinegar; 1 tablespoon

•Lemon juice; 1/2 teaspoon

•1 tablespoon of honey

•Onion powder; 1/4 teaspoon

•Garlic powder; 1/4 teaspoon

•Poppyseeds

**Directions:**

1.Whisk the dressing ingredients together until well mixed, then leave to cool in the fridge.

2.Slice the chicken breasts.

3.Divide 2 bowls of spinach, slaw, and strawberries.

4.Cover with a sliced breast of chicken (4 oz. each), then scatter with almonds.

5.Divide the dressing between the two bowls and drizzle.
**Nutrition:**
Calories: 340 Cal
Fats: 13.6 g
Saturated Fat: 6.2 g

## 499.Green Beans

**Preparation Time**: 5 minutes
**Cooking Time:** 13 minutes
**Servings:** 4
**Ingredients:**
•1-pound green beans
•¾ teaspoon garlic powder
•¾ teaspoon ground black pepper
•1 ¼ teaspoon salt
•½ teaspoon paprika
**Directions:**
1.Turn on the fryer, insert the basket, grease with olive oil, close the lid, set the fryer at 400 degrees F, and preheat for 5 minutes.
2.Meanwhile, put the beans in a bowl, sprinkle generously with olive oil, sprinkle with garlic powder, black pepper, salt, and paprika and stir until well coated.
3.Open the air fryer, add the green beans, close with the lid and cook for 8 minutes until golden and crisp, stirring halfway through the frying process.
4.When the fryer beeps, open the lid, transfer the green beans to a serving plate and serve.
**Nutrition:**
Calories: 45
Carbs: 2 g
Fat: 11 g
Protein: 4 g
Fiber: 3 g

## 500.Bean Potato Spread

**Preparation Time:** 25 minutes
**Cooking Time:** 0 minutes
**Servings:** 7-8
**Ingredients:**
•2 tablespoons lime juice
•1 tablespoon olive oil
•5 garlic cloves, minced
•1 cup garbanzo beans, drained and rinsed
•4 cups cooked sweet potatoes, peeled and chopped
•¼ cup sesame paste
•½ teaspoon cumin, ground
•2 tablespoons water
•A pinch of salt
**Directions:**
1.In a blender, put all together the ingredients and blend to make a smooth mix.
2.Transfer to a bowl.
3.Serve with carrot, celery, or veggie sticks.
**Nutrition:**
Calories 156
Fat 3g
 Carbohydrates 10g
Fiber 6g
 Protein 8g

## 501.Cashew Ginger Dip

**Preparation Time:** 5 minutes
**Cooking Time:** 0 minutes
**Servings:** 1
**Ingredients:**
•1 tablespoon extra-virgin olive oil
•2 teaspoons coconut aminos
•1 cup cashews, soaked in water for 20-25 minutes and drained
•2 garlic cloves
•¼ cup filtered water
•1 teaspoon lemon juice
•½ teaspoon ground ginger

•¼ teaspoon salt

•Pinch cayenne pepper

**Directions:**

1.In a blender or food processor, put together the cashews, garlic, water, olive oil, aminos, lemon juice, ginger, salt, and cayenne pepper.

2.Add the mix in a bowl.

3.Cover and refrigerate until chilled. You can use store it for 4-5 days in the refrigerator.

**Nutrition:**

Calories 124

 Fat 9g

Carbohydrates 5g

Fiber 1g

 Protein 3g

# Vegan Recipes

### 502.Roasted Cauliflower with Pepper Jack Cheese

**Preparation Time:** 4 minutes
**Cooking Time:** 21 minutes
**Servings:** 2
**Ingredients:**
•1/3 teaspoon shallot powder
•1 teaspoon ground black pepper
•1 ½ large-sized heads of cauliflower, broken into florets
•1/4 teaspoon cumin powder
•½ teaspoon garlic salt
•1/4 cup Pepper Jack cheese, grated
•1 ½ tablespoons vegetable oil
•1/3 teaspoon paprika
**Directions:**
1.Boil cauliflower in a large pan of salted water approximately 5 minutes. After that, drain the cauliflower florets; now, transfer them to a baking dish.
2.Toss the cauliflower florets with the rest of the above ingredients.
3.Roast at 395 degrees F for 16 minutes, turn them halfway through the process. Enjoy!
**Nutrition:**
Calories: 271
Fat: 23g
Carbs: 8.9g
Protein: 9.8g
Sugars: 2.8g
Fiber: 4.5g

### 503.Grilled Eggplants

**Preparation Time**: 10 minutes
**Cooking Time:** 10 minutes
**Servings:** 4
**Ingredients:**
•1 large eggplant, cut into thick circles
•Salt and pepper to taste
•1 tsp. smoked paprika
•1 tbsp. coconut flour
•1 tsp. lime juice
•1 tbsp. olive oil
**Directions:**
1.Coat the eggplants in smoked paprika, salt, pepper, lime juice, coconut flour, and let it sit for 10 minutes.
2.In a grilling pan, add the olive oil.
3.Grill the eggplants for 3 minutes on each side.
4.Serve.
**Nutrition:**
Fat: 0.1 g
Sodium: 1.6 mg
Carbohydrates: 4.8 g
Fiber: 2.4 g
Sugars: 2.9 g
Protein: 0.8 g

### 504.Asparagus Avocado Soup

**Preparation Time**: 10 minutes
**Cooking Time:** 20 minutes
**Servings:** 4
**Ingredients:**
•1 avocado, peeled, pitted, cubed
•12 ounces asparagus
•½ teaspoon ground black pepper
•1 teaspoon garlic powder
•1 teaspoon sea salt
•2 tablespoons olive oil, divided
•1/2 of a lemon, juiced
•2 cups vegetable stock
**Directions:**
1.Switch on the air fryer, insert fryer basket, grease it with olive oil, then shut with its lid,

set the fryer at 425 degrees F, and preheat for 5 minutes.

2.Meanwhile, place asparagus in a shallow dish, drizzle with 1tablespoon oil, sprinkle with garlic powder, salt, and black pepper, and toss until well mixed.

3.Open the fryer, add asparagus in it, close with its lid and cook for 10 minutes until nicely golden and roasted, shaking halfway through the frying.

4.When the air fryer beeps, open its lid and transfer asparagus to a food processor.

5.Add remaining ingredients into a food processor and pulse until well combined and smooth.

6.Tip the soup in a saucepan, pour in water if the soup is too thick, and heat it over medium-low heat for 5 minutes until thoroughly heated.

7.Ladle soup into bowls and serve.

**Nutrition:**
Calories: 208
Carbs: 2 g
Fat: 11 g
Protein: 4 g
Fiber: 5 g

### 505.Vegetables in Air Fryer

**Preparation Time**: 20 minutes
**Cooking Time:** 30 minutes
**Servings:** 2
**Ingredients:**
•2 potatoes
•1 zucchini
•1 onion
•1 red pepper
•1 green pepper
**Directions:**
1.Cut the potatoes into slices.
2.Cut the onion into rings.
3.Cut the zucchini slices
4.Cut the peppers into strips.
5.Put all the ingredients in the bowl and add a little salt, ground pepper and some extra virgin olive oil.
6.Mix well.
7.Pass to the basket of the air fryer.
8.Select 1600C, 30 minutes.
9.Check that the vegetables are to your liking.

**Nutrition:**
Calories: 135
Carbs: 2 g
Fat: 11 g
Protein: 4 g
Fiber: 05g

### 506.Sweet Potato Chips

**Preparation Time**: 5 minutes
**Cooking Time:** 10 minutes
**Servings:** 4
**Ingredients:**
•2 large sweet potatoes
•15 ml. of oil
•10 g of salt
•2 g black pepper
•2 g of paprika
•2 g garlic powder
•2 g onion powder
**Directions:**
1.Cut the sweet potatoes into strips 25 mm. thick.
2.Preheat the air fryer for a few minutes.
3.Add the cut sweet potatoes to a large bowl and mix with the oil until the potatoes are all evenly coated.
4.Sprinkle salt, black pepper, paprika, garlic powder, and onion powder. Mix well.
5.Place the French fries in the preheated baskets and cook for 10 minutes at 205°C. Be

sure to shake the baskets halfway through cooking.

**Nutrition:**

Calories: 123

Carbs: 2 g

Fat: 11 g

Protein: 4 g

Fiber: 0 g

### 507.Green Pea Guacamole

**Preparation Time**: 15 minutes

**Cooking Time:** 35 minutes

**Servings:** 4

**Ingredients:**

•1 teaspoon of crushed garlic

•1 chopped tomato

•3 cups of frozen green peas (chopped)

•5 green chopped onions

•1/6 teaspoon of hot sauce

•1/2 teaspoon of grounded cumin

•1/2 cup of lime juice

**Directions:**

1.Blend the peas, garlic, lime juice, and cumin until it is smoothened.

2.Stir in the tomatoes, green onion, and hot sauce into the mixture.

3.Then add salt to taste.

4.Cover it and put it into the refrigerator for a minimum of 30 minutes. This will allow the flavor to blend very well.

**Nutrition:**

Calories: 40.7 Cal

Fat: 0.2 g

Cholesterol: 0.0 mg

Sodium: 157.4 mg

Carbohydrates: 7.6 g

Dietary Fiber: 1.7 g

Protein: 2.7 g

### 508.Rosemary Garlic Potatoes

**Preparation Time:** 5 minutes

**Cooking Time:** 30 minutes

**Servings:** 2

**Ingredients:**

•5 red new potatoes, chopped

•¼ cup olive oil

•2–3 cloves of minced garlic

•1 tablespoon rosemary

**Directions:**

1.Preheat oven to 425 degrees.

2.Stir all ingredients together in a bowl. Pour onto a baking sheet and bake for 30 minutes.

**Nutrition:**

Calories: 176

Protein: 5g

Carbohydrate: 30g

Fat: 2 g

### 509.Sweet and Sour Cabbage

**Preparation Time:** 5 minutes

**Cooking Time:** 15 minutes

**Servings:** 2

**Ingredients:**

•1 tablespoon honey or maple syrup

•1 teaspoon baking stevia

•2 tablespoons water

•1 tablespoon olive oil

•¼ teaspoon caraway seeds

•¼ teaspoon salt

•1/8 teaspoon pepper

•2 cups chopped red cabbage

•1 diced apple

**Directions:**

1.Cook all ingredients in a covered saucepan on the stove for 15 minutes.

**Nutrition:**

Calories: 170

Protein: 17g

Carbohydrate: 20g

Fat: 8 g

### 510. Beet
**Preparation Time:** 5 minutes
**Cooking Time:** 0 minutes
**Servings:** 2
**Ingredients:**
- 2–3 fresh, raw beets grated or shredded in food processor
- 3 tablespoons olive oil
- 2 tablespoons balsamic vinegar
- ¼ teaspoon salt
- 1/3 teaspoon cumin
- Dash stevia powder or liquid
- Dash pepper

**Directions:**
1. Mix all ingredients together for the best raw beet salad.

**Nutrition:**
Calories: 156
Protein: 8g
Carbohydrate: 40g
Fat: 5 g

### 511. Taste of Normandy
**Preparation Time:** 25 minutes
**Cooking Time:** 5 minutes
**Servings:** 4 to 6
**Ingredients:**
For the walnuts:
- 2 tablespoons butter
- ¼ cup sugar or stevia
- 1 cup walnut pieces
- ½ teaspoon kosher salt
- For the dressing
- 3 tablespoons extra-virgin olive oil
- 1½ tablespoons champagne vinegar
- 1½ tablespoons Dijon mustard
- ¼ teaspoon kosher salt

For the salad:
- 1 head red leaf lettuce, torn into pieces
- 3 heads endive, ends trimmed and leaves separated
- 2 apples, cored and cut into thin wedges
- 1 (8-ounce) Camembert wheel, cut into thin wedges

**Directions:**
1. To make the walnuts
2. In a skillet over medium-high heat, melt the butter. Stir in the sugar and cook until it dissolves. Add the walnuts and cook for about 5 minutes, stirring, until toasty. Season with salt and transfer to a plate to cool.
3. To make the dressing
4. In a large bowl, whisk the oil, vinegar, mustard, and salt until combined.
5. To make the salad
6. Add the lettuce and endive to the bowl with the dressing and toss to coat. Transfer to a serving platter.
7. Decoratively arrange the apple and Camembert wedges over the lettuce and scatter the walnuts on top. Serve immediately.

**Nutrition:**
Calories: 699;
Total fat: 52g;
Total carbs: 44g;
Cholesterol: 60mg;
Fiber: 17g;
Protein: 23g;
Sodium: 1170mg

### 512. Smoked Salmon, Cucumber, Egg, and Asparagus
**Preparation Time:** 20 minutes
**Cooking Time:** 5 minutes
**Servings:** 4
**Ingredients:**
- For the vinaigrette

•3 tablespoons walnut oil
•2 tablespoons champagne vinegar
•1 tablespoon chopped fresh dill
•½ teaspoon kosher salt
•¼ teaspoon ground mustard
•Freshly ground black pepper
For the salad:
•Handful green beans, trimmed
•1 (3- to 4-ounce) package spring greens
•12 spears pickled asparagus
•4 large soft-boiled eggs, halved
•8 ounces smoked salmon, thinly sliced
•1 cucumber, thinly sliced
•1 lemon, quartered

**Directions:**
1.To make the dressing
2.In a small bowl, whisk the oil, vinegar, dill, salt, ground mustard, and a few grinds of pepper until emulsified. Set aside.
3.To make the salad
4.Start by blanching the green beans: Bring a pot of salted water to a boil. Drop in the beans. Cook or 1 to 2 minutes until they turn bright green, then immediately drain and rinse under cold water. Set aside.
5.Divide the spring greens among 4 plates. Toss each serving with dressing to taste. Arrange 3 asparagus spears, 1 egg, 2 ounces of salmon, one-fourth of the cucumber slices, and a lemon wedge on each plate. Serve immediately.

**Nutrition:**
Calories: 257;
Total fat: 18g;
Total carbs: 6g;
Cholesterol: 199mg;
Fiber: 2g;
Protein: 19g;
Sodium: 603m

## 513.Barley and Lentil
**Preparation Time:** 5 minutes
**Cooking Time:** 0 minutes
**Servings:** 2
**Ingredients:**
•1 head romaine lettuce
•¾ cup cooked barley
•2 cups cooked lentils
•1 diced carrot
•¼ chopped red onion
•¼ cup olives
•½ chopped cucumber
•3 tablespoons olive oil
•2 tablespoons fresh lemon juice

**Directions:**
8.Mix all ingredients together. Add kosher salt and black pepper to taste.

**Nutrition:**
Calories: 213
Protein: 21g
Carbohydrate: 6g
Fat: 9 g

## 514.Asian Slaw
**Preparation Time:** 5 minutes
**Cooking Time:** 5 minutes
**Servings:** 2
**Ingredients:**
•1 cabbage head, shredded
•4 chopped green onions
•½ cup slivered or sliced almonds
Dressing:
•½ cup olive oil
•¼ cup tamari or soy sauce
•1 tablespoon honey or maple syrup
•1 tablespoon baking stevia

**Directions:**
1.Heat up dressing ingredients in a saucepan on the stove until thoroughly mixed.

2.Mix all ingredients when you are ready to serve.

**Nutrition:**
Calories: 205
Protein: 27g
Carbohydrate: 12g
Fat: 10 g

### 515.Mixed Potato Gratin

**Preparation Time**: 20 minutes
**Cooking Time:** 7 to 9 hours
**Servings:** 8
**Ingredients:**
•6 Yukon Gold potatoes, thinly sliced
•3 sweet potatoes, peeled and thinly sliced
•2 onions, thinly sliced
•4 garlic cloves, minced
•3 tablespoons whole-wheat flour
•4 cups 2% milk, divided
•11/2 cups roasted vegetable broth
•3 tablespoons melted butter
•1 teaspoon dried thyme leaves
•11/2 cups shredded Havarti cheese
**Directions:**
1.Grease a 6-quart slow cooker with straight vegetable oil.
2.In the slow cooker, layer the potatoes, onions, and garlic.
3.In a large bowl, mix the flour with 1/2 cup of the milk until well combined.
4.Gradually add the remaining milk, stirring with a wire whisk to avoid lumps.
5.Stir in the vegetable broth, melted butter, and thyme leaves.
6.Pour the milk mixture over the potatoes in the slow cooker and top with the cheese.
7.Cover and cook on low for 7 to 9 hours, or until the potatoes are tender when pierced with a fork.
**Nutrition:**

Calories: 415 Cal
Carbohydrates: 42 g
Sugar: 10 g
Fiber: 3 g
Fat: 22 g
Saturated Fat: 13 g
Protein: 17 g
Sodium: 431 mg

### 516.Broccoli

**Preparation Time:** 5 minutes
**Cooking Time:** 0 minutes
**Servings:** 2
**Ingredients:**
•1 head broccoli, chopped
•2–3 slices of fried bacon, crumbled
•1 diced green onion
•½ cup raisins or craisins
•½–1 cup of chopped pecans
•¾ cup sunflower seeds
•½ cup of pomegranate
Dressing:
•1 cup organic mayonnaise
•¼ cup baking stevia
•2 teaspoons white vinegar
**Directions:**
1.Mix all ingredients together. Mix dressing and fold into salad.
**Nutrition:**
Calories: 239
Protein: 10g
Carbohydrate: 33g
Fat: 2 g

### 517.Fennel and Arugula Salad with Fig Vinaigrette

**Preparation Time**: 15 minutes
**Cooking Time:** 10 minutes
**Servings:** 6

**Ingredients:**
- 5 ounces of washed and dried arugula
- 1 small fennel bulb, it can be either shaved or tiny sliced
- 2 tablespoons of extra virgin oil or any cooking oil
- 1 teaspoon of lemon zest
- 1/2 teaspoon of salt
- Pepper (freshly ground)
- Pecorino

**Directions:**
1. Mix the arugula and shaved fennel in a serving bowl.
2. On another bowl, mix the olive oil or cooking oil, lemon zest, salt, and pepper
3. Shake together until it becomes creamy and smooth.
4. Pour and dress over the salad, tossing gently for it to combine.
5. Peel or shave out some slices of pecorino and put it on top of the salad.
6. Serve immediately.

**Nutrition:**
Protein: 2.1 g
Carbohydrates: 14.3 g
Dietary Fiber: 3.4 g
Sugars: 9.1 g
Fat: 9.7 g

## 518.Mushrooms Stuffed with Tomato

**Preparation Time**: 5 minutes
**Cooking Time:** 50 minutes
**Servings:** 4
**Ingredients:**
- 8 large mushrooms
- 250 g of minced meat
- 4 cloves of garlic
- Extra virgin olive oil
- Salt
- Ground pepper
- Flour, beaten egg, and breadcrumbs
- Frying oil
- Fried tomato sauce

**Directions:**
1. Remove the stem from the mushrooms and chop it. Peel the garlic and chop. Put some extra virgin olive oil in a pan and add the garlic and mushroom stems.
2. Sauté and add the minced meat. Sauté well until the meat is well-cooked and season.
3. Fill the mushrooms with the minced meat.
4. Press well and take to the freezer for 30 minutes.
5. Pass the mushrooms with flour, beaten egg, and breadcrumbs.
6. Place the mushrooms in the basket of the air fryer.
7. Select 20 minutes, 1800C.
8. Distribute the mushrooms once cooked in the dishes.
9. Heat the tomato sauce and cover the stuffed mushrooms.

**Nutrition:**
Calories: 160
Carbs: 2 g
Fat: 11 g
Protein: 4 g
Fiber: 0 g

## 519.Delicious Zucchini Quiche

**Preparation Time**: 15 minutes
**Cooking Time:** 60 minutes
**Servings:** 8
Ingredients
- 6 eggs
- 2 medium zucchinis, shredded
- 1/2 tsp. dried basil
- 2 garlic cloves, minced
- 1 tbsp. dry onion, minced

•2 tbsp. parmesan cheese, grated

•2 tbsp. fresh parsley, chopped

•1/2 cup olive oil

•1 cup cheddar cheese, shredded

•1/4 cup coconut flour

•3/4 cup almond flour

•1/2 tsp. salt

**Directions:**

1.Preheat the oven to 350 F.

2.Grease 9-inch pie dish and set aside.

3.Squeeze out excess liquid from zucchini.

4.Add all ingredients into the large bowl and mix until well combined.

5.Pour into the prepared pie dish.

6.Bake in preheated oven for 45-60 minutes or until set.

7.Remove from the oven and let it cool completely.

8.Slice and serve.

**Nutrition:**

Calories: 288 Cal

Fat: 26.3 g

Carbohydrates: 5 g

Sugar: 1.6 g

Protein: 11 g

Cholesterol: 139 mg

### 520.Crispy Rye Bread Snacks with Guacamole and Anchovies

**Preparation Time**: 10 minutes

**Cooking Time:** 10 minutes

**Servings:** 4

**Ingredients:**

•4 slices of rye bread

•Guacamole

•Anchovies in oil

**Directions:**

1.Cut each slice of bread into three strips of bread.

2.Place in the basket of the air fryer, without piling up, and go in batches giving it the touch you want to give it. You can select 1800C, 10 minutes.

3.When you have all the crusty rye bread strips, put a layer of guacamole on top, whether homemade or commercial.

4.In each bread, place two anchovies on the guacamole.

5.Serve and enjoy!

**Nutrition:**

Calories: 180

Carbs: 4 g

Fat: 11 g

Protein: 4 g

Fiber: 09 g

# Sauce, Soup and Stew Recipes

### 521. Garlic Sauce

**Preparation Time:** 5 minutes
**Cooking Time:** 5 minutes
**Servings:** 2
**Ingredients:**
- 1 cup water, divided as explained in **Directions:** below
- 4 tbsp. chopped garlic
- 4 cups heavy cream
- 2 tbsp. chopped fresh parsley
- 4 tbsp. cornstarch
- Salt and pepper to taste

**Directions:**
1. Put half the water, garlic, cream, salt, and pepper in the Instant Pot.
2. Secure the lid and turn the pressure release handle to the "sealed" position.
3. Select the MANUAL functions, set to HIGH PRESSURE, and adjust the timer to 3 minutes.
4. After the beep, "quick-release" the steam and remove the lid.
5. Mix the cornstarch with the remaining water. Add this slurry to the garlic sauce.
6. Stir in the parsley and serve.

**Nutrition:**
Calories: 231
Fat: 22 g
Carbs: 3 g
Protein: 7 g

### 522. Cranberry Sauce

**Preparation Time:** 5 minutes
**Cooking Time:** 8 minutes
**Servings:** 2
**Ingredients:**
- ¾ cup fresh cranberries
- 2 tbsp. raw honey
- ½ cup pure squeezed orange juice
- ½ tsp. cinnamon
- 1 tbsp. stevia

**Directions:**
1. Put all the **Ingredients:** in the Instant Pot.
2. Secure the lid and turn the pressure release handle to the "sealed" position.
3. Select the MANUAL functions, set to HIGH PRESSURE, and adjust the timer to 8 minutes.
4. After the beep, "QUICK-RELEASE" the steam and remove the lid.
5. Serve when cool, or save in a bottle for later use.

**Nutrition:**
Calories: 62
Fat: 0 g
Carbohydrate: 17 g
Protein: 0.1 g

### 523. Béarnaise Sauce

**Preparation Time:** 5 minutes
**Cooking Time:** 3 minutes
**Servings:** 2
**Ingredients:**
- ½ cup butter
- 2 egg yolks, beaten
- 2 tsp. lemon juice, freshly squeezed
- ¼ tsp. onion powder
- 2 tbsp. fresh tarragon

**Directions:**
1. Press the SAUTÉ button on the Instant Pot.
2. Melt the butter for 3 minutes and transfer it into a mixing bowl.
3. While whisking the melted butter, slowly add the egg yolks.
4. Continue stirring so that no lumps form.
5. Add the lemon juice, onion powder, and fresh tarragon.
6. Serve.

**Nutrition:**
Calories: 603
Fat: 62 g

Carbs: 4 g

Protein: 5 g

### 524.Chili Sauce

**Preparation Time:** 8 minutes

**Cooking Time:** 15 minutes

**Servings:** 2

**Ingredients:**

- 2 oz. hot peppers
- 2 cups of apple cider vinegar
- 1 tsp. salt

**Directions:**

1.Trim away the stems from the peppers and chop.

2.Add all **Ingredients:** to the Instant Pot.

3.Secure the lid and MANUALLY set the timer to 15 minutes under HIGH pressure.

4.Quick-release the pressure and serve the sauce into bowls.

**Nutrition:**

Calories: 2

Fat: 0 g

Carbs: 0.7 g

Protein: 1 g

### 525.Vanilla Caramel Sauce

**Preparation Time:** 5 minutes

**Cooking Time:** 13 minutes

**Servings:** 2

**Ingredients:**

- 2 tbsp. coconut oil
- 1 cup sugar or stevia
- 1 tsp vanilla extract
- 1/3 cup condensed coconut milk
- 1/3 cup water

**Directions:**

1.Warm up the Instant Pot using the SAUTÉ function.

2.Add the water and sugar, then stir and sauté for 13 minutes.

3.Stir in the milk, coconut oil, and vanilla.

4.Whisk until creamy and add to a glass container.

5.Cool completely and serve when ready.

**Nutrition:**

Calories: 80

Carbs: 14 g

Fat: 5 g

Protein: 0 g

### 526.Delicious Chicken Soup

**Preparation Time:** 10 minutes

**Cooking Time:** 4 hours 30 minutes

**Servings:** 4

**Ingredients:**

- 1 lb chicken breasts, boneless and skinless
- 2 Tbsp fresh basil, chopped
- 1 1/2 cups mozzarella cheese, shredded
- 2 garlic cloves, minced
- 1 Tbsp Parmesan cheese, grated
- 2 Tbsp dried basil
- 2 cups chicken stock
- 28 oz tomatoes, diced
- 1/4 tsp pepper
- 1/2 tsp salt

**Directions:**

1.Add chicken, Parmesan cheese, dried basil, tomatoes, garlic, pepper, and salt to a crock pot and stir well to combine.

2.Cover and cook on low for 4 hours.

3.Add fresh basil and mozzarella cheese and stir well.

4.Cover again and cook for 30 more minutes or until cheese is melted.

5.Remove chicken from the crock pot and shred using forks.

6.Return shredded chicken to the crock pot and stir to mix.

7.Serve and enjoy.

### 527.Flavorful Broccoli Soup

**Preparation Time:** 10 minutes
**Cooking Time:** 4 hours 15 minutes
**Servings:** 6
**Ingredients:**
- 20 oz broccoli florets
- 4 oz cream cheese
- 8 oz cheddar cheese, shredded
- 1/2 tsp paprika
- 1/2 tsp ground mustard
- 3 cups chicken stock
- 2 garlic cloves, chopped
- 1 onion, diced
- 1 cup carrots, shredded
- 1/4 tsp baking soda
- 1/4 tsp salt

**Directions:**
1. Add all ingredients except cream cheese and cheddar cheese to a crock pot and stir well.
2. Cover and cook on low for 4 hours.
3. Purée the soup using an immersion blender until smooth.
4. Stir in the cream cheese and cheddar cheese.
5. Cover and cook on low for 15 minutes longer.
6. Season with pepper and salt.
7. Serve and enjoy.

**Nutrition:**
Calories 275
Fat 19 g

Carbohydrates 19 g
Sugar 4 g
Protein 14 g
Cholesterol 60 mg

### 528.Healthy Spinach Soup

**Preparation Time:** 10 minutes
**Cooking Time:** 3 hours
**Servings:** 8
**Ingredients:**
- 3 cups frozen spinach, chopped, thawed and drained
- 8 oz cheddar cheese, shredded
- 1 egg, lightly beaten
- 10 oz can cream of chicken soup
- 8 oz cream cheese, softened

**Directions:**
1. Add spinach to a large bowl. Purée the spinach.
2. Add egg, chicken soup, cream cheese, and pepper to the spinach purée and mix well.
3. Transfer spinach mixture to a crock pot.
4. Cover and cook on low for 3 hours.
5. Stir in cheddar cheese and serve.

**Nutrition:**
Calories 256
Fat 29 g
Carbohydrates 1 g
Sugar 0.5 g
Protein 11 g
Cholesterol 84 mg

### 529.Healthy Chicken Kale Soup

**Preparation Time:** 10 minutes
**Cooking Time:** 6 hours 15 minutes
**Servings:** 6
**Ingredients:**
- 2 lb chicken breasts, skinless and boneless
- 1/4 cup fresh lemon juice
- 5 oz baby kale
- 32 oz chicken stock

•1/2 cup olive oil

•1 large onion, sliced

•14 oz chicken broth

•1 Tbsp extra-virgin olive oil

•Salt

**Directions:**

1.Heat the extra-virgin olive oil in a pan over medium heat.

2.Season chicken with salt and place in the hot pan.

3.Cover pan and cook chicken for 15 minutes.

4.Remove chicken from the pan and shred it using forks.

5.Add shredded chicken to a crock pot.

6.Add sliced onion, olive oil, and broth to a blender and blend until combined.

7.Pour blended mixture into the crock pot.

8.Add remaining ingredients to the crock pot and stir well.

9.Cover and cook on low for 6 hours.

10.Stir well and serve.

**Nutrition:**

Calories 493

Fat 33 g

Carbohydrates 8 g

Sugar 9 g

Protein 47 g

Cholesterol 135 mg

### 530.Spicy Chicken Pepper Stew

**Preparation Time:** 10 minutes

**Cooking Time:** 6 hours

**Servings:** 6

**Ingredients:**

•3 chicken breasts, skinless and boneless, cut into small pieces

•1 tsp garlic, minced

•1 tsp ground ginger

•2 tsp olive oil

•2 tsp soy sauce

•1 Tbsp fresh lemon juice

•1/2 cup green onions, sliced

•1 Tbsp crushed red pepper

•8 oz chicken stock

•1 bell pepper, chopped

•1 green chili pepper, sliced

•2 jalapeño peppers, sliced

•1/2 tsp black pepper

•1/4 tsp sea salt

**Directions:**

1.Add all ingredients to a large mixing bowl and mix well. Place in the refrigerator overnight.

2.Pour marinated chicken mixture into a crock pot.

3.Cover and cook on low for 6 hours.

4.Stir well and serve.

**Nutrition:**

Calories 171

Fat 4 g

Carbohydrates 7 g

Sugar 7 g

Protein 22 g

Cholesterol 65 mg

### 531.Creamy Broccoli Cauliflower Soup

**Preparation Time:** 10 minutes

**Cooking Time:** 6 hours

**Servings:** 6

**Ingredients:**

•2 cups cauliflower florets, chopped

•3 cups broccoli florets, chopped

•3 1/2 cups chicken stock

•1 large carrot, diced

•1/2 cup shallots, diced

•2 garlic cloves, minced

•1 cup plain yogurt

•6 oz cheddar cheese, shredded

•1 cup coconut milk
•Pepper
•Salt

**Directions:**

1.Add all ingredients except milk, cheese, and yogurt to a crock pot and stir well.

2.Cover and cook on low for 6 hours.

3.Purée the soup using an immersion blender until smooth.

4.Add cheese, milk, and yogurt and blend until smooth and creamy.

5.Season with pepper and salt.

6.Serve and enjoy.

**Nutrition:**

Calories 281

Fat 20 g

Carbohydrates 14 g

Sugar 9 g

Protein 11 g

Cholesterol 32 mg

## 532.Mexican Chicken Soup

**Preparation Time:** 10 minutes

**Cooking Time:** 4 hours

**Servings:** 6

**Ingredients:**

•1 1/2 lb chicken thighs, skinless and boneless
•14 oz chicken stock
•14 oz salsa
•8 oz Monterey Jack cheese, shredded

**Directions:**

1.Place chicken into a crock pot.

2.Pour remaining ingredients over the chicken.

3.Cover and cook on high for 4 hours.

4.Remove chicken from crock pot and shred using forks.

5.Return shredded chicken to the crock pot and stir well.

6.Serve and enjoy.

**Nutrition:**

Calories 371

Fat 15 g

Carbohydrates 7 g

Sugar 2 g

Protein 41 g

Cholesterol 135 mg

## 533.Beef Stew

**Preparation Time:** 10 minutes

**Cooking Time:** 5 hours 5 minutes

**Servings:** 8

**Ingredients:**

•3 lb beef stew meat, trimmed
•1/2 cup red curry paste
•1/3 cup tomato paste
•13 oz can coconut milk
•2 tsp ginger, minced
•2 garlic cloves, minced
•1 medium onion, sliced
•2 Tbsp olive oil
•2 cups carrots, julienned
•2 cups broccoli florets
•2 tsp fresh lime juice
•2 Tbsp fish sauce
•2 tsp sea salt

**Directions:**

1.Heat 1 tablespoon of oil in a pan over medium heat.

2.Brown the meat on all sides in the pan.

3.Add brown meat to a crock pot.

4.Add remaining oil to the same pan and sauté the ginger, garlic, and onion over medium-high heat for 5 minutes.

5.Add coconut milk and stir well.

6.Transfer pan mixture to the crock pot.

7.Add remaining ingredients except for carrots and broccoli.

8.Cover and cook on high for 5 hours.

9.Add carrots and broccoli during the last 30 minutes of cooking.

10.Serve and enjoy.

**Nutrition:**

Calories 537

Fat 26 g

Carbohydrates 13 g

Sugar 16 g

Protein 54 g

Cholesterol 152 mg

## 534.Basil Tomato Soup

**Preparation Time:** 10 minutes

**Cooking Time:** 6 hours

**Servings:** 6

**Ingredients:**

- 28 oz can whole peeled tomatoes
- 1/2 cup fresh basil leaves
- 4 cups chicken stock
- 1 tsp red pepper flakes
- 3 garlic cloves, peeled
- 2 onions, diced
- 3 carrots, peeled and diced
- 3 Tbsp olive oil
- 1 tsp salt

**Directions:**

1.Add all ingredients to a crock pot and stir well.

2.Cover and cook on low for 6 hours.

3.Purée the soup until smooth using an immersion blender.

4.Season soup with pepper and salt.

5.Serve and enjoy.

**Nutrition:**

Calories 126

Fat 5 g

Carbohydrates 13 g

Sugar 7 g

Protein 5 g

Cholesterol 0 mg

## 535.Beef Chili

**Preparation Time:** 10 minutes

**Cooking Time:** 8 hours

**Servings:** 6

**Ingredients:**

- 1 lb ground beef
- 1 tsp garlic powder
- 1 tsp paprika
- 3 tsp chili powder
- 1 Tbsp Worcestershire sauce
- 1 Tbsp fresh parsley, chopped
- 1 tsp onion powder
- 25 oz tomatoes, chopped
- 4 carrots, chopped
- 1 onion, diced
- 1 bell pepper, diced
- 1/2 tsp sea salt

**Directions:**

1.Brown the ground meat in a pan over high heat until meat is no longer pink.

2.Transfer meat to a crock pot.

3.Add bell pepper, tomatoes, carrots, and onion to the crock pot and stir well.

4.Add remaining ingredients and stir well.

5.Cover and cook on low for 8 hours.

6.Serve and enjoy.

**Nutrition:**

Calories 152

Fat 4 g

Carbohydrates 4 g

Sugar 8 g

Protein 18 g

Cholesterol 51 mg

## 536.Squash Soup

**Preparation Time:** 10 minutes

**Cooking Time:** 8 hours

**Servings:** 6

**Ingredients:**

- 2 lb butternut squash, peeled, chopped into chunks
- 1 tsp ginger, minced
- 1/4 tsp cinnamon
- 1 Tbsp curry powder
- 2 bay leaves
- 1 tsp black pepper
- 1/2 cup heavy cream
- 2 cups chicken stock
- 1 Tbsp garlic, minced
- 2 carrots, cut into chunks
- 2 apples, peeled, cored and diced
- 1 large onion, diced
- 1 tsp salt

**Directions:**

1. Spray a crock pot inside with cooking spray.
2. Add all ingredients except cream to the crock pot and stir well.
3. Cover and cook on low for 8 hours.
4. Purée the soup using an immersion blender until smooth and creamy.
5. Stir in heavy cream and season soup with pepper and salt.
6. Serve and enjoy.

**Nutrition:**

Calories 170

Fat 4 g

Carbohydrates 34 g

Sugar 14g

Protein 9 g

Cholesterol 14 mg

## 537.Herb Tomato Soup

**Preparation Time:** 10 minutes

**Cooking Time:** 6 hours

**Servings:** 8

**Ingredients:**

- 55 oz can tomatoes, diced
- 1/2 onion, minced
- 2 cups chicken stock
- 1 cup half and half
- 4 Tbsp butter
- 1 bay leaf
- 1/2 tsp black pepper
- 1/2 tsp garlic powder
- 1 tsp oregano
- 1 tsp dried thyme
- 1 cup carrots, diced
- 1/4 tsp black pepper
- 1/2 tsp salt

**Directions:**

1. Add all ingredients to a crock pot and stir well.
2. Cover and cook on low for 6 hours.
3. Discard bay leaf and purée the soup using an immersion blender until smooth.
4. Serve and enjoy.

**Nutrition:**

Calories 145

Fat 4 g

Carbohydrates 19 g

Sugar 9 g

Protein 2 g

Cholesterol 26 mg

## 538.Easy Beef Mushroom Stew

**Preparation Time:** 10 minutes

**Cooking Time:** 8 hours

**Servings:** 8

**Ingredients:**

- 2 lb stewing beef, cubed
- 1 packet dry onion soup mix
- 4 oz can mushrooms, sliced
- 14 oz can cream of mushroom soup
- 1/2 cup water
- 1/4 tsp black pepper
- 1/2 tsp salt

**Directions:**

1. Spray a crock pot inside with cooking spray.

2.Add all ingredients into the crock pot and stir well.

3.Cover and cook on low for 8 hours.

4.Stir well and serve.

**Nutrition:**

Calories 237

Fat 5 g

Carbohydrates 7 g

Sugar 0.4 g

Protein 31 g

Cholesterol 101 mg

### 539.Goulash

**Preparation Time:** 15 minutes

**Cooking Time:** 55 minutes

**Servings:** 6

**Ingredients:**

•½ cup all-purpose flour

•1 tablespoon kosher salt

•½ teaspoon freshly ground black pepper

•2 pounds' beef stew meat

•2 tablespoons canola oil

•1 medium red bell pepper, seeded and chopped

•4 garlic cloves, minced

•1 large yellow onion, diced

•2 tablespoons smoked paprika

•1½ pounds small Yukon gold potatoes, halved

•2 cups beef broth

•2 tablespoons tomato paste

•¼ cup sour cream

•Fresh parsley, for garnish

**Directions:**

1.Select burn/sauté and set to howdy. Select beginning/stop to start. Let preheat for 5 minutes.

2.Mix together the flour, salt, and pepper in a small bowl. Dip the pieces of beef into the flour mixture, shaking off any extra flour.

3.Add the oil and let heat for 1 minute. Place the beef in the pot and brown it on all sides, about 10 minutes.

4.Add the bell pepper, garlic, onion, and smoked paprika. Sauté for about 8 minutes or until the onion is translucent.

5.Add the potatoes, beef broth, and tomato paste and stir.

6.Select pressure and set to lo. Set time to 30 minutes. Select start/stop to begin.

7.At the point when pressure cooking is finished, brisk delivery the pressure by moving the pressure discharge valve to the vent position. Cautiously eliminate cover when unit has got done with delivering pressure.

8.Add the sour cream and mix thoroughly. Garnish with parsley, if desired, and serve immediately.

**Nutrition:**

Calories: 413

Fat: 13g

Saturated fat: 4g

Cholesterol: 98mg

Sodium: 432mg

Carbohydrates: 64g

Fiber: 5g

Protein: 37g

### 540.Loaded Potato Soup

**Preparation Time:** 15 minutes

**Cooking Time:** 30 minutes

**Servings:** 6

**Ingredients:**

•5 slices bacon, chopped

•1 onion, chopped

•3 garlic cloves, minced

•4 pounds' russet potatoes, peeled and chopped

•4 cups chicken broth

•1 cup whole milk

•½ teaspoon sea salt

•½ teaspoon freshly ground black pepper

•1½ cups shredded cheddar cheese

•Sour cream, for serving (optional)

•Chopped fresh chives, for serving (optional)

**Directions:**

1.Preheat for 5 minutes.

2.Add the bacon, onion, and garlic. Cook, stirring occasionally, for 5 minutes. Set aside some of the bacon for garnish.

3.Add the potatoes and chicken broth. Assemble pressure lid, making sure the pressure release valve is in the seal position.

4.Select pressure and set to hi. Set time to 10 minutes, then select start/stop to begin.

5.At the point when pressure cooking is finished, fast delivery the pressure by moving the weight discharge valve to the vent position. Cautiously eliminate top when unit has got done with delivering pressure.

6.Add the milk and mash the ingredients until the soup reaches your desired consistency. Season with the salt and black pepper. Sprinkle the cheese evenly over the top of the soup. Close crisping lid.

7.Select broil and set time to 5 minutes. Select start/stop to begin.

8.When cooking is complete, top with the reserved crispy bacon and serve with sour cream and chives (if using).

**Nutrition:**

Calories: 468

Total fat: 19g

Saturated fat: 9g

Cholesterol: 51mg

Sodium: 1041mg

Carbohydrates: 53g

Fiber: 8g

Protein: 23g



# 541.Butternut Squash, Apple, Bacon and Orzo Soup

**Preparation Time:** 10 minutes

**Cooking Time:** 28 minutes

**Servings:** 8

**Ingredients:**

•4 slices uncooked bacon, cut into ½-inch pieces

•12 ounces' butternut squash, peeled and cubed

•1 green apple, cut into small cubes

•Kosher salt

•Freshly ground black pepper

•1 tablespoon minced fresh oregano

•2 quarts (64 ounces) chicken stock

•1 cup orzo

**Directions:**

1.Select sear/sauté and set temperature to hi. Select start/stop to begin. Let preheat for 5 minutes.

2.Place the bacon in the pot and cook, stirring frequently, about 5 minutes, or until fat is rendered and the bacon starts to brown. Using a slotted spoon, transfer the bacon to a paper towel-lined plate to drain, leaving the rendered bacon fat in the pot.

3.Add the butternut squash, apple, salt, and pepper and sauté until partially soft, about 5 minutes. Stir in the oregano.

4.Add the bacon back into the pot along with the chicken stock. Bring to a boil for about 10 minutes, then add the orzo. Cook for about 8 minutes, until the orzo is tender. Serve.

**Nutrition:**

Calories: 247

Total Fat: 7g

Saturated Fat: 2g

Cholesterol: 17mg

Sodium: 563mg

Carbohydrates: 33g

Fiber: 3g
Protein: 12g

### 542.Coconut and Shrimp Bisque

**Preparation Time:** 10 minutes
**Cooking Time:** 15 minutes
**Servings:** 4
**Ingredients:**

•¼ cup red curry paste
•2 tablespoons water
•1 tablespoon extra-virgin olive oil
•1 bunch scallions, sliced
•1-pound medium (21-30 count) shrimp, peeled and deveined
•1 cup frozen peas
•1 red bell pepper, diced
•1 (14-ounce) can full-fat coconut milk
•Kosher salt

**Directions:**

1.In a small bowl, whisk together the red curry paste and water. Set aside.
2.Select sear/sauté and set to med. Select start/stop to begin. Let preheat for 3 minutes.
3.Add the oil and scallions. Cook for 2 minutes.
4.Add the shrimp, peas, and bell pepper. Stir well to combine. Stir in the red curry paste. Cook for 5 minutes, until the peas are tender.
5.Stir in coconut milk and cook for an additional 5 minutes until shrimp is cooked through and the bisque is thoroughly heated.
6.Season with salt and serve immediately.

**Nutrition:**

Calories: 460
Total Fat: 32g
Saturated Fat: 23g
Cholesterol: 223mg
Sodium: 902mg
Carbohydrates: 16g
Fiber: 5g

Protein: 29g

### 543.Roasted Tomato and Seafood Stew

**Preparation Time:** 10 minutes
**Cooking Time:** 46 minutes
**Servings:** 6
**Ingredients:**

•2 tablespoons extra-virgin olive oil
•1 yellow onion, diced
•1 fennel bulb, tops removed and bulb diced
•3 garlic cloves, minced
•1 cup dry white wine
•2 (14.5-ounce) cans fire-roasted tomatoes
•2 cups chicken stock
•1-pound medium (21-30 count) shrimp, peeled and deveined
•1-pound raw white fish (cod or haddock), cubed
•Salt
•Freshly ground black pepper
•Fresh basil, torn, for garnish

**Directions:**

1.Select sear/sauté and set to med. Select start/stop to begin. Let preheat for 3 minutes.
2.Add the olive oil, onions, fennel, and garlic. Cook for about 3 minutes, until translucent.
3.Add the white wine and deglaze, scraping any stuck bits from the bottom of the pot using a silicone spatula. Add the roasted tomatoes and chicken stock. Simmer for 25 to 30 minutes. Add the shrimp and white fish.
4.Select sear/sauté and set to md: lo. Select start/stop to begin.
5.Simmer for 10 minutes, stirring frequently, until the shrimp and fish are cooked through. Season with salt and pepper.
6.Ladle into bowl and serve topped with torn basil.

**Nutrition:**
Calories: 301
Total fat: 8g
Saturated Fat: 1g
Cholesterol: 99mg
Sodium: 808mg
Carbohydrates: 21g
Fiber: 4g
Protein: 26g

# Meat Recipes

### 544. Low Carb Pork Dumplings with Dipping Sauce

**Difficulty:** Difficult
**Preparation Time:** 30 minutes
**Cooking Time:** 20 minutes
**Servings:** 6
**Ingredients**
18 dumpling wrappers (1 healthy fat)
One teaspoon olive oil (1/4 condiment)
Bok choy: 4 cups(chopped) (2 leans)
Rice vinegar: 2 tablespoons (1/2 condiment)
Diced ginger: 1 tablespoon (1/4 condiment)
Crushed red pepper: 1/4 teaspoon (1/2 green)
Diced garlic: 1 tablespoon (1/2 condiment)
Lean ground pork: 1/2 cup (2 leans)
Lite soy sauce: 2 teaspoons (1/2 condiment)
Honey: 1/2 tsp. (1/4 healthy fat)
Toasted sesame oil: 1 teaspoon (1/4 condiment)
Finely chopped scallions (1 green)
**Directions**
In a large skillet, heat the olive oil, add the bok choy, cook for 6 minutes and add the garlic, ginger and cook for one minute.
Transfer this mixture to a paper towel and pat dry any excess oil
In a bowl, add the mixture of bok choy, chopped chili and lean ground pork and mix well.
Place gnocchi wrap on a plate and add a spoon to fill half of the wrapper. With water, seal the edges and fold them.
Spray air fryer basket with air, add dumplings into air fryer basket, and cook at 375 F for 12 minutes or until golden brown.

Meanwhile, to make the sauce, combine the sesame oil, rice vinegar, shallot, soy sauce and honey in a mixing bowl.
Serve the gnocchi with the sauce.
**Nutrition:**
140 Calories
5g Fat
12g Protein

### 545. Gluten-Free Air Fryer Chicken Fried Brown Rice

**Difficulty:** Average
**Preparation Time:** 10 minutes
**Cooking Time:** 20 minutes
**Servings:** 2
**Ingredients**
Chicken Breast: 1 Cup (1 lean)
White Onion: 1/4 cup chopped (1/2 green)
Celery: 1/4 Cup chopped (1/2 green)
Cooked brown rice: 4 Cups (2 healthy fat)
Carrots: 1/4 cup chopped (1/2 green)
**Directions**
Place the foil on the air fryer basket, make sure to leave room for airflow, roll up on the sides
Spray the film with olive oil. Mix all the ingredients.
On top of the foil, add all the ingredients to the air fryer basket.
Give a splash of olive oil in the mixture.
Cook for five minutes at 390 ° F.
Open the air fryer and give the mixture a spin cook for another five minutes at 390 ° F.
Remove from air fryer and serve hot.
**Nutrition**
350 Calories
6g Fat
22g Protein

### 546. Air Fryer Cheesy Pork Chops

**Difficulty:** Average
**Preparation Time:** 5 minutes
**Cooking Time:** 8 minutes
**Servings:** 2
**Ingredients**
4 lean pork chops (2 leans)
Salt: half tsp. (1/4 condiment)
Garlic powder: ½ tsp. (1/4 condiment)
Shredded cheese: 4 tbsp. (1 healthy fat)
Chopped cilantro (1 green)
**Direction**
Let the air fryer preheat to 350 degrees.
With garlic, coriander and salt, rub the pork
chops. Put the air fryer on. Let it cook for four
minutes. Turn them over and then cook for
extra two minutes.
Drizzle the cheese on top and cook for
another two minutes or until the cheese has
melted.
Serve with salad.
**Nutrition**
467 Calories
61g Protein
22g Fat

### 547. Air Fryer Pork Chop & Broccoli

**Difficulty:** Average
**Preparation Time:** 20 minutes
**Cooking Time:** 20 minutes
**Servings:** 2
**Ingredients**
Broccoli florets: 2 cups (1 green)
Bone-in pork chop: 2 pieces (1 lean)
Paprika: 1/2 tsp. (1/4 condiment)
Avocado oil: 2 tbsp. (1 healthy fat)
Garlic powder: 1/2 tsp. (1/4 condiment)
Onion powder: 1/2 tsp. (1/4 condiment)
Two cloves of crushed garlic (1/4 condiment)
Salt: 1 teaspoon divided (1/4 condiment)

**Direction**
Let the air fryer preheat to 350 degrees.
Spray the basket with cooking oil
Add a spoon. Oil, onion powder, half a
teaspoon. of salt, garlic powder and paprika
in a bowl mix well, rub this spice mixture on
the sides of the pork chop
Add the pork chops to the fryer basket and
cook for five minutes
Meanwhile, add a teaspoon. oil, garlic, half a
teaspoon of salt and broccoli in a bowl and
coat them well
Turn the pork chop and add the broccoli, let it
cook for another five minutes.
Remove from air fryer and serve.
**Nutrition**
483 Calories
20g Fat
23g Protein

### 548. Mustard Glazed Air Fryer Pork Tenderloin

**Difficulty:** Average
**Preparation Time:** 10 minutes
**Cooking Time:** 18 minutes
**Servings:** 4
**Ingredients**
Yellow mustard: ¼ cup (1/2 green)
One pork tenderloin (1 lean)
Salt: ¼ tsp (1/4 condiment)
Honey: 3 Tbsp. (1/2 healthy fat)
black pepper: 1/8 tsp (1/4 condiment)
Minced garlic: 1 Tbsp. (1/4 condiment)
Dried rosemary: 1 tsp (1/4 green)
Italian seasoning: 1 tsp (1/8 condiment)
**Direction**
Using a knife, cut the top of the pork
tenderloin. Add the garlic (minced) into the
cuts. Then sprinkle with kosher salt and
pepper.

In a bowl, add the honey, mustard, rosemary, and Italian seasoning mixture until well blended. Rub this mustard mix all over the pork.

Leave to marinate in the refrigerator for at least two hours.

Place the pork tenderloin in the basket of the air fryer. Cook for 18-20 minutes at 400 F.

With an instant read thermometer, verify that the internal temperature of the pig should be 145 F.

Remove from air fryer and serve with a side of salad.

**Nutrition**

390 Calories

59g Protein

11g Fat

### 549.Air Fryer Pork Taquitos

**Difficulty:** Average

**Preparation Time:** 10 minutes

**Cooking Time:** 20 minutes

**Servings:** 10

**Ingredients**

Pork tenderloin: 3 cups, cooked & shredded (2 leans)

Shredded mozzarella: 2 and 1/2 cups, fat-free (1 healthy fat)

10 small tortillas (1 healthy fat)

Salsa for dipping (1 condiment)

1 juice of a lime (1/4 condiment)

**Direction**

Allow the air fryer to preheat to 380 F.

Add the lime juice to the pork and mix well

With a damp towel over the tortilla, microwave for ten seconds to soften it

Add the pork filling and cheese on top, in a tortilla, roll the tortilla tightly.

Situate the tortillas on a greased baking sheet

Sprinkle oil on the tortillas. Bake for 7-10 minutes or until the tortillas are golden, turn them halfway.

Serve with salad.

**Nutrition**

253 Calories

18g Fat

20g Protein

### 550.Pork Rind Nachos

**Difficulty:** Average

**Preparation Time:** 5 minutes

**Cooking Time:** 5 minutes

**Servings:** 2

**Ingredients**

2 tbsp. of pork rinds (1 lean)

1/4 cup shredded cooked chicken (1/2 lean)

1/2 cup shredded Monterey jack cheese (1/4 healthy fat)

1/4 cup sliced pickled jalapeños (1/4 green)

1/4 cup guacamole (1/4 healthy fat)

1/4 cup full-fat sour cream (1/4 healthy fat)

**Direction**

Place the pork rinds in a 6-inch round pan. Fill with grilled chicken and Monterey jack cheese. Place the pan in the basket with the air fryer.

Set the temperature to 370 ° F and set the timer for 5 minutes or until the cheese has melted.

Eat immediately with jalapeños, guacamole, and sour cream.

**Nutrition**

295 calories

30g protein

27g fat

### 551.Air Fried Jamaican Jerk Pork

**Difficulty:** Difficult

**Preparation Time:** 10 minutes

**Cooking Time:** 20 minutes

**Servings:** 4
**Ingredients**
Pork, cut into three-inch pieces (1 lean)
Jerk paste: ¼ cup (1/4 condiment)
**Direction**
Rub the jerk dough on all the pork pieces.
Chill to marinate for 4 hours in the
refrigerator.
Allow the air fryer to preheat to 390 F. Spray
with olive oil
Before placing it in the air fryer, allow the
meat to rest for 20 minutes at room
temperature.
Cook for 20 minutes at 390 ° F in the air fryer,
turn halfway.
Remove from air fryer and let sit for ten
minutes before slicing.
Serve with microgreens.
**Nutrition**
234 Calories
31g Protein
9g Fat

### 552.Air Fryer Whole Wheat Crusted Pork Chops

**Difficulty:** Average
**Preparation Time:** 10 minutes
**Cooking Time:** 12 minutes
**Servings:** 4
**Ingredients**
Whole-wheat breadcrumbs: 1 cup (1/2
healthy fat)
Salt: ¼ teaspoon (1/4 condiment)
Pork chops: 2-4 pieces (center cut and
boneless) (2 leans)
Chili powder: half teaspoon (1/4 condiment)
Parmesan cheese: 1 tablespoon (1/4 healthy
fat)
Paprika: 1½ teaspoons (1/2 condiment)
One egg beaten (1 healthy fat)
Onion powder: half teaspoon (1/4 condiment)

Granulated garlic: half teaspoon (1/4
condiment)
**Direction**
Allow the air fryer to preheat to 400 F.
rub kosher salt on each side of the pork
chops, let it rest
Add the beaten egg to a large bowl
Add the parmesan, breadcrumbs, garlic,
pepper, paprika, chili powder and onion
powder to a bowl and mix well
Dip the pork chop in the egg and then in the
breadcrumbs
Put it in the air fryer and spray it with oil.
Leave to cook for 12 minutes at 400 F. Turn it
upside down halfway through cooking. Cook
for another six minutes.
Serve with salad.
**Nutrition**
425 calories
20g fat
31g protein

### 553.Air Fried Philly Cheesesteak Taquitos

**Difficulty:** Average
**Preparation Time:** 20 minutes
**Cooking Time:** 6-8 hours
**Servings:** 6
**Ingredients**
Dry Italian dressing mix: one package (1
condiment)
Super Soft Corn Tortillas: one pack (1 healthy
fat)
Green peppers: two pieces, chopped (1/2
green)
12 cups of lean beef steak strips (3 leans)
Beef stock: 2 cups (1 condiment)
Lettuce shredded, one cup (1/2 green)
Provolone cheese: ten slices (1 healthy fat)
**Direction**

In a slow cooker, add onion, beef, broth, pepper and seasonings.
Cover then cook at low heat for 6 or 8 hours.
Heat the tortillas for two minutes in the microwave.
Allow the air fryer to preheat to 350F.
Remove the cheesesteak from the slow cooker, add 2-3 tablespoons of steak to the tortilla.
Add some cheese, roll the tortilla well, and place in a deep fryer basket.
Make all the tortillas you want.
Lightly brush with olive oil
Cook for 6-8 minutes.
Flip the tortillas over and brush more oil as needed.
Serve with chopped lettuce and enjoy

**Nutrition**
220 calories
21g protein
16g fat

### 554.Beef Lunch Meatballs

**Difficulty:** Easy
**Preparation Time:** 10 minutes
**Cooking Time:** 15 minutes
**Servings:** 4
**Ingredients:**
½ pound beef, ground (1/2 lean)
½ pound Italian sausage, chopped (1/2 lean)
½ tsp. garlic powder (1/4 condiment)
½ tsp. onion powder (1/4 condiment)
Salt and black pepper to the taste (1/4 condiment)
½ cup cheddar cheese, grated (1/2 healthy fat)
Mashed potatoes for serving (1/2 healthy fat)
**Directions:**
In a bowl, mix the beef with the sausage, garlic powder, onion powder, salt, pepper and cheese, mix well and form 16 meatballs with this mixture.
Situate the meatballs in your air fryer and cook them at 370 ° F for 15 minutes.
Serve the meatballs with some mashed potatoes on the side.
**Nutrition:**
132 Calories
6.7g Fat
5.5g Protein

### 555.Roasted Garlic Bacon and Potatoes

**Difficulty:** Easy
**Preparation Time:** 5 minutes
**Cooking Time:** 25 minutes
**Servings:** 4
**Ingredients:**
4 medium-sized potatoes (1 healthy fat)
4 strips of streaky bacon (1 lean)
2 sprigs of rosemary (1 green)
6 cloves of garlic, smashed, unpeeled (1/2 condiment)
3 tsp of vegetable oil (1/2 condiment)
**Directions:**
Preheat Air fryer to 390°F.
Put the smashed garlic, bacon, potatoes, rosemary, and then the oil in a bowl. Stir thoroughly.
Place into air fryer basket and roast until golden for about 25 minutes.
**Nutrition:**
114 Calories
8.1g Fat
6.2g Protein

### 556.Teriyaki Glazed Halibut Steak

**Difficulty:** Average
**Preparation Time:** 30 minutes
**Cooking Time:** 10-15 minutes

**Servings:** 3
**Ingredients**
1-pound halibut steak (1 lean)
**For the Marinade:**
3 oz. soy sauce, low sodium (1/4 condiment)
½ cup mirin (1/4 condiment)
2 tbsp. lime juice (1/8 condiment)
¼ cup sugar (1/8 condiment)
¼ cup orange juice (1/8 condiment)
¼ tsp. ginger ground (1/8 condiment)
¼ tsp. crushed red pepper flakes (1/8 condiment)
1 each garlic clove (smashed) (1/8 condiment)
**Direction**
Place all ingredients for the teriyaki glaze/marinade in a saucepan. Bring to a boil and reduce by half, then allow to cool.
When it cools, pour half of the icing/marinade into a zip-up bag along with the halibut, then refrigerate for 30 minutes.
Preheat Air fryer to 390 ° F. Place marinated halibut in the Air fryer and cook 10-12 minutes. Rub some of the remaining glaze on the halibut steak.
Spread on white rice with basil/mint chutney.
**Nutrition**
116 Calories
7g Fat
7.2g Protein

### 557.Pancetta Chops with Pineapple-Jalapeno Salsa

**Difficulty:** Average
**Preparation Time:** 20 minutes
**Cooking Time:** 20 minutes
**Servings:** 3
**Ingredients**
3 pieces of Pancetta Chops (roughly 10 ounces each) (1 lean)
2 tablespoons parsley (1/2 green)

1 tablespoon of ground Coriander (1/4 condiment)
¾ cup of olive oil (1/4 condiment)
1 tablespoon of finely chopped rosemary (1/4 green)
4 ounces of tomatoes, diced (1/4 green)
2 cloves of garlic, chopped (1/4 condiment)
4 ounces of pineapple, diced (1/2 healthy fat)
8 Jalapenos (1/2 green)
3 tsps. of Dijon Mustard (1/4 condiment)
1½ tsp. of sugar (1/8 condiment)
4 ounces of lemon juice (1/8 condiment)
3 tbsp. of finely chopped Cilantro (1/2 green)
2½ tsp. of salt (1/8 condiment)
**Direction**
Place the rosemary, sugar, mustard, coriander, ¼ cup of olive oil, 1 tablespoon of coriander, 1 ½ teaspoons of salt and 1 tablespoon of parsley in a mixing bowl and mix thoroughly. Add the bacon cutlets and mix.
Fill in marinade into a resealable plastic bag and refrigerate for about 3 hours.
Heat your deep fryer to 390 ° F.
Place the jalapenos in a bowl and season with 1 tsp. of oil to cover them evenly. Transfer the jalapenos to the air fryer and cook for about 7 minutes. Remove from the deep fryer and set aside to cool.
Once cooled, peel, remove the seeds and chop the jalapenos into small pieces and transfer them to a bowl. Add the pineapple, tomatoes, garlic and lemon juice, the rest of the oil, parsley, coriander and salt. Stir and set the sauce aside.
Remove the bacon chops from the refrigerator and allow to rest for 30 minutes at room temperature before cooking.
Place the ribs in the air fryer and roast at 390 ° F for about 12 minutes. The bacon cutlets

are well cooked when the internal temperature is 140 ° F.

**Nutrition**
104 Calories
8.7g Fat
6.7g Protein

### 558.Peppery Roasted Potatoes with Smoked Bacon

**Difficulty:** Average
**Preparation Time:** 15 minutes
**Cooking Time:** 11 minutes
**Servings:** 2
**Ingredients**
5 small rashers smoked bacon (1 lean)
1/3 tsp. garlic powder (1/4 condiment)
1 tsp. sea salt (1/4 condiment)
2 tsp. paprika (1/4 condiment)
1/3 tsp. ground black pepper (1/4 condiment)
1 bell pepper (1/2 green)
1 tsp. mustard (1/4 condiment)
2 habanero peppers, halved (1/2 green)
**Direction**
Simply toss all the ingredients in a mixing dish; then transfer them to your air fryer's basket.
Air-fry at 375F for 10 minutes. Serve warm.
**Nutrition**
122 Calories
9g Fat
10g Protein

### 559.Cornbread with Pulled Pancetta

**Difficulty:** Easy
**Preparation Time:** 24 minutes
**Cooking Time:** 19 minutes
**Servings:** 2
**Ingredients**
2½ cups pulled Pancetta (1 lean)

1 tsp. dried rosemary (1/4 green)
1/2 tsp. chili powder (1/4 condiment)
3 cloves garlic (1/4 condiment)
1/2 recipe cornbread (1 healthy fat)
1/2 tablespoon brown sugar (1/4 condiment)
1/3 cup scallions, thinly sliced (1/2 green)
1 tsp. sea salt (1/8 condiment)
**Direction**
Preheat a large non-stick pan over medium heat; now cook the shallots together with the garlic and the pulled bacon.
Next, add the sugar, chili powder, rosemary and salt. Cook, stirring regularly until thickened.
Preheat your air fryer to 335 ° F. Now, coat two mini loaf pans with cooking spray. Add the pulled bacon mixture and spread over the bottom with a spatula.
Spread the previously prepared cornbread batter over the spicy pulled bacon mixture. Bake this cornbread in a preheated air fryer until a centered tester is clean, or for 18 minutes.
**Nutrition**
117 Calories
9.4g Fat
11g Protein

### 560.Bacon and Garlic Pizzas

**Difficulty:** Easy
**Preparation Time:** 10 minutes
**Cooking Time:** 10 minutes
**Servings:** 4
**Ingredients:**
4 dinner rolls, frozen
4 garlic cloves minced
½ tsp. oregano dried
½ tsp. garlic powder
1 cup ketchup
8 bacon slices, cooked and chopped

1 and ¼ cups cheddar cheese, grated
**Directions:**
Place the rolls on a work surface and press them to obtain 4 ovals.
Spray each oval with cooking spray, transfer them to the air fryer and cook at 370 ° F for 2 minutes.
Spread the ketchup on each oval, divide the garlic, sprinkle with oregano and garlic powder and garnish with bacon and cheese. Return the pizzas to your hot air fryer and cook them at 370 ° F for another 8 minutes. Serve hot for lunch.
**Nutrition**
104 Calories
9g Fat
8.5g Protein

### 561.Stuffed Meatballs

**Difficulty:** Average
**Preparation Time:** 10 minutes
**Cooking Time:** 10 minutes
**Servings:** 4
**Ingredients:**
1/3 cup bread crumbs (1 healthy fat)
3 tbsp. milk (1/2 condiment)
1 tablespoon ketchup (1/4 condiment)
1 egg (1 healthy fat)
½ tsp. marjoram, dried (1/4 condiment)
Salt and black pepper to the taste (1/8 condiment)
1-pound lean beef, ground (1 lean)
20 cheddar cheese cubes (1/2 healthy fat)
1 tablespoon olive oil (1/8 condiment)
**Direction**
In a bowl, mix the breadcrumbs with ketchup, milk, marjoram, salt, pepper and egg and beat well.
Add the beef, mix and form 20 meatballs with this mixture.

Shape each meatball around a cube of cheese, sprinkle with oil and rub.
Place all the meatballs in your preheated air fryer and cook at 390 ° F for 10 minutes.
Serve them for lunch with a side of salad.
**Nutrition**
112 Calories
8.2g Fat
7.7g Protein

### 562.Steaks and Cabbage

**Difficulty:** Easy
**Preparation Time:** 10 minutes
**Cooking Time:** 10 minutes
**Servings:** 4
**Ingredients:**
½ pound sirloin steak, cut into strips (1 lean)
2 tsp. cornstarch (1/8 condiment)
1 tablespoon peanut oil (1/8 condiment)
2 cups green cabbage, chopped (1 green)
1 yellow bell pepper (1/2 green)
2 garlic cloves, minced (1/8 condiment)
Salt and black pepper to the taste (1/8 condiment)
**Directions:**
In a bowl, mix the cabbage with salt, pepper and peanut oil, mix, transfer to air fryer basket, cook at 370 ° F for 4 minutes and transfer to the bowl.
Add the steak strips to the air fryer, also add bell pepper, garlic, salt and pepper, stir and cook for 5 minutes.
Add the cabbage on top, mix, divide into plates and serve for lunch. To enjoy!
**Nutrition**
111 Calories
7.2g Fat
8.7g Protein

### 563.Air Fryer Meat Loaf

**Difficulty:** Easy

**Preparation Time:** 11 minutes
**Cooking Time:** 20 minutes
**Servings:** 4
**Ingredients:**
1 pound 99% lean ground beef (1 lean)
½ teaspoon garlic powder (1/4 condiment)
3 egg whites, beaten (1 healthy fat)
1 cup grated kohlrabi (1 healthy fat)
Salt and pepper to taste (1/4 condiment)
**Directions:**
Preheat the air fryer to 350F for five minutes.
In a bowl, mix all ingredients until well combined.
Pour the mixture into a greased loaf pan that will fit inside the air fryer. Cover with aluminum foil on top.
Place inside the preheated air fryer and cook for 35 to 45 minutes until the meat is cooked through.
Allow the meatloaf to cool before slicing.
**Nutrition:**
270 Calories
34g Protein
10g Fat

### 564.Air Fryer Roasted Beef

**Difficulty:** Average
**Preparation Time:** 8 minutes
**Cooking Time:** 60 minutes
**Servings:** 8
**Ingredients:**
4 pounds beef roast (1 lean)
2 teaspoons garlic powder (1/4 condiment)
½ teaspoon salt (1/8 condiment)
½ teaspoon pepper (1/8 condiment)
2 teaspoons thyme (1/4 green)
1 tablespoon olive oil (1/8 condiment)
**Directions:**
Preheat the air fryer to 350F for five minutes.

Pat dry the beef and place it on a working surface.
In a small bowl, combine the condiments and spices to form a dry rub.
Massage the beef with the dry rub all over the beef.
Place the seasoned beef inside the preheated air fryer and cook for 60 minutes.
Allow the beef to rest before slicing.
**Nutrition:**
434 Calories
61g Protein
12g Fat

### 565.Air Fried Burger Patties

**Difficulty:** Easy
**Preparation Time:** 8 minutes
**Cooking Time:** 15 minutes
**Servings:** 4
**Ingredients:**
1 teaspoon liquid smoke (1/8 condiment)
½ teaspoon garlic powder (1/8 condiment)
½ teaspoon salt (1/8 condiment)
½ teaspoon ground black pepper (1/8 condiment)
1 pound 99% lean ground beef (1 lean)
1 teaspoon parsley (1/2 green)
**Directions:**
Preheat the air fryer to 350F for five minutes.
Place all ingredients in a bowl.
Mix until well combined.
Form four burger patties from the mixture using your hands.
Place the patties inside the fridge to firm up.
After 2 hours, place the patties inside the air fryer basket.
Cook for 15 minutes.
**Nutrition:**
246 Calories
31g Protein

13g Fat

### 566.Air Fried Rib Eye Steak

**Difficulty:** Average
**Preparation Time:** 18 minutes
**Cooking Time:** 15 minutes
**Servings:** 1
**Ingredients:**
½ pound red eye steak, fat-trimmed
½ teaspoon salt
¾ teaspoon ground pepper
½ teaspoon garlic powder
¾ teaspoon steak seasoning
**Directions:**
Preheat the air fryer to 350F for five minutes.
Season the steak with the spices.
Situate in the air fryer and cook for 15 minutes.
Allow to rest before serving.
**Nutrition:**
540 Calories
44g Protein
28g Fat

### 567.Air Fryer Steak Bites and Mushrooms

**Difficulty:** Average
**Preparation Time:** 9 minutes
**Cooking Time:** 25 minutes
**Servings:** 4
**Ingredients:**
1 pound 99% lean steak (fat trimmed), cut into cubes (1 lean)
8 ounces mushrooms, sliced (1 healthy fat)
1 teaspoon melted butter (1/4 healthy fat)
½ teaspoon garlic powder (1/8 condiment)
Salt and pepper to taste (1/8 condiment)
**Directions:**
Preheat the air fryer to 350F for five minutes.
Prep the bottom of the air fryer with foil.

Place all ingredients in a bowl. Toss to coat the beef and mushrooms with the seasoning.
Place the seasoned beef and mushrooms inside the foil-lined fryer basket.
Cook for 20 to 25 minutes.
Halfway through the cooking time, open the fryer basket and give a good shake for even cooking.
**Nutrition:**
299 Calories
14g Protein
5g Fat

### 568.Air Fried Lamb Chops

**Difficulty:** Difficult
**Preparation Time:** 12 minutes
**Cooking Time:** 25 minutes
**Servings:** 2
**Ingredients:**
5 cloves of garlic, sliced (1/8 condiment)
1 teaspoon garam masala (1/8 condiment)
1 teaspoon ground cinnamon (1/8 condiment)
½ teaspoon cayenne powder (1/8 condiment)
½ teaspoon salt (1/8 condiment)
1-pound lamb chops, fat trimmed (1 lean)
**Directions:**
Preheat the air fryer to 350F for five minutes.
Prep bottom of the air fryer with foil.
Place the garlic, garam masala, cinnamon, cayenne pepper, and salt. Mix to create the spice rub.
Massage the lamb chops with the spice rub.
Place inside the air fryer basket.
Cook for 20 to 25 minutes.
**Nutrition:**
338 Calories
46g Protein
12g Fat

### 569. Air Fried Roasted Lamb

**Difficulty:** Difficult
**Preparation Time:** 14 minutes
**Cooking Time:** 25 minutes
**Servings:** 1
**Ingredients:**
10 ounces butterflied lamb leg roast, fat trimmed (2 lean)
1 tablespoon olive oil (1/4 condiment)
1 teaspoon rosemary (1/4 green)
1 teaspoon thyme (1/4 green)
¼ teaspoon salt (1/8 condiment)
½ teaspoon black pepper (1/8 condiment)
**Directions:**
Preheat the air fryer to 360F for five minutes. Prepare the bottom of the air fryer with foil. Season the lamb leg roast with spices and condiments.
Place in the air fryer and cook for 15 to 20 minutes.
**Nutrition:**
181 Calories
18g Protein
3g Fat

### 570. Roast Lamb Rack

**Difficulty:** Difficult
**Preparation Time:** 12 minutes
**Cooking Time:** 30 minutes
**Servings:** 3
**Ingredients:**
1 ½ pounds rack of lamb (1 lean)
Salt and pepper to taste (1/4 condiment)
1 teaspoon grated garlic (1/8 condiment)
1 teaspoon cumin seeds (1/4 healthy fat)
1 teaspoon olive oil (1/8 condiment)
**Directions:**
Preheat the air fryer to 350F for five minutes. Coat the bottom of the air fryer with foil. Season the rack of lamb with the spices.

Place in the air fryer and cook for 25 to 30 minutes.
**Nutrition:**
386 Calories
47.3g Protein
12g Fat

### 571. Air Fried Masala Chops

**Difficulty:** Easy
**Preparation Time:** 9 minutes
**Cooking Time:** 30 minutes
**Servings:** 1
**Ingredients:**
½ pound lamb chop, trimmed from fat (1 lean)
2 tablespoon ginger paste (1/4 condiment)
½ tablespoon red chili powder (1/4 condiment)
1 tablespoon garam masala (1/4 condiment)
½ teaspoon salt (1/4 condiment)
**Directions:**
Preheat the air fryer to 350F for five minutes. Seal the bottom of the air fryer with foil. Season the lamb chops with the spices.
Place inside the air fryer and cook for 25 to 30 minutes
**Nutrition:**
343 Calories
46g Protein
15g Fat

### 572. Mutton Chops

**Difficulty:** Average
**Preparation Time:** 11 minutes
**Cooking Time:** 25 minutes
**Servings:** 8
**Ingredients:**
8 mutton chops, trimmed from fat (2 lean)
1 tablespoon crushed garlic (1/4 condiment)
Salt and pepper to taste (1/4 condiment)
½ teaspoon cumin (1/4 condiment)

**Directions:**
Preheat the air fryer to 350F for five minutes.
Seal the bottom of the air fryer with foil.
Season the mutton chops with spices.
Place in the air fryer basket and cook for 25 minutes.
Cook in batches if necessary.
**Nutrition:**
168 Calories
23g Protein
8g Fat

## 573.Rosemary Crusted Lamb Chops

**Difficulty:** Difficult
**Preparation Time:** 13 minutes
**Cooking Time:** 25 minutes
**Servings:** 2
**Ingredients:**
1-pound lamb chops, trimmed of fat (1 lean)
2 tablespoons fresh rosemary (1/4 green)
½ teaspoon salt (1/8 condiment)
1 teaspoon ground black pepper (1/8 condiment)
3 cloves garlic, minced (1/4 condiment)
**Directions:**
Preheat the air fryer to 350F for five minutes.
Seal the bottom of the air fryer with foil.
Season the lamb chops with the spices and condiments.
Place inside the air fryer basket.
Cook for 25 minutes until golden.
**Nutrition:**
335 Calories
45g Protein
15.7g Fat

## 574.Air Fryer Pork Chops

**Difficulty:** Average
**Preparation Time:** 6 minutes
**Cooking Time:** 25 minutes
**Servings:** 4
**Ingredients:**
1 tablespoon paprika (1/8 condiment)
1 ½ teaspoon salt (1/4 condiment)
1 teaspoon ground mustard (1/8 condiment)
¼ teaspoon garlic powder (1/8 condiment)
4 center cut bone-in pork chops, trimmed from fat (2 lean)
**Directions:**
Preheat the air fryer to 350F for five minutes.
Seal the bottom of the air fryer with foil.
Mix together the paprika, salt, mustard, and garlic powder to create a spice rub.
Massage the pork chops with the spice rub.
Place the seasoned pork chops inside the air fryer and cook for 20 to 25 minutes.
**Nutrition:**
234 Calories
40g Protein
7g Fat

## 575.Air Fryer Pork Tenderloin

**Difficulty:** Average
**Preparation Time:** 13 minutes
**Cooking Time:** 25 minutes
**Servings:** 4
**Ingredients:**
½ teaspoon black pepper (1/8 condiment)
¼ teaspoon garlic powder (1/8 condiment)
¼ teaspoon salt (1/8 condiment)
2 pounds pork tenderloin, trimmed from excess fat (1 lean)
**Directions:**
Preheat the air fryer to 350F for five minutes.
Seal the bottom of the air fryer with foil.
Mix together the black pepper, garlic powder, and salt to create a spice rub.
Massage the pork with the spice rub.
Place the seasoned pork tenderloin inside the air fryer and cook for 20 to 25 minutes.

**Nutrition:**
266 Calories
59g Protein
7g Fat

### 576.Mustard Pork Chops

**Difficulty:** Easy
**Preparation Time:** 11 minutes
**Cooking Time:** 20 minutes
**Servings:** 4
**Ingredients:**
4 tablespoons mustard (1/8 condiment)
2 tablespoons minced garlic (1/4 condiment)
½ teaspoon salt (1/8 condiment)
1 teaspoon ground black pepper (1/8 condiment)
4 pork chops, trimmed from fat (2 lean)
**Directions:**
Preheat the air fryer to 350F for five minutes. Seal the bottom of the air fryer with foil. Place the mustard, garlic, salt, and black pepper in a bowl. Mix until well combined. Massage the pork chops with the spice rub. Place seasoned pork chops inside the air fryer and cook for 20 minutes.
**Nutrition:**
346 Calories
41g Protein
17.9g Fat

### 577.Air Fryer Italian Pork Chops

**Difficulty:** Difficult
**Preparation Time:** 9 minutes
**Cooking Time:** 25 minutes
**Servings:** 2
**Ingredients:**
2 boneless pork loin chops, trimmed from fat (1 lean)
¼ teaspoon salt (1/8 condiment)
1 teaspoon Italian herb seasoning (1/8 condiment)

**Directions:**
Preheat the air fryer to 350F for five minutes. Wrap the bottom of the air fryer with foil. Season the pork loin chops with the spices and seasoning. Place inside the air fryer basket and cook for 20 to 25 minutes.
**Nutrition:**
235 Calories
41g Protein
3g Fat

### 578.Air Fried Riblets

**Difficulty:** Easy
**Preparation Time:** 9 minutes
**Cooking Time:** 25 minutes
**Servings:** 2
**Ingredients:**
1-pound pork riblets (1 lean)
1 teaspoon salt (1/8 condiment)
6 cloves of garlic, minced (1/4 condiment)
**Directions:**
Preheat the air fryer to 350F for five minutes. Wrap the bottom of the air fryer with foil. Season the pork riblets with salt and garlic. Place inside the air fryer and cook for 20 to 25 minutes.
**Nutrition:**
288 Calories
39g Protein
12g Fat

### 579.Pork Tenderloin with Fried Bell Peppers

**Difficulty:** Average
**Preparation Time:** 18 minutes
**Cooking Time:** 20 minutes
**Servings:** 4

**Ingredients:**
2 large bell peppers, seeded and julienned (1 green)
10 ounces Cremini mushrooms, diced (2 healthy fats)
1-pound pork tenderloin (1 lean)
Salt and pepper to taste (1/8 condiment)
**Directions:**
Preheat the air fryer to 350F for five minutes.
Line the bottom of the air fryer with foil.
Place all ingredients in a bowl and toss to coat everything with the seasonings.
Place inside the air fryer basket and cook for 20 minutes.
Halfway through the cooking time, give the fryer basket a shake for even cooking.
**Nutrition:**
385 Calories
37g Protein
4.7g Fat

## 580.Air Fried Beef Jerky

**Difficulty:** Easy
**Preparation Time:** 11 minutes
**Cooking Time:** 15 minutes
**Servings:** 2
**Ingredients:**
12 ounces, sirloin beef, sliced (2 lean)
1 clove of garlic, minced (1/2 condiment)
Salt and pepper to taste (1/2 condiment)
**Directions:**
Preheat the air fryer to 350F for five minutes.
Line the bottom of the air fryer with foil.
Place all ingredients in a bowl and toss to coat the beef slices with the seasoning.
Place beef slices in the air fryer and cook for 15 minutes.
**Nutrition:**
333 Calories
35g Protein
14g Fat

## 581.Air Fried Pot Roast

**Difficulty:** Average
**Preparation Time:** 12 minutes
**Cooking Time:** 60 minutes
**Servings:** 8
**Ingredients:**
4 pounds beef chuck roast (2 lean)
Salt and pepper to taste (1/2 condiment)
5 cloves garlic, minced (1/2 condiment)
1 teaspoon thyme (1/2 green)
**Directions:**
Preheat the air fryer to 350F for five minutes.
Line the bottom of the air fryer with foil.
Score the beef using a knife.
Season the pot roast with the seasoning.
Place inside the air fryer basket and cook for 60 minutes.
**Nutrition:**
420 Calories
61g Protein
16g Fat

## 582.Air Fried Mongolian Beef

**Difficulty:** Average
**Preparation Time:** 9 minutes
**Cooking Time:** 20 minutes
**Servings:** 4
**Ingredients:**
2 cloves garlic, minced (1/4 condiment)
1 cup chopped scallions (1/2 green)
½ teaspoon minced ginger (1/4 condiment)
1 ½ pounds flank steak, thinly sliced (1 lean)
1 teaspoon sesame oil (1/4 condiment)
Salt and pepper to taste (1/4 condiment)
**Directions:**
Preheat the air fryer to 350F for five minutes.
Line the bottom of the air fryer with foil.
Place all ingredients in a bowl. Toss to coat beef with the condiments.
Place inside the air fryer basket.
Cook for 15 to 20 minutes.

**Nutrition:**
258 Calories
37g Protein
9.7g Fat

# Seafood Recipes

### 583.Salmon Burgers

**Preparation Time:** 10 minutes
**Cooking Time:** 15 minutes
**Servings:** 4
**Ingredients:**
- 1 lb. salmon fillets
- 1 onion
- ¼ dill fronds
- 1 tablespoon honey
- 1 tablespoon horseradish
- 1 tablespoon mustard
- 1 tablespoon olive oil
- 2 toasted split rolls
- 1 avocado

**Directions:**
1.Place salmon fillets in a blender and blend until smooth, transfer to a bowl, add onion, dill, honey, horseradish and mix well
2.Add salt and pepper and form 4 patties
3.In a bowl combine mustard, honey, mayonnaise and dill
4.In a skillet heat oil add salmon patties and cook for 2-3 minutes per side
5.When ready remove from heat
6.Divided lettuce and onion between the buns
7.Place salmon patty on top and spoon mustard mixture and avocado slices
8.Serve when ready

**Nutrition:**
Calories: 189
Total Carbohydrate: 6 g
Cholesterol: 3 mg
Total Fat: 7 g
Fiber: 4 g
Protein: 12 g
Sodium: 293 mg

### 584.Tuna Noodle Casserole

**Preparation Time:** 15 minutes
**Cooking Time:** 20 minutes
**Servings:** 4
**Ingredients:**
- 2 oz. egg noodles
- 4 oz. fraiche
- 1 egg
- 1 teaspoon cornstarch
- 1 tablespoon juice from 1 lemon
- 1 can tuna
- 1 cup peas
- ¼ cup parsley

**Directions:**
1.Place noodles in a saucepan with water and bring to a boil
2.In a bowl combine egg, crème fraiche and lemon juice, whisk well
3.When noodles are cooked add crème fraiche mixture to skillet and mix well
4.Add tuna, peas, parsley lemon juice and mix well
5.When ready remove from heat and serve

**Nutrition:**
Calories: 214
Total Carbohydrate: 2 g
Cholesterol: 73 mg
Total Fat: 7 g
Fiber: 2g
Protein: 19 g
Sodium: 308 g

### 585.Sabich Sandwich

**Preparation Time:** 5 minutes
**Cooking Time:** 15 minutes
**Servings:** 2
**Ingredients:**
- 2 tomatoes
- Olive oil
- ½ lb. eggplant

•¼ cucumber

•1 tablespoon lemon

•1 tablespoon parsley

•¼ head cabbage

•2 tablespoons wine vinegar

•2 pita bread

•½ cup hummus

•¼ tahini sauce

•2 hard-boiled eggs

**Directions:**

1.In a skillet fry eggplant slices until tender

2.In a bowl add tomatoes, cucumber, parsley, lemon juice and season salad

3.In another bowl toss cabbage with vinegar

4.In each pita pocket add hummus, eggplant and drizzle tahini sauce

5.Top with eggs, tahini sauce

**Nutrition:**

Calories: 269

Total Carbohydrate: 2 g

Cholesterol: 3 mg

Total Fat: 14 g

Fiber: 2 g

Protein: 7 g

Sodium: 183 mg

### 586.Crispy Fish

**Preparation Time:** 5 minutes

**Cooking Time:** 15 minutes

**Servings:** 4

**Ingredients:**

•Thick fish fillets

•¼ cup all-purpose flour

•1 egg

•1 cup bread crumbs

•2 tablespoons vegetables

•Lemon wedge

**Directions:**

1.In a dish add flour, egg, breadcrumbs in different dishes and set aside

2.Dip each fish fillet into the flour, egg and then bread crumbs bowl

3.Place each fish fillet in a heated skillet and cook for 4-5 minutes per side

4.When ready remove from pan and serve with lemon wedges

**Nutrition:**

Calories: 189

Total Carbohydrate: 2 g

Cholesterol: 73 mg

Total Fat: 17 g

Fiber: 0 g

Protein: 7 g

Sodium: 163 mg Salmon with Vegetables

**Preparation Time:** 10 minutes

**Cooking Time:** 15 minutes

**Servings:** 4

**Ingredients:**

•2 tablespoons olive oil

•2 carrots

•1 head fennel

•2 squash

•¼ onion

•1-inch ginger

•1 cup white wine

•2 cups water

•2 parsley sprigs

•2 tarragon sprigs

•6 oz. salmon fillets

•1 cup cherry tomatoes

•1 scallion

**Directions:**

1.In a skillet heat olive oil, add fennel, squash, onion, ginger, carrot and cook until vegetables are soft

2.Add wine, water, parsley and cook for another 4-5 minutes
3.Season salmon fillets and place in the pan
4.Cook for 5 minutes per side or until is ready
5.Transfer salmon to a bowl, spoon tomatoes and scallion around salmon and serve

**Nutrition:**
Calories: 301
Total Carbohydrate: 2 g
Cholesterol: 13 mg
Total Fat: 17 g
Fiber: 4 g
Protein: 8 g
Sodium: 201 mg

## 587.Arugula and Sweet Potato Salad

**Preparation Time:** 10 minutes
**Cooking Time:** 20 minutes
**Servings:** 4
**Ingredients:**
- 1 lb. sweet potatoes
- 1 cup walnuts
- 1 tablespoon olive oil
- 1 cup water
- 1 tablespoon soy sauce
- 3 cups arugula

**Directions:**
1.Bake potatoes at 400 F until tender, remove and set aside
2.In a bowl drizzle, walnuts with olive oil and microwave for 2-3 minutes or until toasted
3.In a bowl combine all salad ingredients and mix well
4.Pour over soy sauce and serve

**Nutrition:**
Calories: 189
Total Carbohydrate: 2 g
Cholesterol: 13 mg
Total Fat: 7 g
Fiber: 2 g

Protein: 10 g
Sodium: 301 mg

## 588.Shrimp with Garlic

**Preparation Time:** 10 minutes
**Cooking Time:** 25 minutes
**Servings:** 2
**Ingredients:**
- 1 lb. shrimp
- ¼ teaspoon baking soda
- 2 tablespoons oil
- 2 teaspoon minced garlic
- ¼ cup vermouth
- 2 tablespoons unsalted butter
- 1 teaspoon parsley

**Directions:**
1.In a bowl toss shrimp with baking soda and salt, let it stand for a couple of minutes
2.In a skillet heat olive oil and add shrimp
3.Add garlic, red pepper flakes and cook for 1-2 minutes
4.Add vermouth and cook for another 4-5 minutes
5.When ready remove from heat and serve

**Nutrition:**
Calories: 289
Total Carbohydrate: 2 g
Cholesterol: 3 mg
Total Fat: 17 g
Fiber: 2 g
Protein: 7 g
Sodium: 163 mg    Moules Marinieres

**Preparation Time:** 10 minutes
**Cooking Time:** 30 minutes
**Servings:** 4
**Ingredients:**
- 2 tablespoons unsalted butter
- 1 leek
- 1 shallot
- 2 cloves garlic

- •2 bay leaves
- •1 cup white win
- •2 lb. mussels
- •2 tablespoons mayonnaise
- •1 tablespoon lemon zest
- •2 tablespoons parsley
- •1 sourdough bread

**Directions:**

1.In a saucepan melt butter, add leeks, garlic, bay leaves, shallot and cook until vegetables are soft

2.Bring to a boil, add mussels, and cook for 1-2 minutes

3.Transfer mussels to a bowl and cover

4.Whisk in remaining butter with mayonnaise and return mussels to pot

5.Add lemon juice, parsley lemon zest and stir to combine

**Nutrition:**

Calories: 321

Total Carbohydrate: 2 g

Cholesterol: 13 mg

Total Fat: 17 g

Fiber: 2 g

Protein: 9 g

Sodium: 312 mg

### 589.Steamed Mussels with Coconut-Curry

**Preparation Time:** 15 minutes

**Cooking Time:** 20 minutes

**Servings:** 4

**Ingredients:**

- •6 sprigs cilantro
- •2 cloves garlic
- •2 shallots
- •¼ teaspoon coriander seeds
- •¼ teaspoon red chili flakes
- •1 teaspoon zest

- •1 can coconut milk
- •1 tablespoon vegetable oil
- •1 tablespoon curry paste
- •1 tablespoon stevia
- •1 tablespoon fish sauce
- •2 lb. mussels

**Directions:**

1.In a bowl combine lime zest, cilantro stems, shallot, garlic, coriander seed, chili and salt

2.In a saucepan heat oil add, garlic, shallots, pounded paste and curry paste

3.Cook for 3-4 minutes, add coconut milk, stevia and fish sauce

4.Bring to a simmer and add mussels

5.Stir in lime juice, cilantro leaves and cook for a couple of more minutes

6.When ready remove from heat and serve

**Nutrition:**

Calories: 209

Total Carbohydrate: 6 g

Cholesterol: 13 mg

Total Fat: 7 g

Fiber: 2 g

Protein: 17 g

Sodium: 193 mg

### 590.Niçoise Salad

**Preparation Time:** 15 minutes

**Cooking Time:** 10 minutes

**Servings:** 4

**Ingredients:**

- •1 oz. red potatoes
- •1 package green beans
- •2 eggs
- •½ cup tomatoes
- •2 tablespoons wine vinegar
- •¼ teaspoon salt
- •½ teaspoon pepper
- •½ teaspoon thyme

•¼ cup olive oil

•6 oz. tuna

•¼ cup Kalamata olives

**Directions:**

1.In a bowl combine all ingredients together

2.Add salad dressing and serve

**Nutrition:**

Calories: 189

Total Carbohydrate: 2 g

Cholesterol: 13 mg

Total Fat: 7 g

Fiber: 2 g

Protein: 15 g

Sodium: 321 mg

## 591.Seared Scallops

**Preparation Time:** 15 minutes

**Cooking Time:** 20 minutes

**Servings:** 4

**Ingredients:**

•1 lb. sea scallops

•1 tablespoon canola oil

**Directions:**

1.Season scallops and refrigerate for a couple of minutes

2.In a skillet heat oil, add scallops and cook for 1-2 minutes per side

3.When ready remove from heat and serve

**Nutrition:**

Calories: 283

Total Carbohydrate: 10 g

Cholesterol: 3 mg

Total Fat: 8 g

Fiber: 2 g

Protein: 9 g

Sodium: 271 mg

## 592.Black COD

**Preparation Time:** 15 minutes

**Cooking Time:** 20 minutes

**Servings:** 4

**Ingredients:**

•¼ cup miso paste

•¼ cup sake

•1 tablespoon mirin

•1 teaspoon soy sauce

•1 tablespoon olive oil

•4 black cod filets

**Directions:**

1.In a bowl combine miso, soy sauce, oil and sake

2.Rub mixture over cod fillets and let it marinade for 20-30 minutes

3.Adjust broiler and broil cod filets for 10-12 minutes

4.When fish is cook remove and serve

**Nutrition:**

Calories: 231

Total Carbohydrate: 2 g

Cholesterol: 13 mg

Total Fat: 15 g

Fiber: 2 g

Protein: 8 g

Sodium: 298 mg

## 593.Salmon Pasta

**Preparation Time:** 10 minutes

**Cooking Time:** 25 minutes

**Servings:** 2

**Ingredients:**

•5 tablespoons butter

•¼ onion

•1 tablespoon all-purpose flour

•1 teaspoon garlic powder

•2 cups skim milk

•¼ cup Romano cheese

•1 cup green peas

•¼ cup canned mushrooms

•8 oz. salmon

•1 package penne pasta

**Directions:**

1.Bring a pot with water to a boil
2.Add pasta and cook for 10-12 minutes
3.In a skillet melt butter, add onion and sauté until tender
4.Stir in garlic powder, flour, milk and cheese
5.Add mushrooms, peas and cook on low heat for 4-5 minutes
6.Toss in salmon and cook for another 2-3 minutes
7.When ready serve with cooked pasta
**Nutrition:**
Calories: 211
Total Carbohydrate: 7 g
Cholesterol: 13 mg
Total Fat: 18 g
Fiber: 3 g
Protein: 17 g
Sodium: 289 mg

## 594.Miso-Glazed Salmon

**Preparation Time:** 10 minutes
**Cooking Time:** 40 minutes
**Servings:** 4
**Ingredients:**
•¼ cup red miso
•¼ cup sake
•1 tablespoon soy sauce
•1 tablespoon vegetable oil
•4 salmon fillets
**Directions:**
1.In a bowl combine sake, oil, soy sauce and miso
2.Rub mixture over salmon fillets and marinade for 20-30 minutes
3.Preheat a broiler
4.Broil salmon for 5-10 minutes
5.When ready remove and serve
**Nutrition:**
Calories: 198
Total Carbohydrate: 5 g

Cholesterol: 12 mg
Total Fat: 10 g
Fiber: 2 g
Protein: 6 g
Sodium: 257 mg

## 595.Crab Legs

**Preparation Time:** 5 minutes
**Cooking Time:** 20 minutes
**Servings:** 3
**Ingredients:**
•3 lb. crab legs
•¼ cup salted butter, melted and divided
•½ lemon, juiced
•¼ tsp. garlic powder
**Directions:**
1.In a bowl, toss the crab legs and two tablespoons of the melted butter together. Place the crab legs in the basket of the fryer.
2.Cook at 400°F for fifteen minutes, giving the basket a good shake halfway through.
3.Combine the remaining butter with the lemon juice and garlic powder.
4.Crack open the cooked crab legs and remove the meat. Serve with the butter dip on the side and enjoy!
**Nutrition:**
Calories: 392
Fat: 10g
Protein: 18g
Sugar: 8g Shrimp Curry
**Preparation Time:** 15 minutes
**Cooking Time:** 20 minutes
**Servings:** 4
**Ingredients:**
•2 tablespoons peanut oil
•¼ onion
•2 cloves garlic
•1 teaspoon ginger
•1 teaspoon cumin

•1 teaspoon turmeric

•1 teaspoon paprika

•¼ red chili powder

•1 can tomatoes

•1 can coconut milk

•1 lb. peeled shrimp

•1 tablespoon cilantro

**Directions:**

1.In a skillet add onion and cook for 4-5 minutes

2.Add ginger, cumin, garlic, chili, paprika and cook on low heat

3.Pour the tomatoes, coconut milk and simmer for 10-12 minutes

4.Stir in shrimp, cilantro, and cook for 2-3 minutes

5.When ready remove and serve

**Nutrition:**

Calories: 178

Total Carbohydrate: 3 g

Cholesterol: 3 mg

Total Fat: 17 g

Fiber:  g

Protein: 9 g

Sodium: 297 mg

### 596.Crusty Pesto Salmon

**Preparation Time:** 5 minutes

**Cooking Time:** 15 minutes

**Servings:** 2

**Ingredients:**

•¼ cup s, roughly chopped

•¼ cup pesto

•2 x 4-oz. salmon fillets

•2 tbsp. unsalted butter, melted

**Directions:**

1.Mix the s and pesto together.

2.Place the salmon fillets in a round baking dish, roughly six inches in diameter.

3.Brush the fillets with butter, followed by the pesto mixture, ensuring to coat both the top and bottom. Put the baking dish inside the fryer.

4.Cook for twelve minutes at 390°F.

5.The salmon is ready when it flakes easily when prodded with a fork. Serve warm.

**Nutrition:**

Calories: 290

Fat: 11g

Protein: 20g

Sugar: 9g

### 597.Buttery Cod

**Preparation Time:** 10 minutes

**Cooking Time:** 12 minutes

**Servings:** 2

**Ingredients:**

•2 x 4-oz. cod fillets

•2 tbsp. salted butter, melted

•1 tsp. Old Bay seasoning

•½ medium lemon, sliced

**Directions:**

1.Place the cod fillets in a skillet.

2.Brush with melted butter, season with Old Bay, and top with a few lemon wedges.

3.Wrap the fish in aluminum foil and place it in your deep fryer.

4.Cook for eight minutes at 350 ° F.

5.The cod is done when it is easily peeled. Serve hot ....

**Nutrition:**

Calories: 394

Fat: 5g

Protein: 12g

Sugar: 4g

### 598.Sesame Tuna Steak

**Preparation Time:** 5 minutes

**Cooking Time:** 12 minutes

**Servings:** 2

**Ingredients:**
- 1 tbsp. coconut oil, melted
- 2 x 6-oz. tuna steaks
- ½ tsp. garlic powder
- 2 tsp. black sesame seeds
- 2 tsp. white sesame seeds

**Directions:**
1. Apply the coconut oil to the tuna steaks with a brunch, then season with garlic powder.
2. Combine the black and white sesame seeds. Embed them in the tuna steaks, covering the fish all over. Place the tuna into your air fryer.
3. Cook for eight minutes at 400°F, turning the fish halfway through.
4. The tuna steaks are ready when they have reached a temperature of 145°F. Serve straightaway.

**Nutrition:**
Calories: 160
Fat: 6g
Protein: 26g
Sugar: 7g

## 599.Lemon Garlic Shrimp

**Preparation Time:** 10 minutes
**Cooking Time:** 15 minutes
**Servings:** 2
**Ingredients:**
- 1 medium lemon
- ½ lb. medium shrimp, shelled and deveined
- ½ tsp. Old Bay seasoning
- 2 tbsp. unsalted butter, melted
- ½ tsp. minced garlic

**Directions:**
1. Grate the rind of the lemon into a bowl. Cut the lemon in half and juice it over the same bowl. Toss in the shrimp, Old Bay, and butter, mixing everything to make sure the shrimp is completely covered.
2. Transfer to a round baking dish roughly six inches wide, then place this dish in your fryer.
3. Cook at 400°F for six minutes. The shrimp is cooked when it turns a bright pink color.
4. Serve hot, drizzling any leftover sauce over the shrimp.

**Nutrition:**
Calories: 490
Fat: 9g
Protein: 12g
Sugar: 11g

## 600.Foil Packet Salmon

**Preparation Time:** 5 minutes
**Cooking Time:** 15 minutes
**Servings:** 2
**Ingredients:**
- 2 x 4-oz. skinless salmon fillets
- 2 tbsp. unsalted butter, melted
- ½ tsp. garlic powder
- 1 medium lemon
- ½ tsp. dried dill

**Directions:**
1. Take a sheet of aluminum foil and cut into two squares measuring roughly 5" x 5". Lay each of the salmon fillets at the center of each piece. Brush both fillets with a tablespoon of bullet and season with a quarter-teaspoon of garlic powder.
2. Halve the lemon and grate the skin of one half over the fish. Cut four half-slices of lemon, using two to top each fillet. Season each fillet with a quarter-teaspoon of dill.
3. Fold the tops and sides of the aluminum foil over the fish to create a kind of packet. Place each one in the fryer.
4. Cook for twelve minutes at 400°F.
5. The salmon is ready when it flakes easily. Serve hot.

**Nutrition:**
Calories: 240
Fat: 13g
Protein: 21g
Sugar: 9g

## 601.Foil Packet Lobster Tail

**Preparation Time:** 5 minutes
**Cooking Time:** 15 minutes
**Servings:** 2
**Ingredients:**
•2 x 6-oz. lobster tail halves
•2 tbsp. salted butter, melted
•½ medium lemon, juiced
•½ tsp. Old Bay seasoning
•1 tsp. dried parsley
**Directions:**
1.Lay each lobster on a sheet of aluminum foil. Pour a light drizzle of melted butter and lemon juice over each one, and season with Old Bay.
2.Fold down the sides and ends of the foil to seal the lobster. Place each one in the fryer.
3.Cook at 375°F for twelve minutes.
4.Just before serving, top the lobster with dried parsley.
**Nutrition:**
Calories: 510
Fat: 18g
Protein: 26g
Sugar: 12g

## 602.Avocado Shrimp

**Preparation Time:** 10 minutes
**Cooking Time:** 20 minutes
**Servings:** 2
**Ingredients:**
•½ cup onion, chopped
•2 lb. shrimp
•1 tbsp. seasoned salt
•1 avocado
•½ cup pecans, chopped
**Directions:**
1.Pre-heat the fryer at 400°F.
2.Put the chopped onion in the basket of the fryer and spritz with some cooking spray. Leave to cook for five minutes.
3.Add the shrimp and set the timer for a further five minutes. Sprinkle with some seasoned salt, then allow to cook for an additional five minutes.
4.During these last five minutes, halve your avocado and remove the pit. Cube each half, then scoop out the flesh.
5.Take care when removing the shrimp from the fryer. Place it on a dish and top with the avocado and the chopped pecans.
**Nutrition:**
Calories: 195
Fat: 14g
Protein: 36g
Sugar: 10g

# 31 DAY MEAL PLAN

| DAY | BREAKFAST | LUNCH | DINNER |
| --- | --- | --- | --- |
| 1 | AIR FRIED CAULIFLOWER RANCH CHIPS | PIZZA HACK | ZUCCHINI SALMOND SALAD |
| 2 | CHEESY BROCCOLI BITES | MINI MAC IN A BOWL | PAN FRIED SALMOND |
| 3 | BRINE& SPINACH EGG MUFFINS AIR FRIED | PLANT-POWERED PANCAKE | WARM CHORIZO CHICKPEA SALAD |
| 4 | CHEDDAR HERB PIZZA BITES | HEMP SEED PORRIDGE | GREEK ROASTED FISH |
| 5 | PUMPKIN CHOCOLATE CHEESECAKE | MUSHROOM & SPINACH OMELET | TOMATOES FISH BAKE |
| 6 | CLOUD GARLIC BREAD BREAKFAST | WALNUT CRUNCH BANANA BREAD | CHICKEN CACCIATORE |
| 7 | PORTABELLA MUSHROOM STUFFED WITH CHEESE | SWEET CASHEW CHEESE SPREAD | SEAFOOD PAELLA |
| 8 | CRIPSY ROASTED BROCCOLI | AVOCADO SHRIMP | SUGAR CARROT STRIPS |
| 9 | AIR FRYER MINT COOKIES | SEARED SCALLOPS | ONION GREEN BEANS |
| 10 | BROWNIE PIES IN PEANUT BUTTER | BLACK COD | LOW CARB CHICKEN NUGGETS |
| 11 | RED PEPPER & KALE EGG MUFFINS AIR FRIED | NICOISE SALAD | LOW CARB AIR FRIED CALZONES |
| 12 | JALAPENO CHEESE BALLS | CRISPY FISH | AIR FRYER POPCORN CHICKEN |
| 13 | CLOUD FOCACCIA BREAD BREAKFAST | MISO GLAZED SALMON | AIR FRYER SWEET & SOUR CHICKEN |
| 14 | ASPARAGUS RISOTTO WITH CHICKEN | CRAB LEG | DELICIOUS CHICKEN SOUP |
| 15 | BELL-PEPPER WRAPPED IN TORTILLA | CRUSTY PESTO SALMON | FENNEL WILD RICE RISOTTO |

| 16 | CRISPY CAULIFLOWER | CRANBERRY SAUCE | CHICKPEA SANDWICH FILLING |
| 17 | CHICKEN CONTINENTAL SALAD | MINI ZUCCHINI BITES | WALNUT AND DATE PORRIDGE |
| 18 | COCONUT BATTERED CAULIFLOWER BITES | SHAKE CAKE FUELLING | SALTY EDAMAME |
| 19 | LEMON GARLIC OREGANO BONELESS CHICKEN | WHOLE WHEAT BLUEBERRY MUFFINS | EGGPLANT RATATOUILLE |
| 20 | FRIED AVOCADO | BISCUIT PIZZA | CREMINI MUSHROOM SATAY |
| 21 | LIME BACON THYME MUFFINS | LEMONY PARMESAN SALMON | CORN ON COBS |
| 22 | OMEGA 3 BREAKFAST SHAKE | MOUTH WATERING TUNA MELTS | CASHEW GINGER DIP |
| 23 | BLUEBERRY CANTALOUPE AVOCADO | ALMOND PANCAKES | TAHINI DIP |
| 24 | FRIED ZUCCHINI | LEAN AND GREEN CHICKEN PESTO PASTA | CUCUMBER AND DILL SAUCE |
| 25 | YUMMY VEGGIE WAFFLES | SESAME TUNA STEAK | SIMPLE GREEN BEANS |
| 26 | COCONUT COFFEE AND GHEE | FOLI PACKET SALMON | ASIAN GREEN BEANS |
| 27 | PUMPKIN SPICE QUINOA | BUFFALO CHICKEN SLIDERS | AIR FRYER TOFU |
| 28 | CREAM CHEESE EGG BREAKFAST | TYPICAL GREENS SMOOTHIE | KALE MASH |
| 29 | MILLET PORRIDGE | VITAMIN C SMOOTHIE CUBES | CHILLI SAUCE |
| 30 | ZUCCHINI MUFFINS | YUMMY SMOKED SALMON | VANILLA CARAMEL SAUCE |
| 31 | AMARANTH PORRIDGE | SPECIAL ALMOND CEREAL | TASTY KALE & CELERY CRACKERS |

# Conclusion

Many people who have diabetes don't necessarily need to lose weight, but they still choose to go on a diet because it's a great way to keep their meals balanced. It's also the perfect way to cleanse the body of toxins, processed foods, sugars, and unnecessary carbohydrates. In fact, the combination of these things is usually the main reason for heart failure, some cancers, diabetes, cholesterol or obesity

When lean and green food is mixed with air frying, it can make this diet much easier to follow and tastier, for people with type 2 diabetes. Air frying cuts the cooking time in half and makes the food more nutritious and tasty.

These dishes are designed specifically for those with diabetes because they practically make the body burn fat much faster.

Of course, a good diet should also be paired with a good amount of physical activity, which will cause blood sugar levels to drop faster and more consistently.

A good half hour workout with weights (even doing it from home, we don't necessarily have to go to the gym), could be a great way to burn fat, sugar and keep fit.

If you don't like weights, you can still dedicate yourself to some free-body exercises, in the tranquility of your home or in the gym.

Another activity, underestimated and rarely taken into account is walking. Walking is perhaps the most important activity to do, because in addition to weight loss gives an infinite number of other benefits: reactivation of the microcirculation, liberation of the airways, cardiac benefits, etc.

In short, the activities to do are endless and the ways to take care of yourself and your mind as well.

Living well with yourself means living well with those around you.

With that said, I wish you the best!

I really hope you found my advice useful and that you enjoyed all the recipes, which will help you live a healthier and more genuine life!